Praying with the Senses

Praying with the Senses

Contemporary Orthodox Christian Spirituality in Practice

Edited by
Sonja Luehrmann

INDIANA UNIVERSITY PRESS

This book is a publication of

INDIANA UNIVERSITY PRESS
Office of Scholarly Publishing
Herman B Wells Library 350
1320 East 10th Street
Bloomington, Indiana 47405 USA

iupress.indiana.edu

© 2018 by Indiana University Press

All rights reserved

No part of this book may be reproduced or utilized in any form or by any means, electronic or mechanical, including photocopying and recording, or by any information storage and retrieval system, without permission in writing from the publisher. The Association of American University Presses' Resolution on Permissions constitutes the only exception to this prohibition.

The paper used in this publication meets the minimum requirements of the American National Standard for Information Sciences—Permanence of Paper for Printed Library Materials, ANSI Z39.48–1992.

Manufactured in the United States of America

Cataloging information is available from the Library of Congress.

ISBN 978-0-253-03165-5 (cloth)
ISBN 978-0-253-03166-2 (pbk.)
ISBN 978-0-253-03167-9 (e-bk.)

1 2 3 4 5   23 22 21 20 19 18

CONTENTS

Acknowledgments · vii

Introduction: The Senses of Prayer in Eastern Orthodox Christianity / Sonja Luehrmann · 1

Part I. Senses

1 Becoming Orthodox: The Mystery and Mastery of a Christian Tradition / Vlad Naumescu · 29

   A Missionary Primer / Ioann Veniaminov · 55

2 Listening and the Sacramental Life: Degrees of Mediation in Greek Orthodox Christianity / Jeffers Engelhardt · 58

   Creating an Image for Prayer / Sonja Luehrmann · 81

3 Imagining Holy Personhood: Anthropological Thresholds of the Icon / Angie Heo · 83

   Syriac as a Lingua Sacra: *Speaking the Language of Christ in India / Vlad Naumescu* · 103

4 Authorizing: The Paradoxes of Praying by the Book / Sonja Luehrmann · 120

Part II. Worlds

5 Inhabiting Orthodox Russia: Religious Nomadism and the Puzzle of Belonging / Jeanne Kormina · 143

   Baraka: Mixing Muslims, Christians, and Jews / Angie Heo · 163

6 Sharing Space: On the Publicity of Prayer, between an Ethiopian Village and the Rest of the World / Tom Boylston · *165*

Prayers for Cars, Weddings, and Well-Being: Orthodox Prayers En Route in Syria / Andreas Bandak · *183*

7 Struggling Bodies at the Crossroads of Economy and Tradition: The Case of Contemporary Russian Convents / Daria Dubovka · *192*

Competing Prayers for Ukraine / Sonja Luehrmann · *213*

8 Orthodox Revivals: Prayer, Charisma, and Liturgical Religion / Simion Pop · *216*

Epilogue: Not-Orthodoxy / Orthodoxy's Others
William A. Christian Jr. · *242*

Glossary · *253*
Index · *259*

ACKNOWLEDGMENTS

This volume grows out of two years of joint research by seven of the authors, conducted in 2012–14 under the auspices of the Social Science Research Council's grant initiative "New Directions in the Study of Prayer." We thank the John Templeton Foundation for funding this initiative and gratefully acknowledge the support and input of members of the New Directions in the Study of Prayer staff, advisory committee, and fellow grantees, especially Courtney Bender, Taline Cox, Thomas Csordas, Parvis Ghassem-Fachandi, Charles Hirschkind, Kevin Ladd, Birgit Meyer, Ebenezer Obadare, Jonathan VanAntwerpen, Peter van der Veer, and Candace West. Sorin Albu, Nektarios Antoniou, Jeffers Engelhardt, Odysseus Linaras, Chrysostome Mbengu, Simion Pop, Annita Tribella, and Dimitris Vlachos made the team meetings in Cluj, Romania, and Thessaloniki, Greece, particularly memorable times. Nadieszda Kizenko and Vera Shevzov read almost all chapters as they were nearing completion, and Catherine Wanner and David Frick provided valuable insights. We are also grateful to Leslie Walker Williams and Julie Bush for superb editing skills and to Dee Mortensen and the staff of Indiana University Press for their enthusiastic support. Most of all, the contributors to this volume would like to thank one another for helping each of us see Orthodox Christianity in ways none of us could have done individually. Thanks also to partners and family members for allowing us the time to get away.

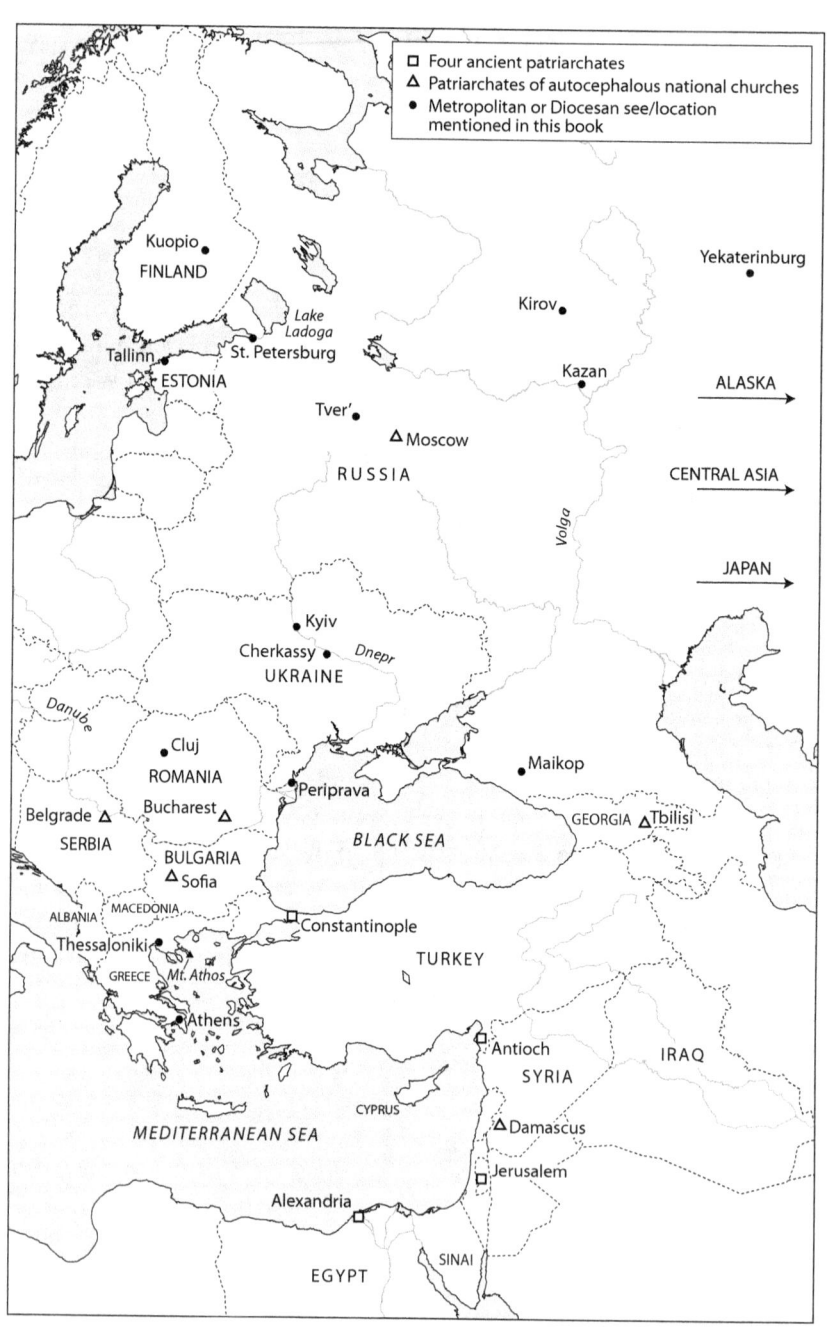

MAP 1. Orthodox churches of Eastern Europe and the Middle East.
Map by Bill Nelson.

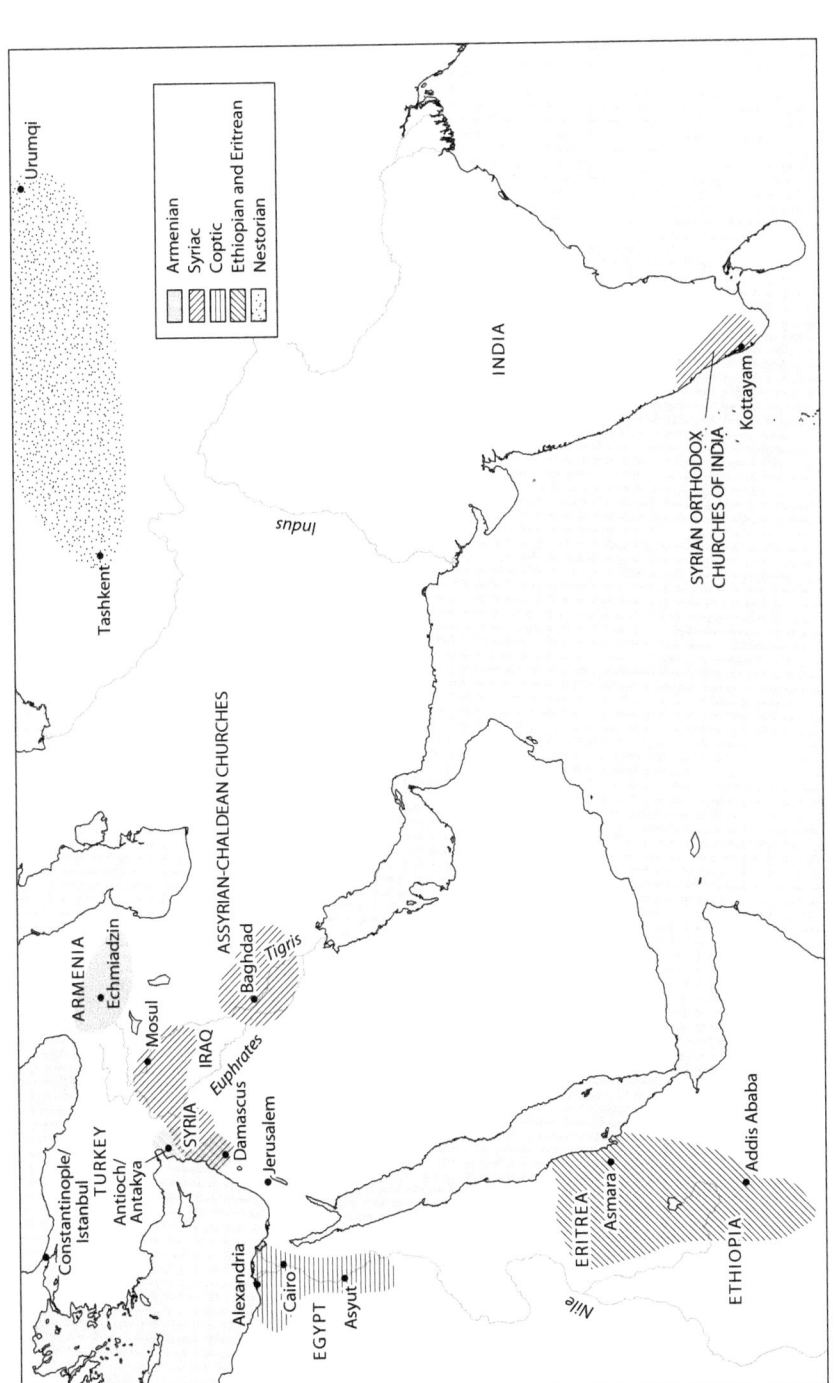

MAP 2. Oriental Orthodox churches of Asia and Northeast Africa. Map by Bill Nelson.

Praying with the Senses

INTRODUCTION

The Senses of Prayer in Eastern Orthodox Christianity

SONJA LUEHRMANN

O<small>NE OF MY FIRST ENCOUNTERS</small> with Orthodox Christian prayer was a Good Friday service in 1993 in the Moscow church of Saint John the Warrior, one of the few churches that had remained open throughout the Soviet period. I remember a gilded, dimly lit interior; the operatic sounds of the academically trained choir; the air heavy from incense, smoke, and the breath of many people; and small old women shoving past me on their way to light candles in front of the icons. I also remember the realization that following along with the movements of others, crossing myself and bowing when they did, was the only way to make it through hours of standing with no place to sit. At some point, my body simply decided to end the experience: my eyes went so black that I could no longer tell if the candle in my hands was burning or extinguished. The friend who had brought me escorted me outside, where we waited for the procession with the *plashchanitsa*, where a black cloth representing the death shroud of Jesus is brought out and carried around the church. My friend, who had been baptized at the age of sixteen in 1991, assured me that she had also felt sick and faint many times as she became used to incense, candles, and overcrowded churches. Her secular Soviet childhood had done as little to prepare her for the body techniques and rhythms of Orthodox prayer and worship as had my German Lutheran upbringing.

Mystery, learning-as-you-go, and physical and mental exertion are constant themes in outsiders' and insiders' discussions of Orthodox prayer. Another constant is the multiplicity of sensory input, the sense of a physical environment in which the prayer takes place and through which the person praying orients his or her own body. This volume grows out of a collaborative effort to understand the sensory worlds of contemporary Eastern Orthodox prayer in their geographic and ethnolinguistic diversity. Over the course of research, each team member tried to look beyond initial impressions of sensory overload and come to a deeper understanding of the hows, whys, and what-fors of the skilled practice that lies behind aesthetically rich rituals as well as more understated occasions. Combining our experiences in different countries and with different degrees of familiarity or distance to Orthodoxy, we were able to see subtle variations across places and times, as well as some of the bonds of style and common tradition that nonetheless make prayer practices mutually recognizable.

One inspiration for such a more closely attuned observation that combines insider knowledge with a stranger's view comes to us from the seventeenth-century Middle East. From 1652 to 1659, a delegation of Arab-speaking Orthodox dignitaries led by Macarius III, patriarch of Antioch and all the East, visited Constantinople, Romania, Moldavia, and Muscovy in the hope of securing economic and political support from Orthodox rulers to help the Arab-speaking Christians in Ottoman-ruled Syria. The patriarch's son, Archdeacon Paul of Aleppo (Bulus Ibn al-Za'im al-Halabi, 1627–69), recorded his impressions in a travel journal. Some of the content revolves around encounters with the rulers of various lands, from the Ottoman sultan Mehmet IV ("may God preserve him!") to the Romanian prince Vasile Lupu ("truly like one of the Byzantine kings of old"). In Moscow the delegation met Tsar Aleksei Mikhailovich, whose piety Paul praised and at whose court the patriarch had to use his halting Greek, rather than the more familiar Turkish, to communicate with interpreters (Feodorov 2014, 258, 262, 266).

Even more often, the journal recounts experiences with prayer and liturgy in various Orthodox lands, where the strange and the familiar blended into one another and were measured by reference to shifting standards of correctness. In the churches of Constantinople, the visitor from ancient but by then provincial Damascus noted, the icon dedicated to the feast that was celebrated that week "is kept on the lectern until the weekend, so that everyone who enters venerates it." Oil lamps were always burning before the iconostasis and the altar door (Feodorov 2014, 260–61). In Romania, the travelers discovered the relics of a saint hitherto unknown to them, Saint Paraskevi the Bulgarian or "the New," looking "as if alive, all covered in veils and silk" (264). In Muscovy, the delegation began an "episode of exertion, toil, labor, and fasting, for everyone in this country, ordinary people as well as monks, eat only once a day, even in the summer, because they never come out of the church service until around the eighth hour [that is, 2 PM], sometimes half an hour later, and their churches are thoroughly deprived of seats" (265).

Muscovite perseverance did not end with the church service, showing a combination of physical fitness and spiritual dedication that seemed unusual even to these high-ranking Orthodox clergy: "After the service they say the prayer of the ninth hour. And all this time they stand like statues, planted in the ground and silent, only bowing for *metanias* [prostrations to the ground], for they are used to keeping quiet and not growing tired. We were astonished, while among them, as we would always leave church with our feet barely carrying us" (Feodorov 2014, 265, brackets by the editor of that publication). The delegation reached Moscow at the height of the liturgical reforms of the Russian patriarch Nikon (1605–81). Conscious of their own tenuous connections to Greek models, the visitors from Damascus noted with approval the attempts to model liturgy, gestures, and iconography after "the Greek people and their ways" (267), as exemplified by the rules of Mount Athos, the monastic republic in northern Greece.

Different from many first-time observers, whose accounts are dominated by an overwhelming sense of emotion and mystery, these travelers from within the Orthodox world brought a sober comparative perspective even to those aspects of Eastern European worship that were strange to them. The visit to Constantinople at the beginning of the journey provided a yardstick by which other practices were measured—icons painted in the Greek manner were more venerable and holy than those painted "after the Franks' and the Poles' model" (268). The long periods of standing in prayer and worship they observed in Muscovy were physically hard for the Syrians but recognizable as authentic expressions of reverence for God and the kind of Athonite, monastic spirit that Patriarch Nikon was trying to introduce.

Finally, as insider-outsiders the travelers from Syria were attuned to the ways in which public, corporate prayer was but the visible tip of an iceberg of spiritual practice that included both invisible, private practices and the ethical regulation of public life. Paul was impressed by the personal piety of Tsar Aleksei, who was known for observing all the saints' feasts of the numerous churches in Moscow. In addition, it was rumored that "in his own palace, with the empress, he behaved more virtuously than a saint, observing the times of worship and prayer in their chapels, even at night" (Feodorov 2014, 268). Patriarch Nikon, in his effort to hold Moscow to Athonite standards, retranslated service books and called upon the authority of the visiting patriarch of Antioch to promote putting three fingers together to make the sign of the cross (as a sign of the Trinity) rather than using just the index and middle finger (as a sign of the dual human-divine nature of Christ). In addition, he strictly regulated public morality through guards roaming the city who, "when they find a drunken clergyman or monk, . . . throw him in prison, in utmost disgrace. Hence, we saw his prisons full of them, in the most wretched state, wearing heavy fetters of wooden blocks around their necks and feet" (267). There is a tone of disapproval in the account here, balanced by admiration for a piety that the visitors recognized as demanding in its asceticism, if sometimes misguided in its zeal.

In this travel report from past centuries, one can glimpse a condensed image of the unity-in-diversity and movement across time and space that defines what we think of as the "aesthetic formation" of Orthodox Christianity (Meyer 2009). Though outsiders to the political struggles of seventeenth-century Muscovy, the Syrian visitors were able to comment on public and private acts of devotion with a sense of recognition and shared standards. The divisions between "Nikonites" and the dissenters who came to be known as Old Believers are still with us today, as are attempts to forge transnational political and economic bonds through appeals to shared adherence to Orthodoxy (Naumescu, this volume; Agadjanian, Roudometof, and Pankhurst 2005). Images from today's Syria also remind us that it is often Orthodox Christians who inhabit the border zones where Christians have been neighbors with members of other faiths for centuries (Bandak 2014). Through a team effort to look at Orthodox Christian prayer in Eastern Europe, Russia, the Middle East, East Africa, and India, this volume seeks to present both the diversity of practices and the shared aesthetic sensibilities that govern how Orthodox spirituality is lived in modern and globalized times.

WHAT IS ORTHODOX CHRISTIANITY?

As has often been pointed out, the Greek-derived word "orthodoxy" means not only "right belief" but also "right praise" or "right worship" (Schmemann 1977). Orthodox churches see themselves as preserving both the teachings of the apostles and their ways of being together and worshipping God. The combination of faithfulness to the apostolic tradition with respect for local politics, language, and aesthetic preferences is inscribed in the self-understanding of Orthodox communities but also bears the traces of passionate and sometimes violent theological controversy. Orthodox Christendom consists of a number of national and regional churches, each with its own hierarchy and order of services, using a variety of liturgical languages. Based on their positions in fifth-century disputes about the nature of Christ and the Virgin Mary, the churches can be divided into so-called Nestorians, Miaphysites, and Chalcedonians, sometimes simplified into a distinction between "Oriental" and "Byzantine" churches. To summarize complicated theological controversies, Nestorians argue that Mary merely gave birth to Christ's human nature, not to his divinity, and therefore ought to be called "Christotokos" (Christ-bearer) rather than "Theotokos" (God-bearer). Their view was defeated at the Council of Ephesus in 431, where Patriarch Nestorius of Constantinople was deposed and exiled, and the title "Theotokos" (in Slavonic, Bogoroditsa; in Arabic, Wālidat Allāh) was made the standard and obligatory reference to Mary. Nestorians remained widespread in Iraq and Persia and were the dominant Christian group in central Asia and northwestern China until the spread of Russian Orthodox missions to these regions in the nineteenth century (Baum and Winkler 2003; Li and Winkler 2013).

In churches of the Byzantine tradition, the well-known hymn "It Is Truly Meet" (in Greek, "Axion Estin"; in Slavonic, "Dostoino est'") still forces worshippers to take a position in this old dispute, whether they realize it or not. Written in the tenth century and incorporating an older praise of the Virgin, it is part of many liturgies and prayer litanies, from matins to the Divine Liturgy (mass), and is also used as a closing prayer for many paraliturgical gatherings of Orthodox Christians, such as parish council meetings, classes for adults and children, and choir practices:

> It is truly meet to bless thee, O Theotokos,
> thou the ever blessed, and most pure, and the Mother of our God.
> Thou the more honorable than the cherubim,
> and beyond compare more glorious than the seraphim,
> who without corruption gavest birth to God the Word,
> thou the true God-Bearer, we magnify thee.

The text is said to have been revealed to a monk on Mount Athos by the archangel Gabriel in the tenth century, although it takes up lines from older liturgical formulas. Like miraculously appeared icons, this prayer-hymn is at once lifted out of the course of human history and seen as an important intervention in it (Shevzov 1999). The impossibility of participating in Orthodox ritual life without affirming Mary as God-bearer shows the polemical side of Orthodoxy, or, in Vlad Naumescu's phrase (this volume, 33), "orthopraxy turning into orthodoxy": right belief (orthodoxy) is defined and refined through controversy about right and wrong ways of worshipping (orthopraxy).

The second significant split occurred at the council following Ephesus, which met at Chalcedon in 451. Here, in part as a concession to Nestorius's sympathizers, the majority of bishops adopted the position that Christ was incarnate "in two natures," divine and human. Followers of Cyril, the patriarch of Alexandria, who had been one of Nestorius's most outspoken critics, rejected this formulation as an undue separation of the mysterious unity of divinity and humanity in Christ. They became known as Monophysites or Miaphysites, those who confessed the "one nature" of Christ. In addition to the Coptic Orthodox Church of Egypt, the Armenian Apostolic Church and the Malankara Church of India are part of the Miaphysite or non-Chalcedonian churches (Noble and Treiger 2014, 8–9; Pelikan 1974, 49–50).

The Chalcedonian churches remained united under the authority of the patriarchs of Constantinople, Jerusalem, and Damascus, a unity that faced its next major challenge in the iconoclastic controversies of the eighth and ninth centuries. These debates also concerned questions of the incarnation of Christ, this time in their consequences for the commandment against making and worshipping graven images: if all Abrahamic faiths forbade the depiction and worship of God in physical form, what was the status of images of Christ, Mary, and saintly human beings? Popular piety had long opted for them as media of memory and presence-making in churches, grave shrines, and homes. Nonetheless, a century of violent destructions and restorations passed before the Council of Nicaea decided that images were worthy of veneration, but not worship, and that "the honor shown to the image ascends to the prototype" (Belting 1994; Bremer 2014, 175). Like the older controversies, this one left enduring traces in Orthodox liturgy and prayer. An entire feast day, the Sunday of Orthodoxy (celebrated on the first Sunday in Lent), is dedicated to commemorating the restoration of icon veneration as a celebration of the church's triumph over all false teachings (Luehrmann 2010; Shevzov 2011). In iconostases across the Orthodox world, an icon of Christ and an icon of Mary with the Christ child flank the altar doors. Their presence is a reference to the arguments about incarnation that eventually made icon veneration not just traditional but also doctrinally right. According to the famous polemics of Saint John of Damascus, another Arab-speaking definer of the Christian faith, denying the possibility of iconographic depictions of Christ would mean denying the incarnation itself, as well as the assertion in Genesis that humans were created in the image and likeness of God (Heo, this volume; Ševčenko 1991).

While some churches were intensely embroiled in these controversies, other ancient centers of the Christian faith remained somewhat removed: Ethiopian

Christianity, established at least since the fourth century, and the Syriac churches in southern India, whose legends refer back to Hindu families converted by the apostle Thomas. Both were Oriental Miaphysite churches that maintained their own traditions of image creation and veneration with intermittent connections to artistic flows from the Christian Mediterranean. Even the Great Schism of 1054, formalizing a gradual drifting apart of the Eastern (Orthodox) and Western (Roman Catholic) parts of Christendom, did not have the same epoch-defining force everywhere. Formally, the churches split over the insertion of the *filioque* clause into the Nicene Creed by the Latin church,[1] the question of the use of leavened or unleavened bread during the Eucharist, and the claims to primacy by the bishop of Rome (the pope). In reality, a gradual divergence of aesthetic and liturgical sensibilities had preceded the formal schism, only to intensify further in its wake (Pelikan 1974, 157–70). Since the Middle Ages, churches in the Christian East have tended to follow a pattern of national or regional churches, while Western Catholicism developed its own centralized, transnational administrative structure.

Often-evoked contrasts between Western Catholicism and Eastern Orthodoxy include use of flat images versus three-dimensional statues, different styles of chant and musical harmony, and different understandings of monastic asceticism and pathways to salvation. Such differences mattered a great deal in the Mediterranean centers but became blurred in the farther reaches of the Eastern Christian world. Catholic traders were as important as Syrian bishops in bringing new impulses to the Christians of the Malabar Coast, and armed servicemen from the Ukrainian Catholic-Orthodox frontier brought three-dimensional statues of Christ with them to the conquest of the Middle Volga, where they are venerated today as some of the oldest tokens of Christian art in the region. In many countries of east-central Europe, Greek Catholic or "Uniate" churches have existed since the seventeenth century. Recognizing the supreme authority of the pope but following the Eastern rite, these groups blur the distinctions even further (Mahieu and Naumescu 2009; Skinner 2009). The Christian West, for its part, went through several phases of intense fascination with Eastern practices such as icon painting and veneration from late medieval Italy to contemporary Anglican Britain (Belting 1994; Woolfenden 2006).

As aesthetic media and spiritual practices travel within and outside the Orthodox world, they are sometimes accepted as a matter of course but sometimes become objects of intense debate. In the absence of common administrative structures, shared sensibilities on how to worship and pray crisscross a diverse world of local and national churches to this day.

WHAT IS PRAYER?

Prayer practices are among the spheres in which Eastern and Western Christendom had begun to drift apart long before the formal schism and where differences, but also dynamic interrelationships, continue until today. Though known in the West for an apophatic mysticism affirming the ultimate unknowability of God and the constant and silent evocation of the name of Christ in the Jesus Prayer (Dubovka, this volume), much of Orthodox prayer is quite routinized and devoid of mystical charisma. "Orthodoxy is all about rhythm," as a priest in the Finnish Orthodox Church put it in a discussion with parishioners, referring to the recurring and ordered nature of ritual life in general and to prayer in particular.

All devout Orthodox persons, ordained and lay, are supposed to perform daily morning, evening, and mealtime prayers and may combine these with other devotions such as reciting special texts to prepare for communion or to do penance after confession. All of these texts are read (often aloud) from a prayer book (Luehrmann 2016 and this volume). Many Orthodox laypeople do not recite such prayers every day but visit a church in times of need to light a candle in front of an icon, request a commemoration of loved ones during the liturgy, or arrange a funeral. They may also participate in pilgrimages or attend special prayer services dedicated to particular needs, such as curing alcoholism or helping in recovery from cancer. Repetition, habitual casual performance, and occasional observance are at least as characteristic of Orthodox prayer as the absorption and spiritual exploits of prayerful virtuosi. Prayer happens in many different places and contexts: at home and at church, as a collective performance and as a personal aside, as an explicit recitation of a canonical text and as a more general attitude of attentiveness.

For the purposes of this volume, we therefore cast a wide net and include a variety of communicative practices under the heading of "prayer": private and collective recitation of texts addressed to saints and divine beings; the performance of praise hymns; the silent or verbalized interaction with sacred media such as icons, relics, and candles; the movement of pilgrimage; and liturgical chanting and engagement with audiovisual media that bring the sounds and sights of Orthodox worship into nonliturgical spaces. As Tom Boylston notes in his chapter, there is always something public about prayer because it is expressed through shared forms. This communal aspect is a crucial meaning of "Orthodox," where acts of prayer are always anchored in, and legitimated by, a tradition that connects a believer to others, even as it can be creatively reinterpreted and individually performed (Bandak and Boylston 2014). Orthodox prayer also tends to combine intercession for others with the ethical aim of changing the self, in which the patience to endure repetition is a crucial tool. In the early twentieth century, the charismatic urban priest and modern Russian saint John of Kronstadt wrote,

> Why is lengthy prayer necessary? In order that by prolonged fervent prayer we may warm our cold hearts, hardened by prolonged vanity. For it is strange to think that the heart, hardened in worldly vanity, can speedily be penetrated during prayer by the warmth of faith and the love of God, and stranger still to demand this of it.... The Lord himself makes clear his will that our prayers should not be short, by giving us for an example the importunate widow who often came to the judge, and troubled him with her requests. (John of Kronstadt 1989, 10)

Prayer in this interpretation is both directed outward as a request and inward as a technology of the self that changes the person who prays. It also has the power to change aspects of the physical and spiritual world, as John explains in his justification of prayers for the dead: those who denigrate the importance of prayers for the dead by claiming that God already knows how to deal with each dead soul "do not realise the importance of every word uttered from a whole heart; they forget that the justice and mercy of God are moved by heartfelt prayer" (20). Salvation comes about through interpersonal ties rather than by individual merit alone, because the dead also pray for the living as members of the same church: "We name them, and they name us. But he who does not lovingly remember his brethren in prayer will not himself be remembered, and does not deserve to be named" (20–21).

"Remembrance" (in Russian, *pominovenie, pamiatovanie*) is a general term that can include explicit intercessory prayer for named individuals, the constant spiritual connection that the person reciting the Jesus Prayer maintains with God, and acts of commemoration such as giving alms in the name of a dead person or lighting a candle (Harmless 2000). It is thus a good way to think of prayer in the widest possible sense: request but also connection, ethical quest but also utilitarian plea, public statement but also a state of mind that may have no visible outside manifestation. Like many social scientists, we are happy to adopt Marcel Mauss's position that prayer is necessarily a social act of communicating with sacred beings ([1909] 2003). But we also recognize that the "society" that Orthodox people seek to partake in may reach beyond the boundaries of what we have access to through observation. Those remembered during prayer include sacred beings and dead ancestors as well as living contemporaries. The oscillation between mundane and transcendent reference points and nearby and remote ends adds a dynamism to prayer as an ethical practice that we seek to understand primarily through its media: the material forms that support prayerful moods and amplify requests, sending them on to relatively less visible and less tangible recipients.

ORTHODOX PRAYER THROUGH AN ANTHROPOLOGICAL LENS: TRADITION, SKILL, AND AESTHETIC FORMATION

This book is the result of several years of collaboration among researchers working in different parts of the Orthodox world, all of whom combine anthropological training with additional fields of expertise. In the individual chapters, readers will see influences from ethnomusicology, comparative religious studies, art history, theology, and psychology. What united us was an interest in what has come to be called sensory ethnography: the study of how the materiality of tangible things and publicly accessible practice shapes subjective experience and emotional engagement with seemingly intangible matters such as religious faith (Houtman and Meyer 2012; Promey 2014). We follow in the footsteps of anthropologists and historians of religion who have investigated visual, aural, and taste-related cultures of Islam, Christianity, and other traditions (Morgan 2012; Hirschkind 2006; Weiner 2014; Bynum 1987, 2011). Like many of them, we are also conscious of one of the dangers of the "sensory turn" that can be observed across disciplines: in investigating subjective experience and taking seriously the aesthetic dimensions of embodied responses to the world, one might be tempted to forget about the institutional framings of this experience. Whereas excessive musings about power and authority can stand in the way of understanding what religious rituals mean to participants, too great a focus on subjective meaning-making bears a risk of confining one's analysis to simply recording those meanings or translating them into different words. No participant (and that includes the participant-observer) can fully grasp everything that goes on during a ritual, and a part that often lies beyond immediate experience is the way in which groups constitute and maintain themselves and hierarchies are buttressed, established, or challenged through ritual action (Rappaport 1999).

Orthodox Christianity is a rich field for investigating the poetics *and* politics of prayer, or rather the political dimensions of aesthetics and the aesthetic dimensions of institutional legitimacy (Hann and Goltz 2010). For an Orthodox believer, the experience of the rightness and efficacy of an act of prayer is always informed by a rich sensory environment, which in turn draws part of its power from perceptions of institutional confirmation. Icons are painted according to transmitted, canonical standards; even more important, they are blessed before use in liturgy or home prayer, allowing a variety of techniques and artistic styles to be united through the "organizational embracement" (Halemba 2015, 9) of the church. Chants in many churches follow historically evolving interpretations of the Byzantine system of eight modes that alternate week by week throughout the church year, giving every liturgy its own feeling and tone. Within and in addition to this system, national churches and individual parishes differ a great deal in what kind of singing feels "right" to them but share a sense of aspiring to a correspondence between musical form and prayerful content, however differently that correspondence might be felt (Engelhardt 2015).

Just as a painted image becomes an icon through an act of blessing, in many parishes participating in the choir or acting as a reader during the service also requires the blessing of the priest. The need to ask for and receive a blessing is an overarching theme that shows the connection between aesthetic rightness and hierarchical order: books with prayers or didactic texts are published by the blessing of a bishop, icons are hung in a church according to the blessing of the rector, people follow particular prayer canons at home after receiving a blessing to do so from their spiritual father. Many Orthodox faithful will also ask for a blessing for apparently secular but potentially risky undertakings, such as going on a trip or undergoing surgery. Daria Dubovka notes that "blessing is on the one hand synonymous with permission, but it is also an order and at the same time a guarantee for the safety of the person who obeys" (2015, 71).

As Dubovka establishes in her chapter on monasticism in this volume, the hierarchical relationships involved in this way of developing faithful selves can be quite constraining. By choosing the language of blessing, Orthodox communities retain a commitment to the theology of free will. Those higher up in the hierarchy do not give orders or grant and withhold permission but bless certain actions as more conducive to individual salvation or communal good than others. In practice, the degree of freedom or constraint involved in a relationship of giving and receiving blessing depends on local sensibilities and personal temperaments, with extremes sometimes becoming the subject of self-critical jokes:

- Father, give me a blessing to spit.
- I bless you.
- What direction do you bless me to spit in, to the right or to the left?

This joke, told among Orthodox Christians in Russia, reflects both the dangers of abdication of responsibility and a shared critique among insiders in a situation of "cultural intimacy" (Herzfeld 1997). The joke works in part because spitting is a profane activity par excellence and perhaps the last thing one would imagine to be regulated through the requesting and granting of spiritual blessings. In contrast to profane spitting, the sacred act of praying is kept apart from everyday activities through its canonical, traditional forms and through the sensory manipulations that accompany it: lighting of candles, physical displacement to nearby or remote sacred places, shutting out external distractions through the use of a prayer book or icons. But the chapters in this book also show close connections between prayer and everyday acts of work, learning, caring for others, and self-expression. This fusion between sacred and profane worlds is sometimes valued by the faithful as a sign that Orthodoxy is a comprehensive lifestyle rather than mere dogma but sometimes frustrates them when sacred bliss fades into mundane tasks.

How to describe the workings of prayer in a tradition where hierarchies and prescriptions matter but where they are deployed through flexible and highly personal relationships? Like other anthropologists who have engaged with Orthodoxy (Hann 2012; Rogers 2010; Boylston 2013), we see the Orthodox orientation toward tradition and its authoritative transmission as an important corrective to studies of Protestant Christianity, where the emphasis is on its connection to modern individualism and dramatic ruptures with the past (Keane 2007; Robbins 2004). But even for Orthodox Christians, authoritative tradition forms complicated bonds with local ways of doing things and with the ethical challenges of the contemporary world. In order to think about the all-encompassing claims of Orthodoxy as well as its locally grounded practices, we draw on three interconnected concepts: Orthodoxy as a discursive tradition; Orthodoxy as an aesthetic formation in which a sense of rightness in prayer is connected to broader sensibilities of style; and prayer as a skill whose mastery depends on practice, disposition, and the relative social positions of those praying, those prayed for, and those who sponsor prayers.

ORTHODOXY AS DISCURSIVE TRADITION

In a famous article, Talal Asad argues that one should not approach Islam from the point of view of institutions, or in terms of contrasts between institutionalized and informal religious knowledge, but as a "discursive tradition." Practices are legitimized by reference to the authority of the Qur'an and the hadith, but this does not translate into rigid regimentation or rote repetition. Rather, it is "practitioners' conceptions of what is apt performance, and how the past is related to present practices, that will be crucial for tradition, not the apparent repetition of an old form" (Asad [1986] 2009, 20–21). Like other scripture-based religions, Orthodox Christianity draws on a diverse body of writings by authoritative figures. These are known collectively as the church fathers. Ranging from third-century desert hermits to nineteenth-century Greek monastics, they wrote across many centuries, lived in different parts of North Africa, Europe, and western Asia, and addressed themselves to a variety of social situations. Like Islam and Judaism but unlike Catholicism, Orthodox Christianity lacks a central authority to interpret these diverse writings and decide what they mean for the present: there is no infallible pope, and the patriarchs of national churches are theoretically first among equals whose opinions do not inherently carry more weight than those of other bishops.

With regard to Judaism and Islam, the dialogue among legal schools and individual rabbis or ulema has long been recognized as providing a measure of freedom and variety, as different authorities offer different views of matters of everyday law and ethics.[2] On the other extreme is the Roman Catholic Church, whose elaborate body of canon law is backed by the "charisma of the office" of a centralized and professionalized hierarchy, with the pope and his cardinals acting as final arbiters for new decisions. From the outside, Orthodox churches may look more like the Catholic Church, with a pronounced clerical hierarchy that is marked by stunning regalia and performed through elaborate terms of address and ritual distinctions. The difference lies in the way spiritual hierarchies translate into organizational structure: "The Orthodox understanding of the church underlines the unity of spirit while accepting a diversity of administrative organization; in the Catholic understanding, the unity of organization serves as visible sign of its spiritual oneness" (Halemba 2015, 146).

Despite the lack of an overarching, transnational structure, organizational hierarchies are fairly rigid within each national Orthodox church and leave their mark on public worship and prayer. Since most parish priests are married and bishops have to come from among celibate monastics, there is no direct career line from priest to bishop, and a liturgy celebrated by a bishop or other member of the upper ecclesial hierarchy takes on a markedly different, festive character from those celebrated by ordinary priests. Litanies in a service always include commemorations of the local bishop or metropolitan and reigning patriarch. Such commemorations take on added significance in regions where different congregations belong to different hierarchies, as in Ukraine and other post-Soviet countries, where some churches belong to the Moscow Patriarchate and others to autonomous national churches (Naumescu 2007; Engelhardt 2015). In the United States and Great Britain, the picture becomes even more complex, as churches of Greek, Antiochian, Ethiopian, Coptic, and Slavic immigrant origin coexist with those of the autonomous Orthodox Church of America. What is more, the ethnic composition of a congregation rarely fully corresponds to its institutional affiliation (Slagle 2011).

Affiliation with an ecclesial hierarchy is part of Orthodox identity and theology. In the writings of Pseudo-Dionysios Aeropagitos, for example, the world becomes aligned with divine will through a system of hierarchical complementarity including Christ, angels, bishops, clergy, and laypeople, where blessing and protection flow down from above and reverence and obedience flow up from below (Goltz 1974). The ritual of greeting a priest or monk and asking his blessing enacts this theology of hierarchy on an everyday basis: on meeting a priest or bishop, the layperson crosses himself or herself, bows, and shapes his or her hands into a cup, which the priest uses as the lowest point of the movement by which he draws a cross across the person's forehead, chest, and shoulders. After receiving the blessing, the layperson kisses the priest's hand, venerating the image of Jesus in him. Such everyday displays of deference and receptivity are one way in which institutional hierarchies pervade the fabric of what it means to live as an Orthodox person.

However, when one looks at how these hierarchies work in practice and how knowledge about right worship and right prayer flows through them, one starts to see how the routinized "charisma of the office" takes second place to the personalized and sometimes idiosyncratic charisma of human relationships (Pop, this volume). Anyone who tries to find out what "the teaching of the Orthodox Church" on a particular issue is will quickly encounter the workings of discursive tradition. During field research on Russian Orthodox views of abortion and contraception in 2010, I asked the priest who was head of the Society of Orthodox Physicians in a large city about the position of the Orthodox Church on the fate of the souls of unbaptized children. A Catholic priest would have quickly answered an analogous question by reference to the catechism, a papal encyclical, or, more recently, the website of the Vatican. My interlocutor, however, said, "Yes, I dealt with this question [*razbiral etot vopros*] in my theology dissertation." He then started to enumerate the views of different church fathers—some thought the children's souls remained in eternal darkness; some thought they were not tortured but also not among the souls who partook of God's glory. In his view, the best-considered position was somewhere in between, where the unbaptized children were in a neutral space of no suffering but also some distance from God. "It's a mystery," he said in closing, articulating what Vlad Naumescu (this volume) calls the "creative uncertainty" of living a tradition made up of many different voices.

As in Islamic jurisprudence and Talmudic scholarship, choosing which textual and live authorities to privilege over others means making judgments by reference to present needs and ethical alternatives. As explained by Talal Asad, tradition involves discourses about "the correct form and purpose of a practice" that relate it "to a *past* (when the practice was instituted, and from which the knowledge of its point and proper performance has been transmitted) and a *future* (how the point of that practice can best be secured in the short or long term, why it should be modified or abandoned), through *a present* (how it is linked to other practices, institutions, and social conditions)" ([1986] 2009, 20). Asad writes with regard to Islam and draws on the British philosopher Alasdair MacIntyre's (1981) concept of tradition as a process of accumulated learning across generations. However, his explanation also resonates quite closely with the Orthodox understanding of tradition as an ongoing process of revelation that did not close with biblical times but continues throughout the history of Christian communities. In the words of Russian émigré theologian Georges Florovsky: "Tradition is not only a protective, conservative principle; it is, primarily, the principle of growth and regeneration. Tradition is not a principle striving to restore the past, using the past as a criterion for the present. . . . Tradition is authority to teach, *potestas magisterii*, authority to bear witness to the truth. The church bears witness to the truth not by reminiscence or from the words of others, but from its own living, unceasing experience" (1972, 47). For Florovsky, the legitimating source of authority was the ongoing presence of the Holy Spirit in the Orthodox Church, connecting past, present, and future. For the layperson who neither knows the origin and history of devotional practices nor consults the works of the church fathers on a daily basis, the authoritative voice of tradition is often the local parish priest, a relative knowledgeable about Orthodoxy, a monastic elder one happened to speak to on a pilgrimage, an Orthodox television or radio program, or the person who answers questions on one's favorite web forum.

As Andreas Bandak and Tom Boylston note, if two authorities disagree or no one can give a definitive answer, it may be that the fullest answer has yet to be revealed: deferral to tradition can be about the future as well as the past. In the "interpretive space" (2014, 34) left in between the multiple sources of tradition, there is room for choice, enabled, but also constrained, by the fiction of the overall spiritual unity of the church. Laypeople choose which parish to attend and how often, which priest to confess to, which internet portals to visit, and whether to prefer the opinion voiced in an Orthodox television show or by a monastic elder over that of one's parish priest. Ethnographic studies of Orthodox spiritual practices such as the ones presented in this volume show people in the midst of making such choices. Decisions involve an eclectic set of personal preferences but are also guided by a general sense of resonance. Does the attitude of the priest and the sound of the choir at a church correspond with someone's overall idea of being Orthodox? Do the services seem too long or too short? Does a way of praying at home or on pilgrimage seem compatible with prayers happening in the church? Is it possible to combine an economic pursuit with the prayerful spirit that is described in the works of the church fathers? For the lay believer, tradition manifests itself most palpably as a style: an overall constellation of aesthetic expressions, attitudes, and ideas in which different individuals may value elements differently while retaining a sense of mutual agreement. To describe this capacity of style to forge connections in the absence of a centralized structure, we adopt the term "aesthetic formation" from the anthropology of sensory experience.

ORTHODOXY AS AESTHETIC FORMATION

As Birgit Meyer writes, religious communities, like nations, need to be imagined through media rather than experienced directly, and attention to the material media of devotion can help us understand how such imaginaries become real and convincing: "In order to become experienced as real, imagined communities need to materialize in the concrete lived environment and be felt in the bones" (Meyer 2009, 5). In order to capture the visceral nature of communities that may not even be held together by a common organizational structure, Meyer coins the term "aesthetic formation." As a way of understanding the importance of aesthetic style for communal belonging, the term acknowledges "the formative impact of a shared aesthetics through which subjects are shaped by tuning their senses, inducing experiences, molding their bodies, and making sense, and which materializes in things" (7). It seems especially fitting for a description of Eastern Orthodox Christianity, where there is no transnational church administration but rather a commitment to recognizable choreographies of gestures, sounds, images, and corresponding attitudes that can produce quite strong distinctions from non-Orthodox outsides. As Meyer notes, style as "forming form" can be an important "marker of distinction" (2009, 11), demarcating communities but also providing criteria by which the "orthodoxy" or "non-orthodoxy" of a prayer practice can be discussed and debated.

One of the findings of our comparative research was the appeal of the idea of Byzantium, or Byzantine roots, as a common reference point in various parts of the Eastern Christian world. Referring to the Christian art and civilization that flourished in the eastern part of the Roman Empire until its fall to the Turks in 1452, "Byzantium" functions as a signifier that can be filled with a variety of meanings. During research group meetings in Cluj, Romania, in 2013 and Thessaloniki, Greece, in 2014, we encountered enthusiasts who were trying to recreate Byzantine liturgical spaces and artistic techniques. What seemed to appeal to them was what they saw as the holistic, *Gesamtkunstwerk* character of Byzantine liturgy, where chants, icons, frescoes, and architectural forms all helped to express a desired correspondence between human and divine movements and purposes. They also emphasized the universality of Byzantine art and its grounding in human nature and the properties of the human body. Sorin, an art historian in Cluj, explained the correspondences between the human forehead and the proportions of the dome of Hagia Sophia, the representative church of the Byzantine emperors that was turned into a mosque in the fifteenth century and into a museum in the twentieth century. Chrysostome, an iconographer in Thessaloniki who was from West Africa and had been educated on Mount Athos, took great pains to demonstrate to us how the Byzantine technique of creating a face through successive applications of darker and lighter paint could be used to represent any human skin tone. And Nektarios, a chanter who guided us around several of Thessaloniki's churches, was researching how the properties of Byzantine architecture served to enhance the sonorous qualities of Byzantine music.

In our individual research in locations as far-flung as India, Egypt, and Russia, we also encountered attempts to rediscover and cultivate "Byzantine" or "Oriental" forms of worship and prayer, conceptualized simultaneously as a return to a historical core of Orthodoxy and an affirmation of its universality, transcending time and place. In the post-Soviet Estonian Orthodox Church that is trying to step out of the shadow of its big neighbor, Russia, musical practices that index Byzantium at once feel arbitrarily foreign and promise "a route of circulation between Estonia and the world of the Ecumenical Patriarchate of Constantinople" (Engelhardt 2015, 75). Filled with slightly different content in different places, Byzantineness is perhaps a style par excellence, where what matters is not so much individual elements such as monophonic chant accompanied by the single-tone deep drone, painting in natural pigments using so-called reverse perspective, or the practice of meditative prayer with short, repetitive formulas known as the Jesus Prayer. Rather, what produces the effect of Byzantineness is the sense that any one element is part of a larger harmonic whole that encompasses verbal, musical, visual, and monumental art. The perceived naturalness of this overarching style moves Orthodoxy beyond particular national histories and historical dependencies and helps set off the Orthodox "East" from the perceived individualism and willfulness of "the West."

Such assertions of the unique capacity of the East to preserve something of original Christian spirituality deny the multiple instances of musical and liturgical borrowing between Eastern and Western Christian worlds across the centuries (Hann 2003, 2014). Asserting the distinctiveness and interconnectedness of Orthodox Christendom seems to become important at moments of historical rupture, as we currently see in the post-Socialist world, but also in response to various waves of globalization. In nineteenth-century Russia, the rediscovery of the writings of Hellenic and Byzantine church fathers and their advice on how to pray and live spiritual lives went along with the rejection of Catholic models of religious education, where catechisms had been translated from Latin and even future priests learned Latin before they learned Greek (Freeze 1983). In today's India, Vlad Naumescu suggests that interest in icons rather than statues and other forms of Byzantification of liturgical environments is a way of asserting an alternative imaginary of transnational connections not associated with the legacies of British colonialism while also exploring pathways of indigenizing spiritual practices that go deeper than Anglican models of enculturation. Meditative body techniques are part of Hinduism as well as Middle Eastern Christian traditions and can breathe new meaning into the name of "Syrian" Christianity.

Byzantification as a pan-Orthodox phenomenon has local equivalents, such as the revival in Russia of medieval monastic *znamenny* chant and the iconography of the fifteenth-century Moscow school. All of these forms of imaginative recuperation point to the importance of material and sensory environments for perceptions of right worship and right prayer. Calling such environments "Byzantine" or "Old Russian" grounds them in the authorizing discourse of a chain of church fathers whose message, though diverse and sometimes contradictory, is understood to express a common spirit that manifests as artistic style. Prayer techniques more narrowly understood also become the object of debates that often pit an Orthodox aesthetic formation against a globalized world whose cultural roots lie in Western Christian norms and forms. Should laypeople or ordinary monastics aspire to the constant recitation of the Jesus Prayer, or is that reserved for the mystics of old (Dubovka and Pop, this volume)? Do warnings of the desert fathers and Byzantine monastics against mental representations during prayer mean that visual imaginaries hinder true prayer, or can the imagination be used as a learning tool in the spirit of the Catholic spiritual exercises of Saint Ignatius of Loyola (Noble 2005)? Where such questions are raised, criticism of Western practices goes along with a concern with prayer as a risky skill, where things can go wrong as well as right.

PRAYER AS SKILL

Prayer, as any human behavior, is learned, and it requires time and practice to develop mastery. As Tanya Luhrmann argues, even the supposed "immediate" experience that North American evangelical Christians have of God becomes possible through training oneself to pay attention to certain thoughts and mental images and not others. God becomes real as someone whom one can casually sit down and chat with through a process of learning that is easier for some than for others, because practice and a proclivity for imaginative absorption both matter (Luhrmann, Nusbaum, and Thisted 2010). In Orthodoxy, where few things are casual, there is a lot to learn, and it is also recognized that prayer is an activity that some people are better at than others. But proclivity for Orthodox prayer is not just a matter of personal psychological characteristics but also of social relationships.

As Vlad Naumescu describes in his chapter, learning to pray often takes place in liturgical and communal contexts. A child may be lifted up to kiss an icon, or a less experienced adult might follow along as others perform habitual actions such as the prayer before a meal or morning and evening prayer. Sunday schools in Russia, India, and Egypt teach children which prayers are appropriate for which situations and ask them to memorize the texts. In many Orthodox churches, learning to pray also means either studying a liturgical language that is different from the modern vernacular or learning to "inhabit" its common phrases without knowing the full meaning of the texts. But beyond the responsibility to learn certain prayers incumbent on all believers, there are the virtuosi whose prayers are believed to have more effect than those of other people and who establish their own special disciplines of prayer. Naumescu calls them "spiritual body-builders" in analogy with evangelical Christians studied by Simon Coleman (2000); Dubovka calls them "urban ascetics," for whom even monastic life might not be prayerful enough. Elsewhere in the literature, we find men and women known as "elders" (in Russian, *startsy*, female *staritsy*) whose intercessory prayers and practical advice are sought out by others because they are considered to have a more direct connection to God (Paert 2010). Prolonged spiritual practice, cultivation of virtues such as humility and love of others, and special gifts make these specialists able to take on the prayer concerns of others (Luehrmann, this volume).

But it is not always practice and experience that counts: the relationship between the person praying and the one prayed for also matters. The oldest female member of a family is often the one with a special responsibility to carry out religious duties and intercede for her relatives (Hirschon 1989, 220–32). I once encountered an elderly lady on a bus in a rural part of Russia who told me that she rarely went to church because when she did she felt obliged to buy and put up a candle for each of her children and grandchildren, and she could not afford to do that very often. As many books sold in Orthodox bookstalls remind their readers, the prayers of a mother for her children are particularly powerful and sometimes miraculous in their effects. In other contexts, the prayers of children might be seen as more efficacious because of their sincerity and presumed lack of self-interest. Requests for saintly intercession also fall into this category of referring one's concerns to those deemed better at praying and closer to God (Heo, this volume). Prayer is thus not necessarily a personal activity but something that can be delegated to others, feeding off of and affirming a web of social relationships and mutual responsibilities (Luehrmann 2016).

It is this idea of prayer as a social practice that can be delegated, shared, and materialized that might be the most fruitful contribution of Orthodox Christianity to a general study of prayer. Although empirical studies of prayer encounter it first as a collective and public practice, social scientists still tend to think of prayer as something people do in person, with particular attitudes, goals, and feelings (Giordan and Woodhead 2015). In the Social Science Research Council project that our research was a part of, this idea of prayer as a personal activity also seemed to predominate, going along with a focus on scriptural religions that offer rules of personal prayer, namely Christianity, Islam, and Judaism. Orthodox Christian practices of delegation and materialization challenge the idea that prayer is a discrete action one undertakes intentionally and open up comparisons to the prayer stones, bands, flags, and mills with which acts of remembering human selves and others to God are materialized and automatized in many religious traditions. Following Webb Keane's idea of the power generated through "semiotic transduction" (2013) from one order of signs to another, one might see this proliferation of materializations as a response to the fundamental dilemma of prayer, which both asserts and expands human agency and explicitly operates at its limits. What happens when prayer is not something people do but a thing they leave behind or buy from others, or a substance that permeates the walls of an old church? This line of inquiry leads away from the idea of mediation between sentient human beings to the possibility that objects remain active even when they are not mediating anything to a present observer. Comparable to the scientists, petri dishes, and germs of actor-network theory (Latour 1993; Roberts 2016), prayer as an object of study can take us to the limits of anthropology and serve as a window where human society opens up onto questions of how human and nonhuman worlds fit together.

THIS VOLUME

The aim of this volume is neither to provide an exhaustive catalog of Orthodox churches worldwide and their prayer practices nor to give a systematic introduction to Orthodox Christian theology (McGuckin 2008; Ware 2015). As anthropologists, we start from close-up investigations of how sensory media are used in prayer and spiritual practice in particular places. But we hope that, put together and enhanced by more general background information, our case studies provide both a sampling of the diversity of Orthodox Christianity in Europe, the Middle East, East Africa, and South Asia and a sense of how bodily practices and sensory media shape personal piety and ethical communities. In the first section ("Senses"), four essays introduce personal spiritual practice and its sensory environments—the gestures, sounds, images, and texts through which people are socialized into an Orthodox community, whether as children or as adult converts. These chapters also introduce some core theological concepts that have resonated across the history of Orthodox theology, such as deification through ethical discipline (Naumescu), the valuing of the human voice over the sounds of musical instruments (Engelhardt), the veneration of holy images and saintly bodies (Heo), and the daily, weekly and yearly liturgical cycles in which prayer at home and in church is embedded (Luehrmann).

In the second section ("Worlds"), we look to the social contexts of prayer, as people seek out good places to pray close to or far away from home (Kormina), come to terms with neighbors of other religions and encounter structures of authority within their own institution (Boylston, Bandak, Dubovka), and articulate wider social and historical visions through changing practices of prayer and confession (Pop). Throughout, we see prayer as something that both constitutes social bonds and forms ethical persons and that can put strain on other ethical commitments. This tension comes out most clearly in Jeanne Kormina's story about pilgrims who seek to be religious while avoiding religious community. It is also visible in the Romanian congregation described by Simion Pop, which creates such dense sociality that it seems unorthodox to some, and among Daria Dubovka's monastics who wander about in search of a monastery that allows for better prayer. In Andreas Bandak's ethnographic vignette about the changing meanings of prayer for Christians in Syria, we are reminded that prayer can both provide stability to embattled communities in times of conflict and become a manifestation of a diminishing sense of strength and security. In all these cases, the quest to be faithful to tradition and find true prayer can generate division as well as bring people together. What would make these communities recognizable to one another are the material and liturgical forms of a common aesthetic formation, without whose unifying frame of reference there could be no controversy over specific practices.

For the reader, we hope to provide a view of the geographical and cultural diversity of the Orthodox Christian world as well as its common features of political and artistic style. While our studies are necessarily selective, we have sought to combine geographic breadth with the depth of ethnographic accounts that are not populated by theologians but by more-or-less-committed Orthodox believers. Despite the image of Orthodoxy as nationalistic and inward-focused, Orthodox communities maintain intense transnational connections with one another and are more likely than those of Catholic and Protestant heartlands to live in close proximity with Muslim, Jewish, Hindu, and indigenous neighbors (Albera and Couroucli 2012; Kan 1999; Pasieka 2015). The short ethnographic vignettes between chapters contain prayer texts and first-hand accounts that show cross-regional parallels, connections, and contrasts within the Orthodox aesthetic formation. Together, the accounts in this book open a window on lived Orthodoxies in the contemporary world, where practicing tradition is always about fears and hopes for the future as much as about belonging to a past.

SONJA LUEHRMANN is Associate Professor of Anthropology at Simon Fraser University in Vancouver, Canada. She is author of *Secularism Soviet Style: Teaching Atheism and Religion in a Volga Republic* (IUP) and *Religion in Secular Archives: Soviet Atheism and Historical Knowledge.*

NOTES

1. The *filioque* (Latin "and from the son") was a clause inserted into the creedal statements about the Holy Spirit: in the original text adopted at the Council of Nicaea,

the Holy Spirit proceeded "from the Father," while Western churches, influenced by Saint Augustine's theology of the Holy Spirit as the love flowing between God the Father and Jesus Christ, started inserting "and from the Son" at some point in the ninth century (Pelikan 1974, 183–85). This difference remains until today and is well known in the Orthodox world as an example of the Western church's disregard for the results of conciliar deliberations.

2. For discussions of parallels between Jewish, Islamic, and Christian orthodoxies, I am indebted to Ayala Fader, Niloofar Haeri, and Jerry Pankhurst.

REFERENCES

Agadjanian, Alexander, Victor Roudometof, and Jerry Pankhurst, eds. 2005. *Eastern Orthodoxy in a Global Age: Tradition Faces the Twenty-First Century*. Walnut Creek, CA: Altamira.

Albera, Dionigi, and Maria Couroucli, eds. 2012. *Sharing Sacred Spaces in the Mediterranean: Christians, Muslims, and Jews at Shrines and Sanctuaries*. Bloomington: Indiana University Press.

Asad, Talal. (1986) 2009. "The Idea of an Anthropology of Islam." *Qui Parle* 17 (2): 1–30.

Bandak, Andreas. 2014. "Of Refrains and Rhythms in Contemporary Damascus: Urban Space and Christian-Muslim Coexistence." *Current Anthropology* 55 (Supplement 10): S248–S261.

Bandak, Andreas, and Tom Boylston. 2014. "The 'Orthodoxy' of Orthodoxy: On Moral Imperfection, Correctness, and Deferral in Religious Worlds." *Religion and Society* 5:25–46.

Baum, Wilhelm, and Dietmar Winkler. 2003. *The Church of the East: A Concise History*. London: Routledge.

Belting, Hans. 1994. *Likeness and Presence: A History of the Image before the Era of Art*. Chicago: University of Chicago Press.

Boylston, Tom. 2013. "Orienting the East: Notes on Anthropology and Orthodox Christianities." *AnthroCyBib*, May. Last accessed September 7, 2015. Retrieved from http://www.blogs.hss.ed.ac.uk/anthrocybib/2013/05/26/orienting-the-east/.

Bremer, Thomas. 2014. *Verehrt wird er in seinem Bilde: Quellenbuch zur Geschichte der Ikonentheologie*. Trier: Paulinus.

Bynum, Caroline Walker. 1987. *Holy Feast and Holy Fast: The Religious Significance of Food for Medieval Women*. Berkeley: University of California Press.

———. 2011. *Christian Materiality: An Essay on Religion in Late Medieval Europe*. Cambridge, MA: Zone Books.

Coleman, Simon. 2000. *The Globalisation of Charismatic Christianity: Spreading the Gospel of Prosperity*. Cambridge: Cambridge University Press.

Dubovka, Daria. 2015. "Poslushanie kak fizicheskii trud i kak dobrodetel': Semioticheskoe nasyshchenie proizvodstva v sovremennykh monastyriakh RPTs." In *Izobretenie religii: Desekuliarizatsiia v postsovetskom kontekste*, edited by Zhanna Kormina, Aleksandr Panchenko, and Sergei Shtyrkov, 63–81. Saint Petersburg: Izdatel'stvo Evropeiskogo universiteta v Sankt-Peterburge.

Engelhardt, Jeffers. 2015. *Singing the Right Way: Orthodox Christians and Secular Enchantment in Estonia*. New York: Oxford University Press.

Feodorov, Ioana, ed. and commentator. 2014. "Paul of Aleppo." In *The Orthodox Church in the Arab World, 700–1700: An Anthology of Sources*, edited by Samuel Noble and Alexander Treiger, 252–75. DeKalb: Northern Illinois University Press.

Florovsky, Georges. 1972. *Bible, Church, Tradition: An Eastern Orthodox View*. Vol. 1 of *Collected Works of Georges Florovsky*. Belmont, MA: Nordland.

Freeze, Gregory. 1983. *The Parish Clergy in Nineteenth-Century Russia: Crisis, Reform, Counter-Reform*. Princeton, NJ: Princeton University Press.

Giordan, Giuseppe, and Linda Woodhead, eds. 2015. *A Sociology of Prayer*. Farnham, UK: Ashgate.

Goltz, Hermann. 1974. *Hiera mesiteia: Zur Theorie der hierarchischen Sozietät im corpus areopagiticum*. Erlangen: Lehrstuhl für Geschichte und Theologie des christlichen Ostens.

Halemba, Agnieszka. 2015. *Negotiating Marian Apparitions: The Politics of Religion in Transcarpathian Ukraine*. Budapest: Central European University Press.

Hann, Chris. 2003. "Creeds, Cultures, and the Witchery of Music." *Journal of the Royal Anthropological Institute* 9 (2): 223–39.

———. 2012. "Personhood, Christianity, Modernity." *Anthropology of this Century* 3. http://aotcpress.com/articles/personhood-christianity-modernity/.

———. 2014. "The Heart of the Matter: Christianity, Materiality, and Modernity." *Current Anthropology* 55 (Supplement 10): S182–S192.

Hann, Chris, and Hermann Goltz. 2010. "Introduction: The Other Christianity?" In *Eastern Christians in Anthropological Perspective*, edited by Chris Hann and Hermann Goltz, 1–29. Berkeley: University of California Press.

Harmless, William. 2000. "Remembering Poemen Remembering: The Desert Fathers and the Spirituality of Memory." *Church History* 69 (3): 483–518.

Herzfeld, Michael. 1997. *Cultural Intimacy: Social Poetics in the Nation State*. New York: Routledge.

Hirschkind, Charles. 2006. *The Ethical Soundscape: Cassette Sermons and Islamic Counterpublics*. New York: Columbia University Press.

Hirschon, Renée. 1989. *Heirs of the Greek Catastrophe: The Social Life of Asia Minor Refugees in Piraeus*. Oxford: Clarendon.

Houtman, Dick, and Birgit Meyer, eds. 2012. *Things: Religion and the Question of Materiality*. New York: Fordham University Press.

John of Kronstadt. 1989. *Spiritual Counsels: Select Passages from My Life in Christ*. Edited by W. Jardine Grisbrooke. Crestwood, NY: St. Vladimir's Seminary Press.

Kan, Sergei. 1999. *Memory Eternal: Tlingit Culture and Orthodox Christianity through Two Centuries*. Seattle: University of Washington Press.

Keane, Webb. 2007. *Christian Moderns: Freedom and Fetish in the Mission Encounter*. Berkeley: University of California Press.

———. 2013. "On Spirit Writing: Materialities of Language and the Religious Work of Transduction." *Journal of the Royal Anthropological Institute* 19 (1): 1–17.

Latour, Bruno. 1993. *We Have Never Been Modern*. Cambridge, MA: Harvard University Press.

Li Tang and Dietmar Winkler, eds. 2013. *From the Oxus River to the Chinese Shores: Studies on East Syriac Christianity in China and Central Asia*. Berlin: LIT.

Luehrmann, Sonja. 2010. "A Dual Quarrel of Images on the Middle Volga: Icon Veneration in the Face of Protestant and Pagan Critique." In *Eastern Christians in Anthro-*

pological Perspective, edited by Chris Hann and Hermann Goltz, 56–78. Berkeley: University of California Press.

———. 2016. "The Politics of Prayer Books: Delegated Intercession, Names, and Community Boundaries in the Russian Orthodox Church." *Journal of Religious and Political Practice* 2 (1): 6–22.

Luhrmann, Tanya, Howard Nusbaum, and Ronald Thisted. 2010. "The Absorption Hypothesis: Learning to Hear God in Evangelical Christianity." *American Anthropologist* 112 (1): 66–78.

MacIntyre, Alasdair. 1981. *After Virtue: A Study in Moral Theory*. London: Duckworth.

Mahieu, Stéphanie, and Vlad Naumescu, eds. 2008. *Churches In-Between: Greek Catholic Churches in Postsocialist Europe*. Berlin: LIT.

Mauss, Marcel. (1909) 2003. *On Prayer*. Edited and with an introduction by W. S. F. Pickering. New York: Berghahn.

McGuckin, John Anthony. 2008. *The Orthodox Church: An Introduction to Its History, Doctrine, and Spiritual Culture*. Oxford: Blackwell.

Meyer, Birgit. 2009. "Introduction: From Imagined Communities to Aesthetic Formations: Religious Mediations, Sensational Forms, and Styles of Binding." In *Aesthetic Formations: Media, Religion, and the Senses*, edited by Birgit Meyer, 1–30. New York: Palgrave Macmillan.

Morgan, David. 2012. *The Embodied Eye: Religious Visual Culture and the Social Life of Feeling*. Berkeley: University of California Press.

Naumescu, Vlad. 2007. *Modes of Religiosity in Eastern Christianity: Religious Processes and Social Change in Ukraine*. Berlin: LIT.

Noble, Alexander, and Samuel Treiger. 2014. Introduction to *The Orthodox Church in the Arab World, 700–1700: An Anthology of Sources*, edited by Samuel Noble and Alexander Treiger, 3–39. DeKalb: Northern Illinois University Press.

Noble, Ivana. 2005. "Religious Experience—Reality or Illusion: Insights from Symeon the New Theologian and Ignatius of Loyola." In *Encountering Transcendence: Contributions to a Theology of Christian Religious Experience*, edited by Lieven Boeve, Hans Geybels, and Stijn van den Bossche, 375–93. Leuven: Peeters.

Paert, Irina. 2010. *Spiritual Elders: Charisma and Tradition in Russian Orthodoxy*. DeKalb: Northern Illinois University Press.

Pasieka, Agnieszka. 2015. *Hierarchy and Pluralism: Living Religious Difference in Catholic Poland*. New York: Palgrave Macmillan.

Pelikan, Yaroslav. 1974. *The Christian Tradition: A History of the Development of Doctrine*. Vol. 2, *The Spirit of Eastern Christendom*. Chicago: University of Chicago Press.

Promey, Sally, ed. 2014. *Sensational Religion: Sensory Cultures in Material Practice*. New Haven: Yale University Press.

Rappaport, Roy A. 1999. *Ritual and Religion in the Making of Humanity*. Cambridge: Cambridge University Press.

Robbins, Joel. 2004. *Becoming Sinners: Christianity and Moral Torment in a Papua New Guinea Society*. Berkeley: University of California Press.

Roberts, Elizabeth. 2016. "Gods, Germs, and Petri Dishes: Toward a Nonsecular Medical Anthropology." *Medical Anthropology* 35 (3): 209–19.

Rogers, Douglas. 2010. "Ex Oriente Lux." In *Eastern Christians in Anthropological Perspective*, edited by Chris Hann and Hermann Goltz, 351–60. Berkeley: University of California Press.

Schmemann, Alexander. 1977. *The Historical Road of Eastern Orthodoxy*. Crestwood, NY: St. Vladimir's Seminary Press.
Ševčenko, Nancy Patterson. 1991. "Icons in the Liturgy." *Dumbarton Oaks Papers* 45:45–57.
Shevzov, Vera. 1999. "Miracle-Working Icons, Laity, and Authority in the Russian Orthodox Church, 1861–1917." *Russian Review* 58 (1): 26–48.
———. 2011. "Between Purity and Pluralism: Icon and Anathema in Modern Russia." In *Alter Icons: The Russian Icon and Modernity*, edited by Jefferson Gattrall and Douglas Greenfield, 50–73. University Park: Pennsylvania State University Press.
Skinner, Barbara. 2009. *The Western Front of the Eastern Church: Uniate and Orthodox Conflict in Eighteenth-Century Poland, Ukraine, Belarus, and Russia*. DeKalb: Northern Illinois University Press.
Slagle, Amy. 2011. *The Eastern Church in the Spiritual Marketplace: American Conversions to Orthodox Christianity*. DeKalb: Northern Illinois University Press.
Ware, Timothy. 2015. *The Orthodox Church: An Introduction to Eastern Christianity*. Revised ed. London: Penguin.
Weiner, Isaac. 2014. *Religion Out Loud: Religious Sound, Public Space, and American Pluralism*. New York: New York University Press.
Woolfenden, Gregory. 2006. "Orthodox Influences on Anglican Liturgy." In *Anglicanism and Orthodoxy: 300 Years after the "Greek College" in Oxford*, edited by Peter Doll, 225–48. New York: Peter Lang.

PART I
SENSES

1 BECOMING ORTHODOX

The Mystery and Mastery of a Christian Tradition

VLAD NAUMESCU

What makes one Orthodox? How does one grow into a faith that weaves its teachings into a rich spiritual tradition, theology, and practice? The sense that one is born Orthodox or grows into it over a long period of time often prevails among observers and believers alike. This view tends to obscure rather than reveal the concrete ways of becoming Orthodox that sustain distinctive and enduring models of ethical life. Even for those who convert to Orthodoxy, motivation varies: aesthetic richness, spiritual depth, or authenticity of prayer is each taken as the most distinctive characteristic of this branch of Christianity. And yet there must be commonly accepted ways to cultivate an Orthodox sensibility that is to be expanded and carried on in life, even beyond loss of belief. As Orthodox-born secular persons often remark, the familiar scents from childhood and images of saints looking back from the icons still move them upon entering a church. This embodied experience of Orthodox spaces and practices leaves a strong imprint on people from very early on. When joining an Orthodox ritual, one can witness children's habituation to the sensory-rich liturgical space, their "hanging around" during services, reciting collective prayers and singing along with the others, joining communal feasts for the dead, and sometimes even playing priest. Surrounded by iconic figures that convey a spiritual presence, they grow into persons within communities of practice centered on sacramental prayer. As adults, they will continue the process of attuning themselves to the rhythms and models of their particular community in pursuit of an Orthodox way of life.

Being "born Orthodox" does not represent a right or an obligation (though it may be presented as such) but is shorthand for a process through which

Orthodox Christians absorb their faith during a long-term involvement that is often diffuse and deferential toward church and tradition. Learning through ritual participation plays a major role as it orients their Christian formation through authorized practice and collective worship. This process is informed by an ideal of human becoming, which entails the fulfillment of one's existence in the image and likeness of God (see Gen. 1:26). *Theosis*, or deification as it is called in Eastern Orthodoxy, conveys a theological anthropology that recognizes in human nature the potential to become like God.[1] Rather than a doctrine, *theosis* represents a "vision of life and grace" (Evdokimov 1990, 50) that sees human flourishing as the realization of God's likeness within each person. The process of growing from mere image to full likeness provides the space for ethical, spiritual, and social engagement in the world, as Father K. M. George, a contemporary Indian Orthodox theologian, remarked in his lecture "The Human Horizon: 'Mystery and Mastery'" (2013).[2] Inspired by a line of theological thinking that goes from fourth-century Saint Gregory of Nyssa to contemporary Orthodox bishop Kallistos Ware, George sees the human person as a mystery: made in the image of God, humans are like God beyond understanding. The human horizon is thus marked by our attempts to master human nature and the recognition that it remains beyond comprehension. For this, Orthodox Christians are encouraged to embrace their humanity, accept its limits and possibilities, and dwell in the world to become like God. "How could you be God when you have not yet become human?" asks Saint Irenaeus of Lyon in his reflections on human becoming (in Vrame 1999, 72).

This chapter employs the terms "mystery" and "mastery" proposed by the Indian theologian to translate the Orthodox path to human flourishing centered on *theosis* into concrete processes of ethical formation. This vision of deification permeates Orthodox epistemologies of revelation, the practice of faith, and the ethical relations between humans and saintly figures, three fields to be explored in this chapter through examples drawn from long-standing research on Eastern Christian traditions in Ukraine, Romania, and South India.[3] For this I take a virtue-ethical approach to religious worlds (see Lambek 2000), which comes closest to the way Orthodox Christians see themselves as being shaped in and through their engagement with the Orthodox tradition. In this perspective, "mastery" represents the practical wisdom or knowing how to do the right thing in a given context, which is so well conveyed by the orthopraxy of Orthodox Christianity. "Mystery," on the other hand, describes an epistemology of revelation and the creative practice that translates the space between image/likeness described by K. M. George into concrete models for Christian life. This space is populated with moral exemplars whose role is to remind Orthodox Christians of core values and virtues and to shape their practice of faith. Here living elders (Russian *startsy*) coexist with the ancient church fathers, national figures with universal Christian saints, to provide models for practice and virtuous life. Their charisma, rooted in a combination of mastery of core techniques and closer access to the mystery of God, gives them the power to actualize church tradition and redefine the criteria for becoming Orthodox. In this way, I will argue, mystery and mastery sustain and transform Orthodoxy and provide the means and ends to human flourishing (Greek *eudaimonia*).

EPISTEMIC HORIZONS: HOLY MYSTERIES AND THE ASPIRATION TO ORTHODOXY

Anthropologists started to explore in recent years how Christianity's central tension between immanence and transcendence plays out in different economies of representation, political theologies, and ethical models. This comparative endeavor has shown how Christian communities manage this tension through different practices and ideologies of mediation, which declare that only "certain words and certain things . . . become privileged channels of divine apprehension" (Engelke 2007, 16; see also Morgan 1999; Keane 2007). Unlike many Christians today who claim a "live and direct" relation with God, Orthodox Christians articulate their relationship in the language of mysteries. Mysteries define the scope and concrete modalities of human apprehension of God, mediating God's presence in the world through church sacraments, also called "holy mysteries" in Orthodoxy (Romanian *taină*, Slavonic *tainstvo*). From the baby receiving communion and chrismation in the baptism ritual, to the Orthodox community jointly proclaiming the mystery of resurrection in the paschal troparion "Christ is risen from the dead! By death he trampled Death; and to those in the tombs he granted life," to the mystical union with God in hesychast prayer, Orthodox Christians discover their faith through the sensory experience of holy mysteries. The initiation into and experience of the sacraments in liturgical practice becomes a heuristic, embodied mode of knowing, which creates tangible evidence without the claim of a full revelation (compare with Pickstock 2010). This corresponds to the Orthodox meaning of "mystery" as "something revealed to our understanding, yet never totally and exhaustively revealed" (Ware 1991, 281). This epistemology of revelation at the core of church tradition makes God accessible to all Christians through liturgical participation and at the same time reminds them of the limits of human comprehension. In an empowering and yet humbling way, the mastery of practice can lead to a better understanding of the mystery of faith but remains ultimately dependent upon the mystery itself. The interplay of mystery and mastery defines the workings of the Orthodox tradition (Slavonic *predanie*, Malayalam *pāramparyṃ*); Orthodox Christians refer to it as a "living tradition" (Greek *parádosis*) constituted through the transmission and practice of mysteries across generations since the times of the apostles. In this way Orthodox tradition aims to preserve the historicity of revelation while providing scope for a creative pursuit of "orthodoxy" in practice (see introduction). This orientation of Orthodox tradition gives a sense of historical continuity and wholeness to what is in reality a very diverse set of communities.

Orthodox Christianity consists of a variety of national and transnational churches rooted in local cultures that share a broad understanding of what Orthodoxy is about and their place in it. To grasp this specificity, one needs to look not only at the ways local Orthodoxies emerged historically but also at how they converge toward an ideal model of being Orthodox: the quest for the "true orthodoxy" of each church and its expression in local traditions (Bandak and Boylston 2014). This quest becomes a vector of change and the measure of what constitutes right worship, leading to a gradual understanding of faith through skilled practice. In practice, the search for orthodoxy materializes into an insistence to do things "the right way": observations or assessments of ritual performance and its efficacy or debates on what constitutes "right worship." Translated in the preoccupation with correct practice (orthopraxy), it also encompasses doubts or uncertainties about the righteousness of one's faith and the hope of salvation. In this sense, "mastery" is a condition not only of orthopraxy but also of successfully managing one's life in light of the aspiration to an ideal orthodoxy.

In the Orthodox world, the aspiration to orthodoxy has been primarily manifested in the formalism of religious practice. It has found a more radical expression in the ritualism of Russian Old Believers, commonly perceived as empty formalism in light of a post-Reformation emphasis on inner faith (see Scheffel 1991, 207). Old Belief emerged in seventeenth-century Russia in response to religious reform within Russian Orthodoxy—a reform that aimed to standardize religious practice by reference to the Greek Byzantine rite that church leaders of the time perceived as the authentic Orthodoxy. Those who fought to maintain the old rite were called Old Believers (Russian *starovery*) or Old Ritualists (Russian *staroobriatsy*) because they argued that any change of ritual form altered their relationship with God and thus their becoming true Christians. In this they translated the ideal of orthodoxy into orthopraxy or right worship, taking the seemingly most trivial details of their practice to matter for their salvation: how to make the sign of the cross, the direction of processions around the church, or the number of "hallelujahs" to be added to the short invocation of the Trinity, "Glory to the Father, and to the Son, and to the Holy Spirit." Seeking to keep what they considered to be the "true faith" pushed Old Believers to pursue continuity in faith, ritual practice, and personhood. The pursuit of continuity became thus a form of virtuous practice that shaped their religious and social life, as we will see in the last section.

Such debates about the orthodoxy of faith do not belong to the past but reemerge again and again in the Orthodox world to mark new boundaries, to legitimate claims to authenticity, and to influence local identity politics. I have encountered them in post-Socialist Ukraine, where one Greek Catholic and three Orthodox churches claimed to be the true inheritor of the church of the tenth-century Kievan Rus (Naumescu 2007), and in South India, where eight Syrian Christian churches dispute the inheritance of the Saint Thomas tradition (Naumescu, forthcoming). In each case the different factions disputed the rightness of the other's faith and ritual practice with arguments resting not only on the exact wording of the creed, the direction of church processions, and whether priests should face east or the congregation but also on which religious and secular authorities to commemorate in prayer. While recurrent divisions within the Orthodox world are usually explained through broader social transformations and political struggles, in Old Belief the schism itself worked throughout centuries as a mechanism for reaffirming the orthodoxy of faith by reinvesting it with new meanings (Humphrey 2014; Naumescu 2011). The importance of religious formalism in this process testifies about the ethical, theological, and political load placed on ritual orthopraxy. In the history of Eastern Christianity, such moments led to orthopraxy (right practice) turning into orthodoxy (right belief) under the threat of heterodoxy (schism or heresy).

One of the most famous cases was the iconoclastic controversy in the eighth and ninth centuries when the popular veneration of icons eventually led to a doctrinal statement that established the theological foundations of this devotional practice (Heo, this volume; Mondzain 2005). More recent examples that illustrate this dynamic can be found in the post-Socialist as well as the postcolonial contexts where I have done research. The Syrian Christian churches in Kerala, for example, emerged out of an indigenous Christian tradition allegedly established by Saint Thomas the Apostle in the first century. Syrian Christians had to reaffirm the orthodoxy of their faith against Portuguese Catholics in the seventeenth century when a major part claimed allegiance to the Syriac Orthodox Church in Antioch. The encounter with Anglican missionaries in the nineteenth century led to further schisms and the establishment of new churches, each professing the "true faith" of the Syrian or Saint Thomas Christians.[4] Among these churches, the attribute "Orthodox" is claimed today only by the Jacobite Syrian Orthodox and the Malankara Syrian Orthodox (also known as Indian Orthodox), but even they try to distinguish themselves from each other by pursuing different forms of orthodoxy (what constitutes right faith). An emerging movement in the Jacobite Church seeks to define its Orthodox character by reaffirming the connection with the Syrian Orthodox Patriarchate in the Middle East. The Indian Orthodox Church, on the other hand, looks for inspiration among Orthodox churches of Byzantine tradition, which have traditionally embraced autocephaly and national traditions. Each church aspires to be Orthodox in a distinct way, but the orientation is common, and so is the churches' return to tradition. Their current attempts to articulate the right faith generate new orthodoxies out of the once shared orthopraxy of Saint Thomas Christians and reinforce the "ortho" in orthodoxy.

The gap between the various modes of practicing Orthodoxy and "orthodoxy" as an aspiration toward the perfection of God (the image/likeness model) brings forth not only the creative production but also the ethical dimension of religious practice: one strives for the good by striving toward right worship. But orthodoxy can be pursued only through claims for continuity, by drawing on the past to affirm and sustain one's practice in the present. The historicity of orthopraxy and the overall aspiration to orthodoxy make the pursuit of continuity both necessary and virtuous, an aspect that singles out Orthodox churches within contemporary Christianity. Tradition provides the historical, social, and ethical grounds for an Orthodox becoming by supplying the models *for* virtuous practice and the inherited models *of* moral exemplarity.

MODELS FOR ORTHODOXY: BECOMING AS LEARNING AND ENSKILMENT

In a popular prayer book for the youth, Paulos Mar Gregorios (2011), late metropolitan of the Indian Orthodox Church, argues that prayer should be central to Christian life because only "by prayer we become like God." He compares prayer to swimming, "a spiritual skill to be acquired by constant practice" but also by letting go: "trust God to support you and teach you how to pray" (2011, 15–16). This analogy grasps well the balance between mastery and mystery required to approach God, the combination between man's own efforts and God's gift. Prayer is "an act of the whole man, body, soul and spirit," Mar Gregorios continues, including posture, gestures, visual focus, speaking, and even wandering thoughts. His words, echoing Marcel Mauss's view of prayer as a technique of the body ([1950] 1979), emphasize that Christian formation is a condition of skilled practice or mastery rather than conviction or adherence to a set of beliefs. It is an outcome of a person's practical knowledge, of knowing what to do in the right context, which enables him or her to participate in collective worship and to dwell in the Orthodox tradition rightfully. This begins with the child being socialized into the liturgical space, raised by his or her parents to reach an icon and kiss it and to make the sign of the cross in front of the iconostasis. It continues throughout the life course, with people being guided by benevolent others in how to approach a miraculous icon or taught the most appropriate akathistos hymn for a particular need. Such gestures reverberate beyond the liturgical context, marking a swift turn toward God in the routine of everyday life. To this day, Orthodox Christians cross themselves when starting an activity, setting on a journey, or passing by a church, a cross, or a small chapel on the side of a road. Once habituated, even such ordinary activities or places come to provide the right contexts for an act of prayer.

Formal religious education gives the same importance to the context of prayer as ritual pedagogies, providing clear instructions on what makes a prayer appropriate. In Indian Orthodox Sunday schools, the very first lesson teaching small children how to pray starts with the right posture, which is supposed to create the space for an encounter with God: "Let us stand with folded hands for a little while. Now we are in the presence of God. Let us close our eyes and pray to God: 'Lord have mercy on me' (thrice)," instructs the Sunday school textbook (Orthodox Syrian Sunday School Association of the East 2012, 60). This is followed by images of different religious and secular contexts for which the child has to find a suitable prayer: Jesus teaching his disciples (for the Lord's Prayer), a child on the way to school, a child next to an ill person, a father leaving for work, and so on (72). Children are supposed to learn prayer as a contextual, relational practice and become aware of the appropriate responses to circumstances that extend beyond the liturgical context. Their religious experience is centered on collective worship since prayer is taught in reference to the liturgy, which constitutes the ideal context for approaching God. The very first lessons are dedicated to short liturgical hymns, which are rehearsed until learned by heart so that children may join the congregation in worship. Pupils learn them in Sunday school and hear them in church, becoming aware of their place in liturgical dynamics. In this way they discover that their own prayers are made meaningful in connection to collective worship and the larger community of practice. The Sunday school textbook affirms that the "believer prays through the church" (7), emphasizing not only that ultimately all prayer is liturgical but also that the church is the ultimate repository of spiritual knowledge. This way one partakes from the legacies of the church and its traditions followed for generations and joins the fellowship of people that make the church—the "great cloud of witnesses" (Malayalam *sakshikaludae valiyoru samooham*; see Heb. 12:1, NIV) who testify to the multiple paths to God. This strong connection between personal prayer and liturgy is central to Orthodoxy, but it is not specific to it. Marcel Mauss observed that prayer is social in content, form, and action, and even in the most individualistic religions collective ritual remains the basis for prayer (Boylston, this volume). The words, gestures, or postures in prayer subscribe to certain prescriptions, and the efficacy of prayer is grounded in the practical tradition and the community of practice that gives its social force (Mauss 2003, 20). Orthodoxy reinforces this relation by emphasizing canonical prayer and the liturgical space as the privileged context for mastering it.

Since Orthodox devotions have been geared toward collective worship, the Orthodox mass or Divine Liturgy became its finest expression, the ritual par excellence perfected throughout time but remaining stable in essence and structure.[5] The apparent immutability of Orthodox liturgy generates a sense of continuity, of an uninterrupted tradition of faith. It also reflects the aspiration to orthodoxy that unites the different Orthodox churches and becomes a model of devotional practice and the expression of the "church" as a liturgical community. Even if the Cherubic Hymn, sung at the beginning of the Eucharistic liturgy, resonates differently in the Syriac liturgy of an Indian Orthodox church or in the Byzantine liturgy sung by Old Believers in Church Slavonic, it still gives the same expression of the extended spiritual community that makes the church. The shared liturgical heritage gives a sense of unity to Orthodox churches despite their cultural specificity, and it provides the measure of right worship for both individual and collective devotion. This has made ritual pedagogy or liturgical catechesis the preferred method of education, as it brings "the individual into the life of the Church" (Schmemann 1993, 11–13) to experience it directly. By joining the liturgical service, Orthodox Christians learn the rite but also the appropriate contexts, relations, emotions, and attitudes associated with the ritual action and accommodate to liturgical rhythms and aesthetics. The choreography of the liturgy creates a movement between active involvement and expectation, which corresponds to the nature of mysteries: a precise tempo of exposure and concealment that marks the position of the believer between the human world and God. For example, the opening and closing of the holy doors of the iconostasis and the liturgical curtain behind them are the most visible aspects of a well-defined context of interaction and participation in the central mysteries of faith. And even activities that may seem peripheral to the liturgical celebration, like icon veneration or lighting candles, belong to the same economy of ritual and its dialogical nature.[6]

Throughout the Orthodox world, liturgical rhythms are markers of spiritual strength and confessional identity. Orthodox Christians like to compare the length of liturgical services in different churches and celebrate the long hours of standing in the church, trusting that this embodied experience proves them spiritually as well. Monasteries and holy places recognized as "spiritual powerhouses" claim their strength from an intense liturgical life. There liturgical services take several hours to complete, marked by a different pace of recitation and singing but also by additional prayers and hymns. Such differences surface in frequent comparisons with other Christian groups whose prayers, more adjusted to the modern condition, seem short and superficial to an Orthodox believer. Their sensitivity to liturgical rhythms is not something articulated easily but surfaces at times, especially when confronted with alternative rhythms of prayer. A Syrian Orthodox friend from the Jacobite Church in Kerala mentioned that upon visiting another Syrian church of Protestant influence, she felt uneasy participating in the liturgical service. It was the same liturgy she was used to, but the service was cut short and some parts were missing. She blamed the discomfort on the different rhythm of worship with which she could not keep up: "I could not finish my full prayer before they moved on. . . . For example when I finish with the Lord's Prayer, I [always] say Hail Mary. But they don't say it . . . it's like it's chopped [referring to the ritual]."

Her observation reveals as much about the embodied dispositions of Orthodox believers and the effect of long-term habit on synchronizing individual and collective rhythms as it does about the politics of small differences that run deep into the history of this fragmented community and its reflections in ritual orthopraxy.[7] Liturgical rhythms are usually picked up through ritual participation and carried on in canonical prayers that stand close to the liturgy as part of the Orthodox service. The prayers gathered in the Indian edition of the Syriac *Book of Common Prayer* (Malayalam *Sh'himo Namaskaram*) extend liturgical worship into the quotidian outside the ritual context. Family prayer, for a long time the most common prayer in every Indian Orthodox home, follows closely the canonical hours for each day of the week. Families gather in the morning and evening to pray together from the *Sh'himo*.[8] The text varies but the structure is the same, and responses are distributed among older and younger generations so that the prayer could maintain the dialogical nature of the liturgy.

Even for spontaneous or extempore prayer, people appeal to canonical forms, despite charismatic and evangelical influences that pervade Keralite Christianity today. This is a common feature of Orthodox worship extending to communities such as Russian Old Believers, for whom there is no prayer outside canonically sanctioned forms. The ongoing correspondence between Divine Liturgy (Qurbana in Malayalam or Qurbono qadisho in Syriac) and prayer (Malayalam *prarthana*) is pursued as well in Indian Orthodox Sunday schools that teach believers to pray through the church. It makes personal devotion converge toward and converse with liturgical worship, whether a prayer, a hymn, or the simplest gesture of acknowledgment. "Sometimes, a look is a prayer," a young Indian Orthodox student remarked when I asked if he uses icons—uncommon in Indian Orthodoxy—for personal devotion. Such embodied dispositions attest to an Orthodox sensibility that extends beyond the liturgical space and blurs the distinction between collective worship and individual prayer.

As the example of the Orthodox woman unable to recognize herself in the Protestant-like worship shows, an Orthodox sensibility cultivated through liturgical participation is tied to the rhythm of speech as much as to the words of the prayer. Language is at the center of Christian prayer, as the formalized speech of creeds, sermons, and testimonies or as the texts and associated reading practices that ground the act of prayer (Luehrmann, this volume). The more puritan forms of Protestant Christianity emphasize words rather than actions as the truthful expression of inner faith.[9] In Orthodoxy, however, the function of speech is less to be understood for its denotative content and more to be valued for its familiar forms. This often happens with liturgical languages where speech is integral to the mystery of faith, articulated in the same rhythm with the whole liturgical performance.

Many Orthodox churches continue to use liturgical languages that are remote from everyday speech, like Syriac in Indian Orthodoxy or Old (Church) Slavonic among Russian Old Believers. Few believers fully understand these sacred languages, but most Orthodox Christians cultivate a certain familiarity with their forms and rhythms; one could say they inhabit rather than know these languages. For Old Believers, the mastery of Church Slavonic is essential because it represents their connection with the pre-schism rite (the "true faith") and the basis of their textual community across time and space. For this reason, children undergo an intense training in reading and writing from the old books, which include liturgical texts and rites, daily prayers, and fasting rules of conduct but also exegetical and apologetic commentaries and histories of the Old Belief. Instruction is formal; small groups are overseen by an elder who emphasizes repetition and correct reading, once children have learned the alphabet. The aim today is to form skilled readers who recite correctly and expressively the religious texts, while in the early days, when literacy rates in the liturgical language were higher, it gave Old Believers the opportunity to engage with their textual tradition actively, debating and reinterpreting its tenets in light of contemporaneous concerns (Naumescu 2011; Rogers 2009, 71–92). The history of Old Belief is marked by believers' quest to maintain the precarious connection to the sacred language and the old texts. Through their exclusive access to the rite and textual tradition, only those Old Believers who mastered the sacred language became priests, deacons, and church readers in their own communities and thus secured the transmission of the "true faith."

Like prayer, sacred literacy is acquired through persistent practice, but it may also come as a divine gift. A story circulating among Russian Old Believers in the community in which I worked in the Romanian Danube Delta told of a child who received at birth the gift of knowing Church Slavonic. That enabled him to fully participate in the liturgical celebration from the first moment he was brought into the church. Such stories cultivate the mystery at the core of Orthodox Christians' attempts at mastery, inviting and acknowledging the role of divine inspiration in their striving for perfection. As much as spiritual skill is a matter of perseverance, as Mar Gregorios advised through his analogy with swimming, skilled practice is not sufficient for spiritual mastery. This is acknowledged not only in popular stories but in mystical teachings as well. Hesychasm, a mystical tradition within Orthodox monasticism, provides one of the most articulate reflections on the relationship between mystery and mastery in spiritual formation. The great mystics who left detailed instructions on the stages of spiritual transformation in the mastery of prayer identify a moment when this process reaches beyond human capacities, what they call "acquiring the knowledge of the heart" (Meyendorff 2002). They differentiate between three stages of prayer—of the lips, of the mind, and of the heart—which correspond to the practice of virtues (praxis), the contemplation of God in nature (theoria), and the knowledge of God (theosis). The practice of virtues, also known as "the purification of the heart," requires a person to redirect his or her passions rather than attempt to suppress or mortify them (Ware 2001, 99). This leads to the development of moral virtues and an acute sensibility that flows onto other people. Famous monks are known to be virtuous, highly spiritual persons who can "see into the heart of people" and heal through prayer (Naumescu 2012). Mastery marks the step from praxis to *theoria* as spiritual fathers not only are skilled practitioners who achieve self-awareness and discernment but also have a deeper understanding of others and the way God works through them. They guide others by virtue of this gift and act upon them sometimes in strange, inexplicable ways, which are meant to further prove the power of their charisma (Dubovka, this volume). This pedagogical relationship developed in the monastic context has spread out in Orthodoxy beyond the monastery walls, reaching deep into society. Today's spiritual fathers mediate Orthodox Christians' interaction with and understanding of tradition and become exemplary figures in the light of it.

The relationship with a spiritual father displays a hierarchy of spiritual power that is often parallel to the institutionalized church and plays out in more efficient modes of charismatic authority and legitimization (Pop, this volume; Forbess 2010). It provides new possibilities for believers to discover and cultivate spiritual relationships that shape their moral being and devotional life in profound, intimate ways. They may develop a special devotion to a saint or spiritual father, testify about his miraculous power, and thus further participate in the development of his charisma. This pedagogical model of monastic origin has helped create new agents of moral transformation and modern types of Orthodox Christians such as the new urban ascetics, whose secular rhythm and family life are discretely marked by ascetic endeavors—an individually tailored prayer program, regular visits to their spiritual fathers, pilgrimages, or monastic retreats. But even this kind of individual mastery through self-cultivation and experimentation with mystical prayer is not cut off from liturgical worship and aesthetics. As Simion Pop (this volume) shows in his work on Romanian Orthodoxy, it has become a driving force in what he calls the charismatization of tradition. The return to church we witness among Orthodox believers is driven by an awareness of the liturgical model as the "right worship" and the need to relate personal devotion to this model (Engelhardt, this volume). This return may be met with an uneven response when the pull of the local parish is much weaker (Kormina, this volume), but as a mode of ethical self-cultivation it functions nonetheless.

There is a visible tension in the attempts of modern believers to cultivate an Orthodox sensibility in a secular environment. Modern ways of life have disrupted traditional rhythms of worship, and church institutions face increasing challenges from various competitors on the emerging religious markets in the post-Socialist and postcolonial contexts. Orthodox churches have adapted differently to these challenges, trying to cope with it not only by inducing more charisma but also by broadening the scope of religious education from ritual participation toward systematic, formal instruction. The shift from practical to didactic has reshaped their relationship to ritual and belief, the learning process and spiritual formation. In post-Socialist countries where Orthodox churches have gained access to public education, they entrust basic moral education to the schools while keeping religious practice under the scrutiny of priests and spiritual fathers. In South India, Orthodox Sunday schools embraced the textbook culture of modern secular education (Kumar 1988) and became ancillary to it. This way the Sunday school came to embody an individualist ethos and to foster moral values and skills that make the younger generation challenge traditional values and the strong kin and intra-caste relations that have been central to the reproduction of the Syrian Christian community in Kerala.

Uncertainties about the future of this Syrian Christian community place more pressure on the youth, with all hopes turned toward them as potential bearers of collective aspirations and the ancient tradition. Paulos Mar Gregorios's prayer instructions evoked in the beginning of this section should be read in this light as a reminder and encouragement for the youth to embrace an Orthodox model of spiritual formation. Addressing a new generation of Orthodox Christians growing up in a divided community and modern Indian society, he restates the Orthodox vision of the image/likeness as a viable model for human realization: "Prayer is thus a way of becoming good by using our freedom to turn towards the good and to will the good. By prayer we become like God" (2011, 10). By reminding them of the mystery that lies within human nature, Mar Gregorios invites the youth to respond to God's gift through the mastery of practice. They have the freedom to accept or refuse this gift, he argues, but once they accept, they need to cultivate it through the virtuous practice of prayer in order to become "whole persons." This vision grounds the act of prayer in a relational ethics where Orthodox Christians engage with the examples and exemplars provided by tradition to explore distinctive paths toward their becoming true Christians.

MODELS OF ORTHODOXY: THE MORALITY OF EXEMPLARS

On the third Sunday after Epiphany, the story of Nicodemus from the Gospel of Saint John (3:1–12) is read during the Divine Liturgy in Indian Orthodox churches. This passage invites the faithful to participate in a conversation between Nicodemus, a member of the Pharisees, and Jesus, who tells him, "No one can see the kingdom of God unless they are born again" (John 3:3, NIV). The term "born-again" is mostly associated today with evangelical Christianity and its distinctive model of spiritual rebirth supposed to turn one into a true Christian. Unlike this model of Christian becoming through individual transformation or rupture with one's (old) self, Orthodoxy has emphasized a model premised on communion (koinonia) and the continuity of faith. This does not mean that change does not occur or that people do not convert to Orthodoxy, but the strong emphasis on continuity in this tradition tends to encompass discontinuities at the personal and collective levels and place them into a broader relational field. The post-Socialist context provides a good contrast between the two modes of spiritual rebirth, the radical conversion of evangelical Christians and the Orthodox making of continuous personhoods out of disruption, confusion, and radical change. The post-Socialist religious revival became an opportunity for the emergence of new Christian communities and the renewal of traditional churches that survived communism. People converted massively to both and started to advocate new moralities that swept across society in full force (Wanner 2003). Much has been said about the growth of evangelical movements during this period, but many people also converted or "returned" to Orthodoxy (Engelhardt 2014). After years of atheist propaganda and secular living, they were suddenly socialized into a world they knew little about: from mass baptisms to public processions and pilgrimages, religion re-entered public life. At the individual level, this process of enchurchment (Russian *votserkovlenie*) entailed (re)discovering Orthodoxy with the aim of "becoming a true Orthodox person" (Zigon 2010, 146). Under these circumstances, the quest for orthodoxy took a full swing, but what a true Orthodox person is remained to be explored.

Ethnographies of post-Socialist religion describe these processes of change and renewal and their effects on individuals, communities, and churches, revealing a fragmented Orthodox landscape (see, for example, Hann and the "Civil Religion" Group 2006; Steinberg and Wanner 2008; Zigon 2012). Besides church schisms, conflicts, and divisions, the post-Socialist revival opened a space for experimentation with religious practice and form, and it challenged existing forms of authority and offered new ones, often based on alternative moral values. An abundance of new moralities, often contradictory, unsettled enduring Orthodox sensibilities with their alternative moral values, discourses, and practices. Some noticed that the neoliberal spirit has entered the religious sphere, turning priests and churches into capitalist entrepreneurs (Köllner 2013; Caldwell 2005) and shaping recent converts into self-monitoring subjects (Zigon 2010). This ambiguity led to confusion, crisis, and moral deliberation—the "ethical moments" anthropologists privileged in their exploration of post-Socialist moralities. In this context, however, prayer or ritual action often constituted an appropriate response for people, a way to reflect on their ordinary actions and debate over idiosyncrasies within their own practice and in relation to alternative values or norms. In a close portrayal of a middle-aged Orthodox woman in post-Soviet Russia, anthropologist Jarrett Zigon (2008) shows how she used petitionary prayer as a mode of moral reasoning to solve simple moral dilemmas, such as traveling on the train without a ticket, but also more consistently as a mode of working on the self toward an Orthodox personhood. Similarly, the potential failure of a funeral ritual among Russian Old Believers in Romania channeled immediate concerns about their precarious post-Socialist condition but also existential doubts about their salvation (Naumescu 2013).

Despite significant variation in forms of moral reasoning and ethical practice, Orthodoxy's consistence as an ethical tradition emerges through numerous efforts to recreate continuity with the past and provides lasting orientations for an Orthodox life. It also appears in popular forms of self-cultivation that are detached from their original source and context but end up sustaining the main orientation of Orthodox tradition. Such is the Jesus Prayer, for example, very popular nowadays especially among the "spiritual bodybuilders." This term, coined by Simon Coleman in his study of the Word of Life Fellowship, an evangelical Christian group in Sweden, shows how self-cultivation works on the "exaggeration principle": that in spiritual growth, one cannot have an "overdose of Jesus's love" (Coleman 2000, 149). Similar to these evangelical Christians, recent Orthodox converts sometimes try a variety of techniques for their spiritual enhancement before their "return" to Orthodoxy. These include yoga, Krishna meditation, or exorcism, until they come to the Jesus Prayer, "the pure prayer" of Orthodox tradition (Ware 1986), which offers a simple but powerful technique to work on the self (Naumescu 2012; Zigon 2010, 123–26; Dubovka, this volume).

While doing fieldwork in western Ukraine in the early 2000s, I joined people on trips to various pilgrimage sites and monasteries that were a testing ground for new devotional forms, spiritual models, and alternative practices to cultivate new moralities. Among them, a newly founded monastery was considered a site of powerful prayer (Ukrainian *silna molitva*) because of a group of young monks who sought to rediscover the tradition of the early church fathers and their empowering prayer practices. They settled upon exorcism as one of the most powerful tools for the transformation of their own selves and of others believed by their families, priests, or even doctors to be possessed and taken to the monastery for healing. The practice of exorcism offered an opportunity for these Ukrainian pilgrims to have a born again–like experience within Orthodoxy and for the monks to train themselves in skilled prayer the hesychast way (Naumescu 2010, 2012). Their mastery of the ancient exorcism ritual proved that they had the power to change individuals and through them the broader society on a scale similar to that brought about by evangelical movements in other parts of the world (compare with Smilde 2007).

Unlike evangelical Christians, though, the monks have reclaimed this idea of personal transformation as source for social change from the Orthodox tradition, especially the teachings of Saint Seraphim of Sarov, a well-known Russian mystic from the nineteenth century. "Acquire inner peace and thousands around you will find salvation," Seraphim advised his disciple seeking to receive the Holy Spirit (quoted in Ware 1986, 30). In this context the idea could have been equally sourced in Soviet atheist pedagogy, which aimed to build a new society through individual transformation. Its modes of working on the self were borrowed from and later successfully transferred back to the religious sphere after the demise of socialism (Luehrmann 2011; Kharkhordin 1999). For the monks, however, the reference to tradition inscribed this mode of ethical cultivation into the pursuit of orthodoxy and assured the authenticity of their experience. Similar to the return to church of Russian Old Believers, contemporary Orthodox Christians take up ancient mystical practices for self-cultivation and by doing so engage with an ethical tradition that offers models of how one ought to live or what kind of person to become.

While some anthropologists have already noticed an increasing individualism penetrating Orthodoxy (Hirschon 2010), its intrinsic relational nature remains central to the Orthodox personhood and the abundant worlds (compare with Orsi 2008) in which Orthodox Christians live. Their embeddedness in webs of relations with the living, the dead, and heavenly others shapes the space of ethical practice defined by the image/likeness ideal. "A *person* emerges in relationship," Father George remarked in his lecture on human becoming (2013), affirming the value of the person (*personne*) over the individual self (*moi*), against the grain of Mauss's observations on the historical evolution of the self ([1938] 1985). This relational model of personhood resonates strongly with the Orthodox idea of communion, the fellowship of people and between people and God justified in Trinitarian theology and the image of the triune God (three persons/hypostases in one). It is translated in practice into relations of deference toward those who know or come to embody the Orthodox tradition. Orthodox Christians defer to the authority of their priests and spiritual fathers, who speak with the voice of the tradition by deferring to church fathers and saints, whose words are sometimes shrouded in mystery (see Bandak and Boylston 2014). This process can produce highly idiosyncratic interpretations of Orthodoxy that speak directly to contemporary believers' concerns while providing the grounds against which their own acts are to be measured.

Tradition functions as the primary source to draw on in order to flourish in the present and provides scope for creativity, expanded agency, and virtuous conduct. Rather than being the main source of ethical action and responsibility, the individual self thus becomes part of a broader ethical field shaped by the pursuit of Christian being and right worship across centuries of religious practice.[10] The life trajectories of Russian Old Believers in the post-Socialist context provide striking examples of the consistency of such ethical practice. Often marked by a return to the church in old age after years of secular dwelling, they testify to a generational specialization that helped the reproduction of this community under adverse circumstances (Rogers 2009). The Old Believers who spent much of their adulthood away from their church and community saw the radical shifts in their lives not as ruptures but as returns to earlier promises or invitations to follow in the path of their ancestors and carry on the old faith. Stemming from a tradition of practice grounded in the pursuit of continuity, their decision to return produced continuous personhoods out of their discontinuous lives and made them potential exemplars to remind others of the virtues pertaining to the Old Belief (Naumescu 2016).

In an Orthodox world where personhood is framed in relational terms, the intentionality of one's acts can extend in time and space: people not only act but can be acted upon, provoked, or invited to (re)act. Tradition can generate continuities in one's life not only through a return to church but also by discerning how others' actions might have led to one's failure, suffering, or salvation. This has often happened in the Ukrainian monastery where, in search for the roots of affliction, monks often attributed intentions to departed relatives or spiritual agents who, through evil action or human deed, produced a "sin" or "virtue" transmittable through generations up to the possessed person. In one of the rare fortunate cases I witnessed, a departed grandfather and martyr of the Ukrainian church interceded from beyond the grave for the salvation of his nephew, a young criminal, helping his conversion to monastic life and thus restoring his Christian personhood (another way of being "born again"). This shows how agency and responsibility extend beyond particular individuals, including those who act upon them, or who are delegated to pray for their sins or ills, to their spiritual fathers in whose care they are and those powerful saints-intercessors who are always at hand. In this process prayer remains central because it brings Orthodox Christians in communion with the living and the dead as part of the extended community of faith that makes the church. Every act of prayer becomes thus an act of recognition, belonging, and affirming the continuity of Orthodox tradition.

The pursuit of continuity that Orthodox Christians entertain through what may often look as idiosyncratic practice is concentrated in certain people (exemplars), functions, and performances that serve to establish criteria for orthodoxy and clarify its significance for everyone. Individual encounters with Orthodox tradition are mediated by exemplary figures, whether saints, martyrs, or spiritual fathers. Novices in the monastery look for guidance in the lives of saints and the writings of church fathers, iconographers search for inspiration in the works and lives of famous Orthodox painters and their icons, and laypeople are nourished by the charisma of their spiritual fathers. Spiritual apprentices are expected to dwell in the tradition of the church fathers, share in the life of those who preceded them, and emulate their practice in order to grow into a Christian person and achieve the knowledge of God.

The actualization of tradition is a matter of everyday practice, whether through performance, entextualization, charismatic inspiration, or personal reflection. People may wonder how Orthodox Christians today can live by the age-old examples of Orthodox tradition or of the fourth or twelfth century church fathers. What makes their stories, written centuries ago for monastic practice, so appealing to laypeople in contemporary Russia or Romania, and how far does this cultural intimacy extend? Similar to the Jesus Prayer and hesychasm, the *Philokalia*, a collection of spiritual writings by the most important church fathers of Eastern Christianity (from the fourth to the fourteenth century), became extremely popular in recent years in the Eastern Orthodox world. Focused on virtuous practice and spiritual growth, this impressive work of spirituality can be found in various languages and formats, freely explored by "churched" people and urban ascetics or more cautiously used by novices and monks under the guidance of their spiritual fathers. A common reference among Orthodox Christians in Romania or Russia, the *Philokalia* was also recently translated into Malayalam with a preface written by the same Paulos Mar Gregorios. Anticipating the strangeness of these spiritual texts for an Indian audience, Mar Gregorios tried to convey the underlying principle, the "love of good" (Malayalam *satpremam*), and to outline the path to it through mastery and inner silence (Greek *hesychia*)—practically emphasizing the two pillars of Orthodox becoming. Ten years past its publication, the book—in both its abridged form (one volume) and extended form (five volumes)—remains accessible only to the learned few, while the majority are still attracted to the most popular Christian figures in South Indian devotional culture, the patriarchs of the Malankara church (*bawas*). More so than in other Orthodox cultures, these "holy men" are "the most powerful spiritual figures in Indian Orthodoxy" whose miraculous powers testify about their sainthood (Visvanathan 1993, 214–61; Dempsey 1999 and 2001). The great festivals on their special days, gravesites, relics, and lives are central to personal and collective devotion, liturgical rhythms, and spiritual formation.

Such holy figures emerge because of their powerful intercessions, while others become exemplars for the ethical virtues their saintly lives embodied. However, both types encourage the cultivation of personal relations and devotions that make the tradition meaningful for Orthodox audiences today. Icons make the ideal illustration of this kind of exemplarity that grounds a relational ethics: they are spiritualized portrayals of concrete human persons who were changed (transfigured) by their experience of God. Their role is to guide and instruct believers in their spiritual quest, inviting them to imitate the virtues rather than the person (Ouspensky 1982, 38; Heo, this volume). The goal of the icon in the eyes of an Orthodox pedagogue is "not to know about the saints but to become saints. . . . It shows the possibility for all humans to achieve deification" (Vrame 1999, 55–56). Transposing the same principle into textual form, the lives of saints are a popular read for the virtues they communicate, providing examples for people to deal with moral dilemmas and personal concerns. Exemplification in liturgical sermons serves a similar purpose, with stories such as the one of Nicodemus that opened this section being read very differently by the Syrian Christians in Kerala or Damascus but offered to both for reflection and guidance in personal lives (see Bandak 2015).

The veneration of saints in Orthodox Christianity is based on the assumption that there is no single path to the formation of Christian personhood and encourages people to search for their own way with the help of moral exemplars. The relationships they establish with such figures create temporal continuities and generate spiritual genealogies that bring together various exemplars in unpredictable ways. Orthodox Christians may successfully bring the hesychast fathers from the *Philokalia* in conversation with a nineteenth-century Russian mystic such as Saint Seraphim of Sarov and with contemporary spiritual fathers (*startsy*) to search for answers to concrete spiritual problems. In doing so they defer to the spiritual knowledge of these figures who speak for the Orthodox tradition and search for new meanings in their words. The morality of exemplars points to the fact that ethical models are always contextualized, interpreted, and deeply embedded in personal experiences and webs of relations that cross time and space. This makes them accessible but also potentially destabilizing, with some exemplars being puzzling or contradictory on purpose to serve a pedagogical goal. Orthodox tradition has long cultivated paradoxical examples and exemplars to destabilize and unsettle the novice, the witness, or the listener and thus prompt their moral transformation (Forbess 2015). Holy foolery has probably been the most articulate manifestation of this tradition in Byzantine and Russian Orthodoxy, with the "fools for Christ" representing not exemplars to emulate but provocateurs who reveal a "deeper truth" about the ills of people and society (Ivanov 2006). Old Believers have also used this model in the seventeenth century to defend the orthodoxy of their faith against the "false orthodoxy" of the Russian church (Hunt 2008). As a pedagogical tool for moral education, the paradox plays the same role that mystery plays in Orthodox theology and practice: revealing the limits of human understanding while maintaining the promise of a fuller revelation.

Through all these different ethical practices, the cultivation of mystery and mastery stands out as a central feature of Orthodox becoming, shared by the various Orthodox traditions beyond their cultural-historical specificity. Similar to the pursuit of continuity, mystery and mastery constitute a vector of ethical formation for the different exemplars out there. Together, they give a sense of sustained direction to what is actually a very diverse field of ethical practice and models for one's striving for the good. While Orthodox Christians seem to pick up values and develop virtues in a more intuitive, exploratory manner, their personal explorations are broadly shaped by these two vectors, which are central to the Orthodox tradition.

In this exploration of the potential paths to Orthodox formation, I have chosen "mystery" and "mastery" over the more familiar anthropological language of ethics and morality since these concepts allow a heuristic approach that remains close to Orthodoxy's own vocabulary and theological reflections on the topic. Father K. M. George, from whom I borrowed the terms, used them in his lecture to explore the horizon of human possibilities today from the perspective of a practicing Orthodox Christian in India. Acknowledging that there is no single answer to this question, he provided a cautious yet optimistic view that stresses the poesis of this religious world: "The important thing is to recognize that the image of God is an open reality. . . . Like the horizon it can be pushed further and further infinitely depending on our spiritual mobility and our capacity for higher vision" (2013). His reflections refer once again to the model of the image/likeness, which allows Orthodox Christians to embrace the diversity of theological interpretations as well as the models and exemplars proposed by church tradition and to seek to shape their own spiritual journey. Such creative uncertainty continues to encourage people today to approach Orthodoxy and engage with its tradition and practice in search of fulfillment in their own lives.

VLAD NAUMESCU is Associate Professor of Anthropology at the Central European University, Budapest. He is author of *Modes of Religiosity in Eastern Christianity: Religious Processes and Social Change in Ukraine* and editor with Stéphanie Mahieu of *Churches In-Between: Greek Catholic Churches in Postsocialist Europe*.

NOTES

1. This holds true for the Eastern Orthodox churches, while others, especially Oriental Orthodox, may take a different view informed by their own position on the nature of Christ (see for example the Coptic Church; Heo, this volume).
2. Father K. M. George, a generous friend and guide into the world of Indian Orthodoxy, has borrowed the phrase "mystery and mastery" from his guru, Paulos Mar Gregorios, late metropolitan of the Indian Orthodox Church. Here I provide an anthropological reading of these terms to explore an ethical tradition that provides vectors of moral formation rather than predetermined paths to an Orthodox becoming.
3. I draw primarily on fieldwork with Russian Old Believers in Romania and Syrian Christians in South India but also reference my earlier work on Orthodox and Greek Catholic Christians in Ukraine together with studies by colleagues working on other Orthodox communities around the world to make the case for a shared ethical repertoire in Orthodox Christianity.
4. This history affected their rites and liturgies, the devotional culture, and institutional formation: out of the eight churches, three are Oriental Orthodox (Antiochian rite), two Catholic (one of them Uniate), one Nestorian (Assyrian Church of the East), one Anglican, and another Reformed Episcopalian. Despite the fragmentation, these churches remain rooted in the same tradition and speak to a shared spiritual heritage that crosses institutional boundaries and political allegiances (see Joseph, Balakrishnan, and Perczel 2014 for an overview).

5. The liturgies of Byzantine and Oriental Orthodox churches (of Saint John Chrysostom, Saint Basil, and Saint James) share a basic structure centered on the Eucharistic celebration, which was formalized in the fourth century.

6. The reverse perspective of icons that implicates the viewer and congregational singing is a further example of the dialogical, relational nature of Orthodox worship (see chapters by Engelhardt and Heo in this volume).

7. The prayer Hail Mary was a point of contention during the nineteenth century reform of the Jacobite Orthodox rite under the influence of the Anglican Church Mission Society in South India. Today such differences mark the distinction between the Orthodox and Protestant churches of Syrian or Saint Thomas Christians.

8. This version is a partial Malayalam translation of the Syriac *Sh'himo* by Konattu Mathen Malpan, authorized by Patriarch Ignatius 'Abded Aloho of Antioch in 1910.

9. Evangelical Christians, for example, take speech as a vehicle of conversion and outward sign of inner sanctification (Harding 1987), while Seventh-day Adventists in Madagascar approach the Bible with intellectual curiosity and a genuine effort to comprehend (Keller 2005).

10. Bandak and Boylston provide a similar view on this aspect, arguing that "in an orthodox religious world, one talks not about the *invention* of tradition but about the *intention* of tradition" (2014, 29; compare with Lambek 2002, 11).

REFERENCES

Bandak, Andreas. 2015. "Exemplary Series and Christian Typology: Modelling on Sainthood in Damascus." *Journal of the Royal Anthropological Institute* 21 (S1): 47–63.

Bandak, Andreas, and Tom Boylston. 2014. "The 'Orthodoxy' of Orthodoxy: On Moral Imperfection, Correctness, and Deferral in Religious Worlds." *Religion and Society: Advances in Research* 5 (1): 25–46.

Caldwell, Melissa. 2005. "A New Role for Religion in Russia's New Consumer Age: The Case of Moscow." *Religion, State and Society* 33 (1):19–34.

Coleman, Simon. 2000. *The Globalisation of Charismatic Christianity: Spreading the Gospel of Prosperity*. Cambridge: Cambridge University Press.

Dempsey, Corinne G. 1999. "Lessons in Miracles from Kerala, South India: Stories of Three 'Christian' Saints." *History of Religions* 39 (2): 150–76.

———. 2001. *Kerala Christian Sainthood: Collisions of Culture and Worldview in South India*. Oxford: Oxford University Press.

Engelhardt, Jeffers. 2014. *Singing the Right Way: Orthodox Christians and Secular Enchantment in Estonia*. New York: Oxford University Press.

Engelke, Matthew. 2007. *A Problem of Presence: Beyond Scripture in an African Church*. Berkeley: University of California Press.

Evdokimov, Paul. 1990. *The Art of the Icon: A Theology of Beauty*. Redondo Beach, CA: Oakwood.

Forbess, Alice. 2010. "The Spirit and the Letter: Monastic Education in a Romanian Orthodox Convent." In *Eastern Christians in Anthropological Perspective*, edited by C. Hann and H. Goltz, 131–54. Berkeley: University of California Press.

———. 2015. "Paradoxical Paradigms: Moral Reasoning, Inspiration, and Problems of Knowing among Orthodox Christian Monastics." *Journal of the Royal Anthropological Institute* 21 (S1): 113–28.

George, K. M. 2013. "The Human Horizon: 'Mystery and Mastery.'" Public lecture, Vichara Academy for Theological Inquiry, Session 2, Kottayam, India, July 23, 2013.

Hann, Chris, and the "Civil Religion" Group. 2006. *The Postsocialist Religious Question: Faith and Power in Central Asia and East-Central Europe*. Berlin: Lit.

Harding, Susan. 1987. "Convicted by the Holy Spirit: The Rhetoric of Fundamental Baptist Conversion." *American Ethnologist* 14 (1): 167–81.

Hirschon, Renée. 2010. "Indigenous Persons and Imported Individuals: Changing Paradigms of Personal Identity in Contemporary Greece." In *Eastern Christians in Anthropological Perspective*, edited by C. Hann and H. Goltz, 289–310. Berkeley: University of California Press.

Humphrey, Caroline. 2014. "Schism, Event and Revolution: The Old Believers of Trans-Baikalia." *Current Anthropology* 55 (S10): S216–225.

Hunt, Priscilla. 2008. "The Foolishness in the Life of the Archpriest Avvakum and the Problem of Innovation." *Russian History* 35 (3–4): 275–308.

Ivanov, Sergey. 2006. *Holy Fools in Byzantium and Beyond*. Translated by Simon Franklin. Oxford: Oxford University Press

Joseph, M. P. Uday Balakrishnan, and Istvan Perczel. 2014. "Syrian Christian Churches in India." In *Eastern Christianity and Politics in the Twenty-First Century*, edited by Lucian N. Leustean, 563–599. London: Routledge.

Keane, Webb. 2007. *Christian Moderns: Freedom and Fetish in the Mission Encounter*. Berkeley: University of California Press.

Keller, Eva. 2005. *The Road to Clarity: Seventh-Day Adventism in Madagascar*. New York: Palgrave Macmillan.

Kharkhordin, Oleg. 1999. *The Collective and the Individual in Russia: A Study of Practices*. Berkeley: University of California Press.

Köllner, Tobias. 2013. *Practising without Belonging? Entrepreneurship, Morality, and Religion in Contemporary Russia*. Berlin: Lit.

Kumar, Krishna. 1988. "Origins of India's 'Textbook Culture.'" *Comparative Education Review* 32 (4): 452–64.

Lambek, Michael. 2000. "The Anthropology of Religion and the Quarrel between Poetry and Philosophy." *Current Anthropology* 41 (3): 309–19.

———. 2002. *The Weight of the Past: Living with History in Mahajanga, Madagascar*. New York: Palgrave Macmillan.

Luehrmann, Sonja. 2011. *Secularism Soviet Style: Teaching Atheism and Religion in a Volga Republic*. Bloomington: Indiana University Press.

Mar Gregorios, Paulos. 2011. "What Is Prayer?" In *Prayer Book for Young People*. Kottayam, India: Malankara Orthodox Church Publications and MGF Orthodox Theological Seminary.

Mauss, Marcel. (1938) 1985. "A Category of the Human Mind: The Notion of the Person; the Notion of Self." In *The Category of the Person: Anthropology, Philosophy, History*, edited by Michael Carrithers, Stephen Collins, and Steven Lukes, 1–25. Cambridge: Cambridge University Press.

———. (1950) 1979. Body Techniques. In *Sociology and Psychology: Essays*, edited by M. Mauss, 95–123. London: Routledge.

———. 2003. *On Prayer: Text and Commentary*. With an introduction by W. S. F. Pickering. Oxford: Berghahn Books.

Meyendorff, Jean. 2002. *Saint Gregoire Palamas et la mystique orthodoxe*. Paris: Editions du Seuil.
Mondzain, Marie-José. 2005. *Image, Icon, Economy: The Byzantine Origins of the Contemporary Imaginary*. Palo Alto: Stanford University Press.
Morgan, David. 1999. *Visual Piety: A History and Theory of Popular Religious Images*. Berkeley: University of California Press.
Naumescu, Vlad. 2007. *Modes of Religiosity in Eastern Christianity: Religious Processes and Social Change in Ukraine*. Berlin: Lit.
———. 2010. "Exorcising Demons in Post-Soviet Ukraine: A Monastic Community and Its Imagistic Practice." In *Eastern Christians in Anthropological Perspective*, edited by C. Hann and H. Goltz, 155–76. Berkeley: University of California Press.
———. 2011. "The Case for Religious Transmission: Time and Transmission in the Anthropology of Christianity." *Religion and Society: Advances in Research* 2:54–71.
———. 2012. "Learning the 'Science of Feelings': Religious Training in Eastern Christian Monasticism." *Ethnos* 77 (2): 227–51.
———. 2013. "Old Believers' Passion Play: The Meaning of Doubt in an Orthodox Ritualist Movement." In *Ethnographies of Doubt: Faith and Uncertainty in Contemporary Societies*, edited by Mathijs Pelkmans, 85–117. London: I. B. Tauris.
———. 2016. "The End Times and the Near Future: The Ethical Engagements of Russian Old Believers in Romania." *Journal of the Royal Anthropological Institute* 22 (2): 314–31.
———. Forthcoming. "Pedagogies of Prayer: Teaching Orthodoxy in the Malankara Church, South India." *Comparative Studies in Society and History*.
Orsi, Robert A. 2008. "Abundant History: Marian Apparitions as Alternative Modernity." *Historically Speaking* 9 (7): 12–16.
Orthodox Syrian Sunday School Association of the East. 2012. *Nazareth Division—Class 1*. Kottayam, India.
Ouspensky, Leonid. 1982. "The Meaning and Language of Icons." In *The Meaning of Icons*, by L. Ouspensky and V. Lossky, 23–50. Crestwood, NY: St. Vladimir's Seminary Press, 23–50.
Pickstock, C. J. C. 2010. "Liturgy and the Senses." *South Atlantic Quarterly* 109 (4): 719–39.
Rogers, Douglas. 2009. *The Old Faith and the Russian Land: An Historical Ethnography of Ethics in the Urals*. Ithaca: Cornell University Press.
Scheffel, David. 1991. *In the Shadow of Antichrist: The Old Believers of Alberta*. Lewiston, NY: Broadview Press.
Schmemann, Alexander. 1993. *Liturgy and Life: Christian Development through Liturgical Experience*. Crestwood, NY: St. Vladimir's Seminary Press.
Smilde, David. 2007. *Reason to Believe: Cultural Agency in Latin American Evangelicalism*. Berkeley: University of California Press.
Steinberg, Mark D., and Catherine Wanner, eds. 2008. *Religion, Morality, and Community in Post-Soviet Societies*. Bloomington: Indiana University Press.
Visvanathan, Susan. 1993. *The Christians of Kerala: History, Belief and Ritual among the Yakoba*. Madras, India: Oxford University Press.
Vrame, Anton C. 1999. *The Educating Icon*. Brookline: Holy Cross Orthodox Press.
Wanner, Catherine. 2003. "Advocating New Moralities: Conversion to Evangelicalism in Ukraine." *Religion, State and Society* 31 (3): 273–87.
Ware, Kallistos. 1986. *The Power of the Name: The Jesus Prayer in Orthodox Spirituality*. Oxford: SLG Press/Sisters of the Love of God Press.

———. 1991. *The Orthodox Church*. Harmondsworth: Penguin Books.
———. 2001. *The Inner Kingdom*. Crestwood, NY: St. Vladimir's Seminary Press.
Zigon, Jarrett. 2008. "Aleksandra Vladimirovna: Moral Narratives of a Russian Orthodox Woman." In *Religion, Morality, and Community in Post-Soviet Societies*, edited by Mark D. Steinberg and Catherine Wanner, 85–113. Bloomington: Indiana University Press.
———. 2010. *HIV Is God's Blessing: Rehabilitating Morality in Neoliberal Russia*. Berkeley: University of California Press.
———, ed. 2012. *Multiple Moralities and Religions in Post-Soviet Russia*. New York: Berghahn.

A MISSIONARY PRIMER

IOANN VENIAMINOV

(Editor's note: The pamphlet *Indication of the Way into the Kingdom of Heaven* was published by the priest Ioann Veniaminov in Unangan [Aleut], one of the indigenous languages of Alaska, in 1833. Later canonized as Saint Innocent, metropolitan of Moscow, Veniaminov served as priest and bishop in Russia's Alaskan colonies between 1824 and 1838. To this day, Orthodox Christianity remains widespread among the Unangan, Alutiiq, and Tlingit of South Alaska.

Veniaminov's explanation of the Christian life was aimed at Unangan converts but later became popular among Russian readers as well, with several Russian-language editions published between 1839 and 1855. It is a good example of a lay-oriented theology of *theosis*, explaining both distance from and closeness to God in very practical, bodily, and emotional terms. The missionary insists on the possibility of gaining salvation while living a worldly life, at least in the male-gendered terms of being a husband and father.)

> The first man, being created in the image and likeness of God, until he had obscured the likeness of God by his self-will, was blessed in that very image and likeness of God. Just as God has no end and is eternal, so too Adam was created immortal. God is all-just, and Adam was created sinless and just. God is all-happy, and Adam was created happy, and his happiness could have increased day by day throughout all eternity.
>
> Adam lived in a most beautiful Paradise, in a garden planted by God Himself, where he was content with everything. He was always healthy and well, and he would never have known any kind of sickness. He was

not afraid of anyone or anything. All the animals and birds obeyed him as their king. He felt neither cold nor heat. And although he labored and worked in Paradise yet he worked with pleasure and delight, and did not find toil burdensome or work tiring.

His heart and soul were full of the knowledge and love of God. He was always quiet and happy, and he never knew and never saw anything unpleasant, upsetting, painful or sad. All his desires were pure, right and in order. His memory, intellect and all the other faculties of his soul were perfect. And being innocent and pure, he always lived with God and conversed with Him, and God loved him as His favorite son. To be brief, Adam was in Paradise, and Paradise was in Adam.

Now, if Adam had not broken the commandment of His Creator, he would have been happy himself and all his descendants would have always been happy too. But Adam sinned before God and broke His law, and the easiest law; and for that reason God banished him from Paradise, because God cannot live with sin or with a sinner.

Adam at once lost the happiness he had enjoyed in Paradise. His soul was darkened, his thoughts or desires were muddled, his imagination and memory began to be clouded. Instead of joy and peace of soul, he saw sorrow, afflictions, troubles, poverty, the most painful labors and every kind of adversity. Finally sickly old age threatened him, and after that—death. But the most horrible thing of all was that the devil, who is consoled by the sufferings of men, gained power over Adam.

The very elements, that is the air, fire, etc., which had previously served Adam and ministered to his pleasure, then became hostile to him. From that time Adam and all his descendants began to feel hunger, heat and the effects of change of winds and weather. Wild animals became savage, and began to look upon people as their enemies and as prey. From that time people began to feel external and internal diseases which in course of time increased in number and severity. Men forgot that they were brothers and began to attack one another, to hate, to deceive, to torture and to kill. And finally, after all kinds of bitter labors and anxieties, they had to die; and as they were sinners they had to be in hell and to be eternally and unceasingly tormented there.

No human being by himself could or can restore what Adam lost. And what would have happened to us if Jesus Christ in His mercy had not redeemed us? What would have happened to the whole human race? God[,] Who loves us far more than we love ourselves, in His great mercy sent us His Son Jesus Christ to save us. Jesus Christ became a man like us, but without sin.

By His teaching Jesus Christ scattered the darkness and errors of the human mind, and enlightened the whole world with the light of the Gospel. Now everyone who wants to can know the will of God and the means and way to happiness. . . .

Some say: "How can we who are so weak and sinful be like the Saints, and how are we to be saved? We live in the world and have various duties." This is not only untrue, but it is blasphemy and an insult to our Creator. . . . Look at the Saints! They were not all hermits; and they were like us at first and were not sinless, and they were also engaged in worldly affairs, cares and duties, and many of them had a family as well. But while doing their worldly occupations and duties, they did not forget at the same time their duties as Christians; and while living in the world, they made their way at the same time into the Kingdom of Heaven and often led others with them as well. In exactly the same way, if we wish, we can be at once good citizens, faithful husbands and good fathers, and also good and faithful Christians.

SOURCE

Saint Innocent of Alaska, *Indication of the Way into the Kingdom of Heaven: An Introduction to Christian Life* (Jordanville, NY: Holy Trinity Publications, 2013).

2 LISTENING AND THE SACRAMENTAL LIFE: DEGREES OF MEDIATION IN GREEK ORTHODOX CHRISTIANITY

JEFFERS ENGELHARDT

THE MEDIA OF ORTHODOX CHRISTIANITY are sensible everywhere—in the materials and prototypes of icons; in the sacred language, script, and chant notation of service books; in the intercessory power of saints; in the bodies and voices of clergy; in the architectural acoustics of churches; in the Eucharist; and, ultimately, in Christ as the hypostatic union of God and humanity.[1] In the case of the iconoclast controversy and the codification of exclusively vocal worship by the church fathers and ecumenical councils, mediatic concerns (with their attendant understandings of personhood and sensory experience) helped to define Orthodoxy as such. This process, I suggest, is ongoing, continually connecting media technologies to ideas about the orthodoxy of Orthodoxy (Bandak and Boylston 2014).

It is not only these "old" media that are essential to the making of Orthodoxy and Orthodox Christians. As they are activated by religious institutions and engaged by believers at "nodes of mediation" (Mazzarella 2004, 352), the "new" technologies mediating Orthodoxy are essential as well—radio and television broadcasts; social media and curated online content; digital recordings of chant and sermons; digitized service and prayer books; the Jesus Prayer, elders' sayings, and *íson* (the vocal drone in Byzantine chant) apps for mobile devices; and mobile devices themselves.

This chapter emerges from fieldwork in and around Thessaloniki in Central Macedonia, Greece, exploring Orthodox Christians' engagement with media technologies "old" and "new." Here, I hope to illuminate how the media turn "away from belief and toward materiality; away from formalism and toward practice; away from religion and the secular toward the postsecular and, in some cases, even back to enchantment" (Engelke 2010, 375) in the study of religion intersects with Orthodox traditions bearing on media and mediation. As its foundational concerns with voice, images, materiality, the body, and the senses show, Orthodox Christianity has long been shaped by rich, reflexive discourse on the nature of religious mediation (Engelhardt 2015, 34–46).

My point of departure here is a conversation I had with Georgios, a twenty-four-year-old student, chanter, and son of a priest. As Georgios talked about his priest, whose pastoral work includes sending targeted e-mails to groups of parishioners with YouTube links and online readings, and his practice of listening to live ("real prayer"), not studio ("artificial perfection"), recordings from the Irmologion ahead of specific feasts, he articulated with particular clarity the mediatic nature and spiritual teleology of contemporary Greek Orthodoxy (my interviews were conducted in English and with a Greek translator):

> Everything about media falls under the three stages of our faith—catharsis, illumination (*theoria*), and *theosis* [deification]. All the hymnody and liturgy and prayers are accessible to everyone, but not everyone needs them in the same way. The church fathers who wrote theology were in a state of illumination; saints are in a state of *theosis*. All may at times use hymnody and music and media, but this is most important for us in the first stage of catharsis. They, as we know from reading their lives, were hesychastic and left behind all media and only focused on the sacraments—receiving the Eucharist, confession, etc. Media are more important for us in this first stage, and the fact that there isn't a sacrament in your room at home is what pushes you back to community and liturgy.

This last thought is essential to an understanding of the nature of media in Orthodoxy. For Georgios, while the church fathers and saints had more immediate knowledge and experience of God, the mediation of texts, sounds, images, objects, and materials was more necessary for those at the purifying stage of catharsis. Orthodox Christians use media to establish and inhabit what they call a "Christocentric everyday" at the junctures of institutions, media technologies, a religiously shaped sensorium, and the living tradition (Greek *parádosis*) of Orthodoxy. The Christocentric everyday is a worldly Orthodox milieu of ethical action and Christlike becoming, a counterpoint to the exemplary monastic version of this struggle that was a constant part of laypeople's lives in and around Thessaloniki, not least because of the city's proximity to Mount Athos. In our conversations, people characterized the Christocentric everyday as a noisy, hectic place juxtaposed with the serene hesychastic meditation of the saints (see Dubovka in this volume). For ordinary believers, listening practices helped navigate family and professional commitments and the encroachments of secularity. Listening filled silences not dedicated to prayer and masked sounds and messages not dedicated to Christocentric living, helping laypeople follow the exemplar of saints by aspiring to pray continually and "remember God."

Orthodox Christian engagements with media technologies at the stage of catharsis aspired ideally (and without paradox) to the immediacy of illumination and *theosis* (see Blanton 2015; Brennan 2012, 2010). As Georgios explained, these engagements continually returned to the authority of liturgical experience—to an Orthodox anthropology of human beings as liturgical beings who are fully realized through worship—and a sacramental theology. In this economy of mediation, the church, not only as institutionalized power but also as the continuity, conciliarity, and communion (koinonia) of Orthodox tradition, is the ultimate authorized mediator. Here, the church is the "community of deferral" (Bandak and Boylston 2014, 26) that is hailed through the understood (but perhaps unarticulated) orthodoxy of people's engagements with media technologies. As Andreas Bandak and Tom Boylston suggest, such forms of deferral to the authority and mystery of the church through open-ended scriptural, aesthetic, and practical traditions are particularly Orthodox, creating "a world in which divine perfection and fallible humanity are able to interrelate" (26).

For those I worked with, attending to Orthodox media and engaging media technologies in an Orthodox way made sense through the experience and memory of liturgy and, ultimately, through the absolute end of Orthodox mediation—the felt immediacy of God's presence and mystery in the sacraments. Electronic, broadcast, and digital media, even when produced and authorized by Orthodox institutions, were *marked* media—the electric currents, code, formats, and technologies that brought sounds and messages beyond the sacramental space of the church heightened the awareness of mediation and sense of remove from the sacramental life of the church. On the other hand, the "natural" media for Orthodox sounds and messages, such as incense-laden air, human voices and bodies, and bells, were *unmarked* media thought of as immediate in the context of liturgical experience and sacramental theology.

Chief among these unmarked media was the human voice, the ideal medium of Orthodox sound that reveals a mystical continuity between the voices of God, celestial beings, and human beings. The voice unites humanity and divinity through Christ, the incarnate Word of God and the second person of the Trinity, whose bodily existence included having a voice. This privileging of the human voice is based on beliefs about its immediate perfection as a source of sound created by God and able to pray, perform scripture, and sing the musical prototypes of celestial beings (Moody 2015). Conversely, the proscription of musical instruments in most parts of the Orthodox world is based on beliefs about their imperfection as human creations alienated from language, incapable of prayer, and associated with pagan ritual and worldly pursuits like dance and work. Although instrumental music is extolled in the Old Testament (for example, in Psalm 150), it is usually considered as one of the many Old Covenant practices not incorporated into what became Orthodox Christianity. The Orthodox voice is pastoral—it leads the church in worship and prayer, not in making music. This immediacy is echoed in Orthodox theological discourse on the voice in which it is described not only as singing or chanting but also as reading, serving, praying, glorifying, and hymning. In Orthodox monastic traditions, the medium of the voice is valued because it is not a possession that ties one to the world as a form of property.

This brings me to an important distinction. The contrast I draw here between marked and unmarked mediation recasts the often-observed capacity of certain forms of religious mediation to transcend themselves through their authorization and sacralization, effacing form and rendering content immediate (Blanton 2015, 27; Brennan 2010, 2012; Eisenlohr 2009; Engelke 2007; Meyer 2009, 12; Oosterbaan 2008; Stolow 2010). This is a contrast between sacramental participation distanced through the objectified, aestheticized (Feaster 2015, 145), disembodied (Feld 1995; Schafer [1977] 1993) qualities of recorded voices, prayers, and messages and the sensed or remembered immediacy of sacramental participation in liturgy. The Orthodox Christian engagements with media technologies did not recognize a Kittler-type (1999) immediacy in decontextualized voices reduced to sound through their technological inscription (a potential powerfully acted upon in other contexts of religious mediation; see Martin 2014). Rather, the prayers and messages people listened to beyond the acoustic, spiritual, and social space of the church were markedly mediatic and ontologically removed from Orthodox sacramental life. For instance, people generally would not cross themselves (as they intuitively would during liturgy) while listening to recordings of prayers and hymns (although I will describe moments of intense bodily and sensory engagement with recorded prayer later on). Gesturing bodies responded differently to the marked media of pastoral voices coming from electronic devices.

While the affordances of electronic and digital media technologies expedited and enriched processes of religious learning (training cantors, studying theology and saints' lives) and extended the scale of religious publics and spiritual fathers' guidance, they necessarily intensified questions of religious authority and discernment. Orthodox radio and television broadcast outlets in Thessaloniki were run by the church, but individually curated YouTube channels and MP3 blogs of sermons and talks were where alternative religious styles, sensibilities, and messages circulated. As Georgios and others shared with me, reflexivity and discernment mattered in making one's way through the media landscapes of contemporary Greek Orthodoxy in terms of understanding church-authorized messages and the clamor of extra-institutional mediation. Parish priests who sent weekly e-mails with links to hymns and sermons, spiritual fathers who maintained blogs and were quick to answer text messages, and chant teachers who shared flash drives full of particular stylistic interpretations played an important role in establishing the Orthodoxy of these marked media.

The Orthodoxy of traditional, unmarked media (bodies and voices, books, icons, relics, bells, the Eucharist) required far less (if any) spiritual discernment, since these were intimately connected to and authorized by the felt immediacy of liturgy and the sacramental life of the church. This sense of immediacy, essentially indistinguishable from Orthodox tradition and the church itself, is what oriented the "push back to the church" that Georgios and others spoke of as the ultimate end of their engagements with media technologies. Practices of listening to chant, prayers, sermons, and religious talks strengthened (or were intended to strengthen) individuals' participation in Orthodox sacramental life (see Harrison 2013). Orthodox media used in Orthodox ways continually invoked the mystery (*mysterion*, the Greek word for sacrament) of divine grace in the sacramental life of the church in the world. This kind of sacramental mystery had everything to do with the degrees of Orthodox mediation and a religiously attuned sensorium: mysteries are commonly described as visible signs of invisible grace (and these signs engage all the other senses as well). They encompass the conventional seven mysteries (baptism, chrismation, Eucharist, confession, marriage, ordination, holy unction) and extend to all of life in its sacramental, Eucharistic sense (see Schmemann 1973). Famously, Saint John Chrysostom writes that mysteries are so called because what is seen is not what is understood or believed. One thing is seen but another perceived, and this, as Chrysostom stresses, depends upon conditions of belief and the capacity to behold signs of mystery. In other words, mystery reaches to the core of Orthodoxy's semiotic ideologies and forms of marked and unmarked media as they are continually located in the church and its tradition (see Bandak and Boylston 2014)—in the "push back to the church."

The engagements with media technologies I explore here were key parts of this movement, imbuing the everyday with Christocentric purpose, sharpening individuals' discernment of correct doctrine and style, leading people in prayer and focusing their attention on the offering of worship, preparing cantors to fulfill their pastoral role, and improving people's spiritual condition. These capacities are not inherent in media technologies or mediatic forms themselves. Rather, this process of mediation relies upon the "ethically responsive sensorium" (Hirschkind 2006, 10) of listeners and their experience and memory of liturgy, as its efficacy depends upon listeners knowing how to receive the right way (see Engelhardt 2015; Luhrmann, Nusbaum, and Thisted 2010; Reinhardt 2014, 323; but see Oosterbaan 2008, 134, for an alternative model of ethical listening and Larkin 2014 on the place of inattention in engaging religious media). While "new" media technologies reshaped and rescaled the circuits through which Orthodoxy took shape (see Carl 2015; Larkin 2009, 118; Stolow 2010), they also led people back to the church and worked to produce and align religious subjects and institutions.

In what follows, then, I situate ethnographically the all-important "push back to the church"—a movement toward immediacy—within a moment of Greek post-crisis neoliberal austerity in 2013. This was not something novel to that moment, however. Rather, it was an instance of a broader dynamic in Orthodox Christianity in which reflexive understandings of religious orthodoxy were mobilized at moments of transition, revival, and renewal in the name of moral and social reform—(re)turning to or restoring "Byzantine" or "medieval" styles of iconography, chant, liturgy, and architecture; (re)converting; composing new prayers and repurposing existing ones; (re)establishing institutions for education and social care; and reimagining or recovering the relationship of Orthodox Christianity to conditions of secularity and plurality. From an Orthodox perspective, these responses to cycles of crisis were not considered innovations but rather clarifying, communally affirmed articulations of the living tradition of Orthodoxy that reorient the church toward its own truth.

MEDIA ENGAGEMENT AND SOCIAL ETHICS

"Don't fear God when it's thundering—God has already decided what to do. Fear God when nothing's happening." This was how Nikos, a diligent Orthodox believer, father, and entrepreneur living in a village outside Thessaloniki, described his experience of post-crisis neoliberal austerity. His point was that the economic and political turmoil of 2013 (manifest most immediately in the unfinished villas dotting the landscape of his village and more broadly in the policies of the European Commission, European Central Bank, and International Monetary Fund "troika"; anti-immigration rhetoric; young-adult economic malaise; and resistance to a secularism identified with the EU) was the outcome of a prior spiritual and social failure. This was a failure to place Orthodoxy at the center of life choices and social ethics and to discern whether the messages of authorized religious voices had valid connections to canonical Orthodoxy and the teachings of the church fathers or were motivated by "personal prejudice and egotistical views." For Nikos, "all political and financial crises are spiritual crises"—a failure to set the sacramental life of the church at the center of one's life, above material success and social status. He cited a recent religious broadcast on the Athens-based Church of Piraeus FM station, which he streamed online on a daily basis. The talk emphasized the causes and dangers of stress in contemporary life, maintaining that stress is a "spiritual ailment because you don't have trust in God, a distraction from the true faith."

Nikos valued these messages because they linked Greek politics and social ethics to Orthodoxy, enabling him and his family to meaningfully relate their media engagements to an experience of post-crisis neoliberal austerity. By listening mainly to broadcast content on official church channels, Nikos and his family opened themselves up to messages not of their own choosing, about which they later consulted trusted online sources and their spiritual fathers. All this was a reminder that "faith is alive and dynamic, and one needs to stay informed about the truth of the faith and the correctness of the faith." For Nikos, Orthodox media were involved both in the etiology of social and political crisis (for not speaking about Orthodox social ethics with sufficient force) and in the overcoming of those crises (by making the church once again central in the life of the nation). Daily media engagements were a means of religious cultivation and political resistance to a host of forces glossed as the EU in the Greek context but that might appear as crises brought about by secularism, atheism, or ecumenism; political oppression; ethno-national conflict; interreligious struggle; or disaffection with mainstream Protestant and evangelical Christianities in other contexts.

Not all Orthodox Christians in and around Thessaloniki engaged media technologies to the same extent and in the same ways, of course. What stood out, however, was that the rhythms of their day or week; the soundscapes they inhabited; their social interactions with family, friends, and strangers; and their lives of prayer were punctuated by purposeful engagements with Orthodox media. They sought sound in the form of chant, prayer, and speech rather than the hesychastic silence idealized in Orthodox monastic tradition. They lived in a world of marked media in an Orthodox way, a counterpoint to the relative immediacy and silence of nearby Mount Athos.

Accessing Byzantine chant, sermons, and religious talks on laptops through institutionally and individually curated YouTube channels was by far the most common practice—something done by older village priests around the table with their families; middle-aged, single professionals living in urban apartments; and students in their early twenties rethinking the role of Orthodoxy in their lives. It was also common for middle-aged professional men and women with families to use physical recordings of Byzantine chant and prayer services in their listening practices (professionally produced CDs and, in some cases, prized vinyl records from the 1970s). These were people with disposable income and the inclination to travel to monasteries and purchase recordings (mostly men), study the styles of renowned cantors for professional and spiritual reasons (mostly men and some women), and shop frequently at church-run media stores selling books, CDs, icons, and other Orthodox material (mostly women). The materiality of these media meant they were in close spatial proximity to other Orthodox media—laminated reproductions of icons of Saint Nicholas the Wonderworker in cars and prayer books and incense burners on bookshelves in homes.

For middle-aged and younger people who used mobile media technologies continually in everyday life, similar Orthodox content was added and edited as MP3 files on a daily or weekly basis. The least common media engagement I found was with broadcast or live-streamed radio and television content (not least because much of this content was available asynchronously online). Those who turned to synchronous broadcasts and live-streaming liturgies and religious talks were, by and large, middle-aged women who did significant amounts of work in the home and men and women with long commutes by car.

In all cases, the Orthodox Christians I worked with were active—if not extremely active—churchgoers who performed the daily prescribed prayers, listened to the particular festal hymns of the day, and worked to deepen their knowledge of Orthodox teaching and tradition through daily media engagements. Their listening practices, in other words, embodied the religiously shaped sensorium and movement toward a felt immediacy that is the end of Orthodox mediation. Moreover, they were people who did not sense an important moral distinction between the marked media of recordings, YouTube, and mobile devices and the unmarked media of voices, books, and icons. On multiple occasions, people shared with me a saying they attributed to Saint John Chrysostom in order to describe their understanding of Orthodox media. The two versions I heard were "A knife can kill or cure, depending on the person" and "A knife can cut bread or cut a throat, depending on who holds it." Media technologies, in this scheme, are morally neutral. They can be used efficaciously, with the discernment of a religiously shaped sensorium and pastoral guidance for spiritual improvement, and to draw closer to the sacramental life of the church. So while specific media technologies shape Orthodoxy, media technologies can also be made Orthodox, so to speak, through specific practices and sensibilities.

In and around Thessaloniki, the Orthodoxy of the soundscape and landscape, the ubiquity of Orthodox media, and the commonplace presence of Orthodoxy in public culture, national identity, and the built environment naturalized the relation of media technologies and Orthodoxy. The amplified voices of male chanters and choirs permeated the urban and suburban spaces around churches and monasteries. Bells and amplified chant and prayer emanating from churches and chapels were unremarkable aspects of urban and suburban life (see Eisenlohr 2012 and Weiner 2014 on media, sound, and religious diversity), and people intuitively crossed themselves upon hearing these Orthodox sounds. This was something I attributed to their unmarked status as the sounding of sacred spaces and the fact that people heard these sounds as indices of worship and prayer rather than as the marked media of a CD or mobile device. For many attending services, electronic amplification was desirable even when it was unnecessary and low quality—an aesthetic norm for mediating the Orthodox voice with a religious signal penetrating through the noise of low-fidelity equipment as people listened through the electrosonic materiality of the voice to the sacramental reality it mediated. Icons of Orthodox saints and graffiti of Byzantine-style angels by the artist Fikos were prominent in all kinds of public spaces, as were miniature, mailbox-sized prayer chapels along roadsides and larger concrete prayer chapels outside corporate buildings and homes. Finally, the intensity of Orthodox life—particularly devout worshippers routinely participated in four-hour Vigils and churches swelled to capacity on Sundays and feast days—was grounded upon the support of the Greek state and a deep connection to tourism and heritage industries.

So who was outside these circuits of Orthodox mediation? Some who were intensely active in church and pursued a life of prayer were outside because of access and religious ideology. In terms of access, it was a matter not only of how generational identity and engagement with media technologies articulated but also of how individuals did or did not encounter models of media engagement through priests' e-mails, family members and friends, and parish communities. In terms of religious ideology, it was a matter of whether or not people sensed a crucial distinction between the marked media of recordings, broadcasts, online content, and mobile devices and the unmarked media—the felt immediacy—of voices, books, and icons. From a "traditionalist" (Fajfer 2012) Orthodox perspective, the electric and electronic can impede spiritual progress by dehumanizing individuals' capacities of attention, discernment, and ascetic struggle (see Larkin 2014). Others were outside for the most obvious of reasons—a lack of religious commitment or interest in creating a Christocentric everyday through their engagements with media.

DEGREES OF MEDIATION IN ORTHODOX LISTENING PRACTICES

I turn now to portraits of four people whose listening practices and engagements with media technologies point to how the "push back to the church" unfolded in individual lives. These stories tease out how the distinctions people made between marked and unmarked media moved between the Christocentric everyday and the sacramental life of the church, affirming the (at times tenuous) centripetal force of the latter in Orthodox mediation. Whether it was using recordings and mobile apps to teach and prepare cantors to sing correctly, prayerfully, and with humility; connecting one's day to the liturgical calendar by listening to daily broadcast services; managing one's immersion in Orthodox discourse by seeking out and downloading sermons and talks by particular priests and spiritual fathers; or preparing oneself to attend liturgy and participate in the sacramental life of the church more fully, these practices captured how Orthodox religious mediation worked.

Manolis

Manolis lives with his wife and small children in a village outside Thessaloniki. He works as a physical therapist, chants in a local parish, and has a passion for winemaking. Now in his late twenties, he began chanting (nearly every word in Orthodox liturgy is mediated by a sung voice) when he was nineteen after making a pilgrimage to Mount Athos for Holy Pascha. There, he sang secular Cypriot songs for some of the monks who were impressed with his voice but admonished him that if one can sing well, it is sinful not to cultivate one's voice to praise God. This resonated with Manolis's understanding of Orthodox personhood, and he quickly sought out a teacher with whom he could study

Byzantine chant. His father-in-law is a priest and gave him the opportunity to be at the chanting stand (analogion) as he was learning. Eventually, Manolis came to lead the chanting in services, which he explained was a means of spiritual and ethical "improvement" because "services aren't just services—they are mysteries":

> We want to be with our God more. When you want to spend more time with a person, you want to become more like them, just like you want to be more like God and more in God's energies and awe in services. Chanting is a way of being thankful and doxologizing—a way of becoming as forgiving and accepting with others as God is with us. I guess that could be *theosis*. And the modes [the melodic patterns and affective forms that are paired with particular liturgical texts and calendric cycles] help with this—they express our emotions to God and make the emotions from outside. Your repentance is shaped by a repentant mode.

Media were an essential part of Manolis's study, and different media technologies assumed different functions in his spiritual and technical "improvement" as a cantor. Manolis amassed a collection of CDs from Orthodox bookstores in Thessaloniki, recordings from Mount Athos and other monasteries he visited, an extensive mental catalog of YouTube videos and channels, and hundreds of MP3 files obtained from his teacher on flash drives. He explained that his CDs were tokens of powerful experiences at monasteries and pilgrimage sites—material artifacts mediating special styles of chanting that were the basis of his affective memories and religious/aesthetic ideals. Manolis used his mental catalog of YouTube videos and channels to prepare for services (like many I spoke with, he did not bookmark YouTube content but kept scores of individual and institutional curators in mind), checking on how to correctly perform more demanding, modally variable hymns like "Axion Estin"—a hymn magnifying the honor and purity of the Theotokos. The MP3 files his teacher passed along on flash drives were different versions of the same daily hymns performed by esteemed cantors. Unlike earlier chant pedagogies using recordings on disks, tapes, or records, this intensified form of teaching and encounter with tradition was enabled by the compression of the MP3 format (see Sterne 2012). Manolis's teacher instructed him to listen critically and comparatively to different realizations of hymns, not only to prepare to sing "in a humble, spiritual way" in services and "make it prayer, not just struggling with the music," but also to shape his sense of style and understanding of ethos (the affective character of a Byzantine mode) and *yphos* (the style of interpreting and performing the neumes or signs of Byzantine notation) (Khalil 2009).

Manolis's "improvement" extended to engagements with media outside of services as well—engagements that helped him "not to be scattered" in preparation for prayer or that were prayer practices in and of themselves. Like candles and incense that, when lit at home, focus the mind and senses into a "prayerful mode" and "cleanse the house from the evil one," Manolis used CDs and MP3s as technologies to enhance his attentiveness and lead him in prayer. He often listened to a recording of the supplicatory canon (*paraklesis*) to the Theotokos sung by the choir of the women's monastery of Ormylia near Thessaloniki—a choir revered locally for the ascetic simplicity of its style, which was based on the tradition of the Simonpetra Monastery on Mount Athos. Manolis used this recorded *paraklesis* in the way others listened to these prayers to the Theotokos and other saints—by following the text in palm-sized booklets accompanying CDs, online, or on a mobile device and in the presence of an icon of the Theotokos or saint (or an image of an icon online or on a mobile device). He would also recite the Jesus Prayer with the help of a prayer rope while playing a *paraklesis* or other recording, creating a polyphony of prayer that rendered the recording as ambient prayerful background rather than the surrogate voice of prayer. The "improvement" afforded by Manolis's everyday practice of the Jesus Prayer was woven into a musical and religious engagement with the urban sonic environment as well. As he traveled from his village into Thessaloniki by bus for work, he would perform the Jesus Prayer in an internal, ersatz Byzantine chant, using the hum of the bus's engine and tires as the *íson* grounding his melodic extemporizations.

Vasilis

In the middle of a conversation with Vasilis, a cantor, choir leader, and teacher in his late twenties from Thessaloniki, we were interrupted by a call on his mobile phone. Vasilis's ringtone was an *apechema*—a solo intonation formula in Byzantine chant used to establish the pitch and modal ethos of a hymn (Lind 2012, 98–100). We had just been talking about the electrosonic materiality of the voice, the liturgical/aesthetic norm of electronic amplification (often low-quality), and the vocal technique of chanting with a microphone in contemporary Greek Orthodoxy (see Harkness 2014), all of which, Vasilis felt, made it necessary to discern spiritually between the voice as object (its status as a marked medium) and the voice as worship and prayer (its status as an unmarked medium gesturing toward immediacy). He explained that because Orthodox canons and traditions were codified before the advent of electronic media technologies, there was much debate in Greece about what proper engagement with media is for Orthodox Christians. Were only the "old" media of icons, books, bells, and voices appropriate, or could the "new" media of mobile devices and websites be used in Orthodox ways? Some bishops and theologians were critical of the ubiquity of broadcast services and liturgies on Greek radio and television (prior to the controversial June 2013 austerity measure of defunding the Hellenic Broadcasting Corporation) since, according to Vasilis, "one could be going about daily business and drinking or smoking or eating and flipping through channels and watching some television magazine and then a liturgy and not change one's behavior in any way." Simply put, a fear in Greece was that with too many easily accessible services and liturgies broadcast on television and radio and available asynchronously online, people would not go to church, signaling the failure of a semiotic ideology (Keane 2007) directed toward the sacraments and mystery of the church. Or if they went, they would attend with the sensory habits and passive spiritual disposition of broadcast services and liturgies—worship and prayer would not be immediate.

Vasilis had a different perspective, inspired in part by a sermon he listened to many times on CD by the revered and extremely popular Metropolitan Athanasius of Cyprus. In the sermon, Metropolitan Athanasius explained that technologies like electric lights, heating, microphones, and loudspeakers were tools that can aid worship "so long as the human person isn't offended—anything that doesn't work against humanity can be used in liturgical life" (but see opposite attitudes in monastic communities on Mount Athos in Fajfer 2012). Vasilis extended this understanding to media technologies as well, paraphrasing the apostle Paul that "we must use whatever means we have to advance our spirituality and knowledge." The recorded sermons of Metropolitan Athanasius and others, recordings or broadcasts of a *paraklesis* to the Theotokos or a saint chanted by extraordinary monastic choirs, and having the Great Compline prayers accessible on mobile devices have "worked miracles" in Vasilis's and others' lives, renewing their faith and "reconverting" them to the church.

As Vasilis finished his call, I asked whether his *apechema* ringtone, heard dozens of times each day in the frenetic bustle of urban life and family routines through the treble-heavy speakers of his mobile phone (see Marshall 2014 on the "treble culture" of mobile devices more generally), contributed to the contemporary problems we were just discussing—the electrosonic objectification of the voice as a shift from prayer to performance, spiritual humility to virtuosic pride, pastoral leadership to individual distinction. He answered as I expected he would, drawing my attention to the picture of his wife and child on the lock screen of his mobile phone: "I put this there because I love them very much. On another day, I will put an icon of Christ there because I love him very much." He went on to liken the sound of recorded chant to mediated images or reproductions of icons, stressing that its incursion into the textures of daily routine was invaluable to Christocentric living and remembering God—in Vasilis's words, the imperative to "always pray," paraphrasing the letter of Paul directed to the Christians of Vasilis's city (1 Thess. 5:17). Vasilis was reflexive about marked media in these examples, knowing that their ends were in participating in the sacramental life of the church.

In his teaching and chanting, Vasilis stressed the value of media technologies in extending the scale of human interaction in lessons and services required to assimilate Byzantine chant (see Summit 2016). This pedagogy of prayer involved imitating recordings of great cantors, creating a recorded archive of lessons and services, and using a digital *íson* for practice and, occasionally, chanting services. (Mobile applications for generating *íson* pitches digitally are controversial in Greece because of the nonhuman ontology of their sound.) These tools intensified the learning process, sensitizing novice cantors to the intricacies of modal ethos and *yphos* to the extent that Vasilis knows "fifteen-year-olds that chant as well as if they'd been studying their whole life, as if they'd been studying sixty years, and not just imitating exactly all the ornaments of great cantors." He quickly added: "Was there a spiritual advantage when it took fifty or sixty years? I can't say because this is how I learned."

The discursive context of Vasilis's embrace of digital media technologies was the strong association of the nonelectric, nonelectronic, and nondigital with immediacy and mystery. He wondered, for instance, what spiritual benefit was lost over the course of years and a lifetime by cantors—whose work is the offering of an ordained ecclesial office—who rely on quickly accessible, digitally compiled texts for services instead of taking the time to immerse themselves in the Typikon (a book of rubrics specifying the correct ordering of services according to Orthodox calendric cycles) and an "ascetic mode" in order to juggle the requisite service books. His answer, emanating nostalgically from the experience of Greek neoliberal austerity (and comparable to a range of traditionalist nostalgias in contexts of modernity), deferred to a mystical, "natural," more immediate mode of prayer and worship:

> On Mount Athos, at Vatopeidi, you have a chorus of fifty people; they use no lights, only lamps and candles—this has an effect and you receive it in a way that goes very deep. The silence of only physical means—it touches deep down in you. So it's about the senses—you have the electric light and it's at

a constant volume, but the candle fluctuates and changes; you have a book and you can touch it and smell it. To a person like me, who is not a saint and very far away from a deep spiritual reality, all this affects me and helps me pray. Nothing bothers a holy person, though—you can have electronic books, a digital drone, and electric lights. This physical reality doesn't get to them and doesn't affect their state of perception. But again I have the question: if we asked a famous elder—take Elder Paisios—and gave him two chapels, one with candles and just books and one with lights and electronic equipment, microphones and iPads and whatnot. Where would he go and attend? He would probably go to the natural one. Is there a reality that we're not perceptive to? Are they more spiritually insightful, that they can understand it differently?

Vasilis teased out a distinction between the mysteries of "natural" (unmarked) media and materials and the practicalities of electronic and digital (marked) media that goes to the core of an individual's spiritual condition. Drawing on an Athonite, ascetic ideal of Orthodox spirituality, he described Elder Paisios's hypothetical choice as the mystical expression of the reality he inhabited immediately, not the means of encountering that reality. Elder Paisios, a monk who died in 1994 and was canonized a saint in 2015, would be untroubled by electronic media because of the fullness of his sacramental mode of living. (This recalls Georgios's thoughts at the outset about media and the stages of faith in which saints "left behind all media and only focused on the sacraments.") Nevertheless, there was something of a romantic link in Vasilis's mind between the unplugged powers of traditional media and their role in perceiving mystery.

In Vasilis's thinking about the mediation of Orthodoxy, media technologies are tools for spiritual advancement when engaged through the desire to humbly love God. He put this bluntly: a prideful cantor will be unchanged by a microphone, and a humble cantor will sing humbly with a microphone. Media technologies themselves have no inherent soteriological capacity, which is why Vasilis could say that "spirituality isn't affected by technology." The sensorium and performative practices through which individuals realized Orthodoxy by engaging media technologies correctly, with discernment, and within tradition (see Engelhardt 2015), continually returned to the authority of liturgical experience and sacramental theology. For Vasilis, this meant there was an absolute end in the mediation of Orthodoxy, and that end was in the sacraments, not in the Christocentric everyday of engaging media technologies: "There is a difference between the spiritual state of a person and salvation. Technology cannot save you; you can become a better person by listening to everything, but if you don't participate in the sacraments you cannot be saved. Technology cannot come and take over or replace the sacraments."

Eleni

Eleni is a music teacher at a school and a mother living in a newly built condominium development (where many of her extended family live) in a village outside Thessaloniki. She is a "sound engineer" in Paul Greene's (1999) sense—someone who uses Orthodox media and media technologies to transform the quotidian textures of daily life into devotion. She explained it this way: "Fifty years ago, what did women do while working to not worry about the house and children and put the mind on higher things? They prayed the Jesus Prayer or they had the time to go to a priest. But I don't have this time." Eleni spent significant amounts of time each day engaging Orthodox media while commuting to work in her car, working at home, and in the late evening before going to sleep. Many times each day, she listened to Lydia FM, a Church of Greece radio station broadcasting from Thessaloniki, or tuned into 4E TV, a Church of Greece satellite channel also based in Thessaloniki, to hear a *paraklesis* and readings for the saint of the day, lectures on social issues and theology, chant from the Simonpetra Monastery on Mount Athos, and stories from the Holy Mountain. In turning to synchronous Orthodox broadcasts at these times, Eleni joined the religious public these broadcasts hailed, which was itself linked to the Orthodox liturgical calendar. At other times, "for something lighter," she listened to the popular Serbian neo-Byzantine singer Divna Ljubojević and the Greek composer and oud player Christos Tsiamoulis.

Eleni did not depend solely on broadcast media programming to transform the everyday. She also invested substantial energy in locating, streaming, and downloading sermons and religious talks by her spiritual father, Archimandrite Stephanos Tolios, on the website www.littlewhitecandle.com and Father Andreas Konanos and other well-known Orthodox speakers on YouTube. In these cases, she followed the online trails of trusted, charismatic clergy rather than turning to church-run media outlets. Eleni would listen to these sermons and talks on a laptop while doing work around the house like ironing, and she characterized herself as someone who engages "a lot of Orthodox media because I don't have time to go to spiritual talks." Her use of nonbroadcast media and curated Orthodox websites was part of an intentional strategy of keeping her mind "from wandering onto everyday things" in moments when it could be turned toward God and her spiritual betterment, and her move over the past decade from playing cassettes and CDs to using online content and downloaded MP3s made this practice "easier and richer." In these moments, Eleni's engagement was far from passive—if she found her mind wandering or did not understand something while listening to sermons and religious talks, she would go back and relisten with full attention, just as she would stop to refocus her mind "when it runs off when I'm doing the Jesus Prayer."

Another technology essential to Eleni's spiritual life was her mobile phone. She would exchange text messages several times each week with her spiritual father, asking him questions about what to read and listen to, church and family life, raising children and personal spiritual struggles, and whether she should receive the Eucharist on a given Sunday. Others, she said, maintained similar relationships with their spiritual fathers over e-mail, navigating the social and spiritual terrain of pre- and post-crisis Greek suburbanization by purposing technologies for Orthodox ends.

Katerina

Katerina is a professional in her mid-forties living in central Thessaloniki with her husband and four girls. Growing up, she did not have a strong connection to the church, but after a cosmopolitan career as a model, she had a reconversion experience and entered the Faculty of Theology at Aristotle University of Thessaloniki, where she studied religious education, concentrating on the use of contemporary media in teaching Orthodox youth. Katerina's engagement with religious media was the most intense of all those I spoke with in and around Thessaloniki. She used radio (Lydia FM), television (4E TV), curated Orthodox websites, and YouTube to listen to, download, and stream sermons, services and liturgies, and talks on pastoral theology and church tradition. On her commute to work, she listened to sermons on her mobile phone through earbuds while riding the bus. Her listening was encyclopedic—she would download fifteen to twenty sermons by the same priest as MP3 files and keep them on her mobile phone (again an affordance of the compressed portability of the MP3 format). When she finished her listening during the morning and afternoon commute, she had the sense that she "had read a chapter of a book."

At home, Katerina always kept her laptop nearby, listening at 3:30 each afternoon to a live stream of the *paraklesis* for the saint of the day and afterward to another archived sermon while preparing dinner. After her daughters went to bed at 10:00, she listened to a live stream of the Great Compline, sitting quietly and reciting the prayers in unison with the priests and cantors or attending to unfinished work, and sometimes she listened to another sermon or religious talk after the Great Compline while going to bed. Katerina's engagement with media was decidedly aural, and she stressed that "my sense of hearing is most important in staying prayerful."

Reflecting on the fact that so much of her day was shaped by media engagement, Katerina described the Christocentric attuning her engagement accomplished:

> It is very important because my work and work at home have an even more special meaning. They have to be done, but they have a more Christocentric perspective, a more Christocentric way of doing things as you're listening. I'm offering something to the people around me—my kids and family—and I'm mindful of that by listening to something that's Christocentric and part of my service, my *diakonia*. My mind is focused and does not wander around to things that have no importance and are not spiritually beneficial.

I asked Katerina how her Christocentric attuning through media engagement related to her life of prayer and participation in liturgy—how it related to a sensorium, spiritual condition, and sacramental theology rooted in the immediacy of worship. She put it this way:

> I would love that my experience in church is heightened because of my listening during the week. I certainly believe that all that has taken place during the week in terms of canons, lectures, and sermons improves me—that I would be in a worse position spiritually if I hadn't done it. At the end of the day, it's only God who knows if all of this is a fruitful endeavor and my church attendance is a more spiritually fruitful experience. My mind says this is the case, though, but God works in a superlogical way, not in an unreasonable way, but a way beyond reason. Only God knows if this is making me a better person.

FROM THE CHRISTOCENTRIC EVERYDAY TO THE SACRAMENTAL LIFE OF ORTHODOXY

Each of these stories circles back to an essential question: if listening and engaging with media technologies cannot save you, since salvation comes through the grace and mystery of God and the sacraments, what is the significance of the Christocentric everyday they help to create? Those I worked with offered answers that, from a variety of perspectives rooted in their experiences of post-crisis austerity in and around Thessaloniki, returned to the co-constitution of the church as an institution and individuals as ethical subjects. The media technologies that listeners engaged isolated, extracted, and objectified the aural aspects of prayer and religious mediation, thereby sharpening reflexivity about what listening in an Orthodox way entailed. Listeners were keenly aware that the technologies they engaged were markedly mediatic, and this attunement was what prompted the "push back to the church," to the perceived immediacy of sacramental participation that was the end of Orthodox mediation. This semiotic ideology meant that religious discernment, the pastoral guidance of priests and spiritual fathers, and an understanding of mystery rooted in the tradition of the church realized the orthodoxy of Orthodoxy through individual listening practices. The Christocentric everyday of engagements with media technologies, in other words, constituted the church when people deferred to and participated in its sacramental life as an outcome of their listening. This was the ultimate context for projects of everyday ethical self-fashioning through Orthodox media.

There is much about this that was particular to the Greek context I explored. The ubiquity of Orthodox media (both marked and unmarked) in the sonic and built environment and the resolute nonsecularity of much public life and discourse fundamentally shaped people's practices and understandings. But perhaps more than anything, it is the word "back" in the phrase "push back to the church" that captured something particular about the moment of post-crisis austerity in 2013 I write about here. "Back" presumed prior experience with and knowledge of a particular Orthodox semiotic ideology—a memory of the felt immediacy of "natural," unmarked media and the mystery of sacraments. "Back" also presumed the default Orthodoxy of Greek cultural and social identity at a time when that identity was felt to be under siege from a host of external forces (the European Commission, European Central Bank, and International Monetary Fund "troika" and the EU). Finally, "back" was a return to Orthodox social ethics in the economic and political life of the nation—an antidote to the failures eventuating in a series of crises after 2009 that was represented metaphorically in the move from "new" digital and electronic media to the "old" media of Orthodox tradition.

My friend Stelios had a different take on this final point. He spoke of a tradition of media engagement among Orthodox faithful, not of media engagement that led back to tradition. In a world where the felt immediacy of liturgical experience had been superseded by "reasoned argument and issues of religious diversity" and where "people are no longer so simple and are open to psychosynthetic challenges," honing one's discernment through media engagement was crucial. For Stelios, a transformed, Christocentric everyday was about substituting a live-stream of the Great Compline for another thirty minutes on Facebook in the evening, a CD purchased at Mount Athos for radio news commentary during the morning commute, or MP3s of an esteemed cantor for the unbeneficial noise of urban life. At the junctures of sensory attunement to marked media, living an Orthodox life, and the church as an institution, the "push back to the church" was about listening to media and their messages (listening in the sense of a willing, moral, obedient activity—*hypakouō*; see Harrison 2013, 219) while orienting oneself to the sacramental life of Orthodox Christianity.

JEFFERS ENGELHARDT is Associate Professor of Music at Amherst College. He is author of *Singing the Right Way: Orthodox Christians and Secular Enchantment in Estonia* and editor with Philip V. Bohlman of *Resounding Transcendence: Transitions in Music, Religion, and Ritual*.

NOTE

1. I would like to thank Sonja Luehrmann, principal investigator for the "Sensory Spirituality: Prayer as Transformative Practice in Eastern Christianity" project, and the SSRC New Directions in the Study of Prayer initiative for making this research possible. Additionally, I extend my thanks to Nektarios Antoniou for his invaluable help with my fieldwork and to Teresa Berger, Daria Dubovka, Angie Heo, Jeanne Kormina, Sonja Luehrmann, Vlad Naumescu, Simion Pop, and two anonymous reviewers for their feedback and insight at different stages in writing this chapter.

REFERENCES

Bandak, Andreas, and Tom Boylston. 2014. "The 'Orthodoxy' of Orthodoxy: On Moral Imperfection, Correctness, and Deferral in Religious Worlds." *Religion and Society* 5:25–46.

Blanton, Anderson. 2015. *Hittin' the Prayer Bones: Materiality of Spirit in the Pentecostal South*. Chapel Hill: University of North Carolina Press.

Brennan, Vicki L. 2010. "Mediating 'The Voice of the Spirit': Musical and Religious Transformations in Nigeria's Oil Boom." *American Ethnologist* 37 (2): 354–70.

———. 2012. "Take Control: The Labor of Immediacy in Yoruba Christian Music." *Journal of Popular Music Studies* 24 (4): 411–29.

Carl, Florian. 2015. "Music, Ritual and Media in Charismatic Religious Experience in Ghana." In *Congregational Music Making and Community in a Mediated Age*, edited by Thomas Wagner and Anna Nekola, 45–60. Farnham, UK: Ashgate.

Eisenlohr, Patrick. 2009. "Technologies of the Spirit: Devotional Islam, Sound Reproduction, and the Dialectics of Mediation and Immediacy in Mauritius." *Anthropological Theory* 9:273–96.

———. 2012. "Media and Religious Diversity." *Annual Review of Anthropology* 41:37–55.

Engelhardt, Jeffers. 2015. *Singing the Right Way: Orthodox Christians and Secular Enchantment in Estonia*. New York: Oxford University Press.

Engelke, Matthew. 2007. *A Problem of Presence: Beyond Scripture in an African Church*. Berkeley: University of California Press.

———. 2010. "Religion and the Media Turn: A Review Essay." *American Ethnologist* 37 (2): 371–79.

Fajfer, Łukasz. 2012. "The 'Garden of the Virgin Mary' Meets the Twenty-First Century: The Challenge of Technology on Mount Athos." *Religion, State and Society* 40 (3–4): 349–62.

Feaster, Patrick. 2015. "Phonography." In *Keywords in Sound*, edited by David Novak and Matt Sakakeeny, 139–50. Durham: Duke University Press.

Feld, Steven. 1995. "From Schizophonia to Schismogenesis: The Discourses and Practices of World Music and World Beat." In *The Traffic in Culture: Refiguring Art and Anthropology*, edited by George E. Marcus and Fred R. Myers, 96–126. Berkeley: University of California Press.

Greene, Paul D. 1999. "Sound Engineering in a Tamil Village: Playing Audio Cassettes as Devotional Performance." *Ethnomusicology* 43 (3): 459–89.

Harkness, Nicholas. 2014. *Songs of Seoul: An Ethnography of Voice and Voicing in Christian South Korea*. Berkeley: University of California Press.

Harrison, Carol. 2006. *The Ethical Soundscape: Cassette Sermons and Islamic Counterpublics*. New York: Columbia University Press.

———. 2013. *The Art of Listening in the Early Church*. New York: Oxford University Press.

Keane, Webb. 2007. *Christian Moderns: Freedom and Fetish in the Mission Encounter*. Berkeley: University of California Press.

Khalil, Alexander Konrad. 2009. *Echoes of Constantinople: Oral and Written Tradition of the Psaltes of the Ecumenical Patriarchate of Constantinople*. PhD diss., UCLA.

Kittler, Friedrich. 1999. *Gramophone, Film, Typewriter*. Translated by Geoffrey Winthrop-Young and Michael Wutz. Palo Alto: Stanford University Press.

Larkin, Brian. 2009. "Islamic Renewal, Radio, and the Surface of Things." In *Aesthetic Formations: Media, Religion, and the Senses*, edited by Birgit Meyer, 117–36. New York: Palgrave Macmillan.

———. 2014. "Techniques of Inattention: The Mediality of Loudspeakers in Nigeria." *Anthropological Quarterly* 87 (4): 989–1015.

Lind, Tore Tvarnø. 2012. *The Past Is Always Present: The Revival of the Byzantine Musical Tradition at Mount Athos*. Lanham, MD: Scarecrow Press.

Luhrmann, T. M., Howard Nusbaum, and Ronald Thisted. 2010. "The Absorption Hypothesis: Learning to Hear God in Evangelical Christianity." *American Anthropologist* 112 (1): 66–78.

Marshall, Wayne. 2014. "Treble Culture." In *The Oxford Handbook of Mobile Music Studies, Vol. 2*, edited by Sumanth Gopinath and Jason Stanyek, 43–76. New York: Oxford University Press.

Martin, Lerone A. 2014. *Preaching on Wax: The Phonograph and the Shaping of Modern African American Religion*. New York: New York University Press.

Mazzarella, William. 2004. "Culture, Globalization, Mediation." *Annual Review of Anthropology* 33:345–67.

Meyer, Birgit. 2009. "Introduction: From Imagined Communities to Aesthetic Formations: Religious Mediations, Sensational Forms, and Styles of Binding." In *Aesthetic Formations: Media, Religion, and the Senses*, edited by Birgit Meyer, 1–28. New York: Palgrave Macmillan.

Moody, Ivan. 2015. "The Seraphim Above: Some Perspectives on the Theology of Orthodox Church Music." *Religions* 6:350–64.
Oosterbaan, Martijn. 2008. "Spiritual Attunement: Pentecostal Radio in the Soundscape of a Favela in Rio de Janeiro." *Social Text* 26 (3): 123–45.
Reinhardt, Bruno. 2014. "Soaking in Tapes: The Haptic Voice of Global Pentecostal Pedagogy in Ghana." *Journal of the Royal Anthropological Institute* 20:315–36.
Schafer, R. Murray. (1977) 1993. *The Soundscape: Our Sonic Environment and the Tuning of the World*. Rochester, VT: Destiny Books.
Schmemann, Alexander. 1973. *For the Life of the World: Sacraments and Orthodoxy*. Crestwood, NY: St. Vladimir's Seminary Press.
Sterne, Jonathan. 2012. *MP3: The Meaning of a Format*. Durham: Duke University Press.
Stolow, Jeremy. 2010. *Orthodox by Design: Judaism, Print Politics, and the ArtScroll Revolution*. Berkeley: University of California Press.
Summit, Jeffrey A. 2016. "Technology and the Transmission of Oral Tradition in the Contemporary Jewish Community." In *Resounding Transcendence: Transitions in Music, Religion, and Ritual*, edited by Jeffers Engelhardt and Philip V. Bohlman, 147–62. New York: Oxford University Press.
Weiner, Isaac. 2014. *Religion Out Loud: Religious Sound, Public Space, and American Pluralism*. New York: New York University Press.

CREATING AN IMAGE FOR PRAYER

SONJA LUEHRMANN

When creating images of saints and biblical stories, iconographers in the Byzantine tradition do not rely on their imagination but on previous icons depicting the same subjects. The idea is to minimize the artist's influence on the experience of the person who will use the icon in prayer, to provide "a vision of spiritual reality that is free of passion," as the priest Oleg Steniaev puts it.[1]

But what if an icon for a saint does not yet exist? In contemporary Russia there are reasons why iconographers need to create new motifs. After seventy years of socialism, iconography is being reinvented. The transmission of knowledge was interrupted, and many iconographers are self-taught, combining elements of different styles into what some call "postmodern icons."

A major force behind iconographic innovation is the canonization of new saints. Between 1989 and 2011, 1,776 "neomartyrs and confessors of Russia" were canonized, and the process is ongoing. These are twentieth-century clerics and laypeople who were either killed by the Bolsheviks for their religious convictions or suffered arrest and deprivations. Careful archival research precedes canonization, to show that the person did not denounce others even under torture and did not renounce his or her faith. Iconographers charged with creating the first icon of a new saint also do their own research, trying to find archival or family photographs. However, an icon is not simply a copy of a photographic likeness. To provide a view of a person's spiritual essence, he or she is often portrayed as neither very young nor very old, with a face that betrays no signs of suffering.

Such spiritual realism has a mystical side: iconographer Elena Utkina had to create an icon of a canonized priest whose only available photograph showed him as a beardless youth. She imagined what he looked like as a mature priest, adding a beard and some wrinkles in the face. Later the family brought another photograph, whose resemblance to the icon confirmed to Elena that her intuition was inspired by the new saint.

One feature that new icons take from older styles is the centrality of the human face: the person who is to be addressed in prayer faces the viewer directly. Iconographer Natalia Maslova explains: "Icons can be devoted to a festival, like the Entry into Jerusalem or the Descent of the Holy Spirit at Pentecost, [or] all the twelve holy days. And then there are prayer icons, which a person puts in front of himself and prays to those saints who are depicted on the icon." To visually participate in an event, it is sufficient to see the characters from the side, but to "stand before" an icon in prayer requires saint and devotee facing one another fully. Where a photograph serves as model, this sometimes means replacing a profile with a frontal view. Purging signs of torture and shifting faces so nothing remains hidden are acts of corrective imagination that bring photographic and visionary realism in line with one another.

NOTE

1. "Komu gorit virtual'naia svecha?," last accessed February 1, 2016, http://www.pravoslavie.ru/86517.html.

3 IMAGINING HOLY PERSONHOOD: ANTHROPOLOGICAL THRESHOLDS OF THE ICON

ANGIE HEO

IMAGINING HOLY PERSONHOOD

On one of Cairo's steamy summer afternoons, my Coptic friend Hanan and I stopped by a Coptic Orthodox church to pray after shopping in the buzzing commercial parts of downtown Shubra. Famous for being the site of the Virgin Mary's appearance back in 1986, the Church of Saint Dimyana in Shubra Babadublu had once attracted thousands to its narrow sanctuary. Finding the church empty this time around, Hanan first paid her greetings to the holy relics of Saint Dimyana the Martyr, the church's fourth-century matron who is honored for refusing to worship idols during the rule of Roman imperial paganism. Saint Dimyana's portrait icon always depicts her surrounded by the forty virgin-martyrs who ended up dying alongside her, crowned with haloes of heavenly sainthood (figure 5). As in most other shrines throughout Coptic Egypt, her icon hangs upright above her physical remains so that visitors can look at her face while contemplating her exemplary deeds and addressing their personal requests to her.

Facing Saint Dimyana's icon, Hanan opened her address to the saint by singing her glorification hymn (Arabic *tamgid al-Shahida Dimyana*). Reading from the lyrics posted next to the icon, she sang about the heroine's life—her virtues of purity and faith, her upbringing and tribulations. As she sang one of the hymn's final stanzas, I heard Hanan's voice quiver and watched tears well up as she imagined the scene of Saint Dimyana's death:

Makatha yu'adhdhib-ha	[The emperor] continued to torture her
Muddat thalatha sanawat	For three years
Kullu yum yutlub-ha	Every day, he asked her

Bi-'abadat al-masnu'at	To worship the idols
Rabat-ha fi adhnab khil	He tied her to the horse's tail
Wa-dar bi-ha haul al-madina	And it ran with her around the city
Wa-nazal damma-ha yigri kal-sil	And her blood fell like a flood
Wal-'adhari 'alayha hazina	And the virgins around her mourned[1]

In the Coptic Orthodox tradition, martyrs (Arabic *al-shahid, al-shuhada'*) hold a high rank in the divine hierarchy of apostles, wonder-workers, and ascetics, their blood frequently referred to as "the seed of the church." The Coptic calendar begins in 284 AD with the onset of Emperor Diocletian's era of persecution, resulting in the deaths of holy figures including Saint Dimyana, Saint Menas, Saint Mercurius, and Saint Abanub. To invoke and call upon Saint Dimyana's powers of intercession, Hanan followed conventions of retrieving the gruesome details of martyrdom and creating an image of the saint. Remembering a holy person with fullest sympathy is a multisensory exercise involving pictures, sounds, smells, postures, and movements. Through commemorative acts of prayer, a devotee might be, in turn, moved to tears or inspired to change his or her life.

Icons have long played a key role in shaping the collective representation of a given holy person's identity. Treasured wall paintings from the Upper Egyptian monastery of Bawit (near present-day Asyut) offer depictions of holy figures like Jesus, Abba Menas, Bishop Abraham, and Abbot Shenoute, which date back to as early as the fourth century. In the Old Church of St. Antony the Hermit on the Red Sea coast, some saintly portraits continue older styles of full frontality and heavy outlining, and others assimilate later twelfth-century influences from Islamic, Byzantine, and Crusader art (Bolman 2002, 77–154). A saint's iconographic representations can also vary significantly from region to region. Unlike most other Eastern Orthodox communities, the Coptic Orthodox Church currently permits more liberal usage of Roman Catholic iconography. It is not uncommon, for example, to find more images of the Paris-originated "Mary of the Miraculous Medal" than one of the Orthodox Theotokos icon styles in Egyptian homes and shrines, as well as in official Coptic high liturgical settings (Finnestad 1996).[2]

Following Eastern Orthodox doctrine, an icon's legitimacy lies in the Incarnation, or the assumption of Christ's person in fleshly, material form. What the icon depicts by analogy is the "holy person" and, ultimately, the redemptive potential for humanity to become divine. In his theological writings on the divine image, the Russian theologian Vladimir Lossky asserts that "personhood belongs to every human being by virtue of a singular and unique relation to God who created him 'in His image'" (1974, 137). An Orthodox imaginary is thus also a theological anthropology, that is, *anthropos* defined in the ontological terms of a human-divine relation.

In everyday practice, this Orthodox imaginary of the icon involves ritual scripts and pedagogies for imagining the relationship with the divine. By drawing on stories of martyrdom and the Orthodox tradition of holy suffering, people remember human capacities to become divine through concrete techniques of the imagination. In narrative perceptions of saints and their glorious deaths, people envision the extraordinary thresholds of humans becoming divine: for example, by reciting the stages of Saint Dimyana's martyrdom, Hanan imagines Saint Dimyana suffering great lengths of torture and also her eventual overcoming of it. Ritual singing of hymnody and praise, in addition to readings from the Holy Synaxarium (detailing the lives of the saints), aids believers in celebrating the divine aspects of heroes and heroines from the past. Theological teachings on image veneration further translate into corporeal, practical techniques for how to pray with icons by focusing on the persons represented. The late Coptic monk Matthew the Poor (1919–2006, known in Arabic as Matta al-Miskin) encouraged ecumenical collaboration with Russian Orthodox lines of thought, instructing the following steps for proper image veneration: "Whenever you meditate on icons (*al-aiqunat*), do not stop at the borders of color or wood, or in the art's beauty or lack of it, but lift your thoughts to what is behind the colors and matter, *to the person who is its owner* [*illa shakhs sahib-ha*]" (Miskin 1952, 576, emphasis mine). While spiritual intellect beyond the icon's physicality may be the desired end goal, acts of sensory perception are integral to imagining a holy person most effectively. "Picture yourself boiling in oil!" the renowned priest Father Daoud Lamaʿi once exhorted in a sermon, directing young Coptic students to feel with corporeal terror and identify closely with the saint's extravagantly painful passions.

Imagining holy personhood is made possible through linkages between various material forms (sensory and technological) and everyday practices of interacting with saints. It is only through social and moral acts of perception that adherents like Hanan feel saints exerting their presence and continuing on as "living" after their deaths. As representations of heavenly characters and their miraculous capacities, icons shape and enable senses of transcendence and transgression. They also direct and constrain ritual imaginaries according to the disciplines and customs prescribed by institutional authorities.

To grasp how images shape the Orthodox imaginary of holy personhood, it is useful to enlarge our notion of what an image is. Following Charles Peirce's well-known typology of signs, the "icon" is a sign that stands in relation to its object by virtue of some resemblance or similarity with it (Peirce 1992). Beyond the portrait image, a more expansive understanding of the image therefore includes other phenomenal forms—sonic images, mimetic acts, namesakes, personal virtues—which evoke semblances of otherworldly presence in the world. Holy persons, inasmuch as they are perceived to be divine likenesses, summon anthropological capacities of extraordinariness, that is, capacities to surpass the material conventions of ordinary life and death.

In this essay, I draw primarily from my fieldwork in Coptic Egypt for over a decade (2004–14) to examine how icons stand for saints in different ways and, more particularly, how imaginings of personhood consolidate the special status of saints. First, I consider the broader historical controversies over image veneration and iconoclasm and point to discourses of idolatry and false imagination in more current contexts. Second, I explore the material means through which saintly contemporaries are canonized and represented as holy icons. Third, I look at the iconizing media of names and virtues, paying special attention to the interactive aspects of witnessing and securing the permanent cult glory of a person.

IMAGE VENERATION AND WARS OF ICONOCLASM

In February 2014, the Evangelical Theological Seminary in Cairo celebrated the complete renovation of its chapel. In addition to wiring new technologies and replacing its aging ceilings and floors, four backlit stained-glass windows were installed in its walls. The windows' images were cause for mild uproar within Egypt's Coptic Protestant community that winter. Designed in the style of modern Coptic Orthodox iconography, with its characteristically austere and abstract qualities, the new narrative portraits of Christ and the disciples rubbed a few pastors the wrong way. These pastors from the rural villages of Upper Egypt expressed disapproval of what they called "icons" (Arabized Coptic *ai-qunat*) and the visual associations with Orthodox Christianity that they invoked. In their opinion, Coptic Evangelical teachings are clearly opposed to the ritual veneration of saints and the use of icons in worship (see also Sedra 2011).[3]

In a public forum held in the chapel, the seminary's president, Atef Gendy, defended the new stained-glass images, pointing out that they were not "icons" but "art." He further explained that the portrait depictions conveyed the deep, rich cultural heritage of the Coptic tradition from which Protestants had no reason to exclude themselves. The short-lived dispute between the Upper Egyptian pastors and the seminary administration revealed some differences in how the chapel's new images were valued and what threats or gifts they posed as a result.

Historically across the North African Mediterranean landscape of saint veneration, Christians, Jews, and Muslims all have grappled with upholding and representing holy women and men in morally acceptable ways (Brown 1981). Apart from heavily rehearsed Orthodox-Protestant clashes surrounding the legitimacy of saints and icons, Protestants in Egypt are also engaged in their own internal battles about what to do with material media of pictorial imagination (see Luehrmann 2010). Gendy's distinction between "icon" and "art" is one way of carving out a more secular value system for appreciating the images as "cultural" and "national" rather than as sacred vehicles of holiness. Such a frame for assessing the value of Coptic icons can lead to particular cultural and national narratives of their various aesthetic histories. It is quite common to hear, from an art historical perspective for instance, that Coptic iconography developed under the influence of Greco-Roman art and pharaonic forms and motifs (Török 2005; Badawy 1978; Wessel 1965). In the somewhat counterintuitive view of theologian and icon-writer Leonid Ouspensky, the fact that elements of the pagan world entered into Christian imaginary aesthetics illustrates "not a 'paganisation of Christian art,' as is often thought, but the Christianization of pagan art" (Ouspensky 1999, 28).

Perhaps the most well examined historical controversies over image veneration are Byzantium's crises of iconoclasm (*eikonoklásía*, Greek for "breaking of icons") in the eighth and ninth centuries. In this controversy, politicians and prelates were not concerned with "art" but rather with the holy legitimacy of imperial representation and action. A hallmark event was Emperor Leo III's edict in 726, which ordered the removal and destruction of icons throughout the empire and provoked letters, treatises, sermons, and critique from clergy such as John of Damascus and Patriarch Nikephoros,[4] who responded with their defenses of image veneration. The controversies ended with the death of Emperor Theophilus in 842, after which the veneration of flat images was restored, while the veneration of three-dimensional statues was defined as a violation of the biblical ban on "graven images." The terms of iconoclastic conflict illustrated the intrinsically political nature of theological and religious matters, such that the "'Caesaro-papalism' of the Iconoclastic emperors was itself a kind of theological doctrine" (Florovsky 1972, 102–103, quoted in Pelikan 1990, 7) that elevated the emperor to the status of the church's supreme head. According to Byzantine social historians Leslie Brubaker and John Haldon, the fact that "the relationship between individuals and the holy was redefined at the same time as that between individuals and their ruler" speaks to changing ties between religion and politics (2011, 10). Escalating tensions between the church and state, as well as a string of military defeats, set the historical stage for new governing rationalities of mediation. Contending dogmas elaborating divine hierarchies of intercession were thus, at their very core, also contending political theories of earthly rule.

As in all image wars, it was the rule of similarity and likeness that determined whether or not the holy icon counted as a true or false representation of divine power. Scholarly writings on the technical fineries of these debates are vast (Grabar 1957; Kitzinger 1958; Elsner 1988; Brubaker and Haldon 2011), and here I will only crudely recount two topics among the many raised by the late ancient and early medieval sciences of iconophilia. First, for defenders of image veneration, Christological personhood was the main source for grasping the divine formula of the holy icon: "since the person of Christ contained the Father as in an image, the Father could be honored in the Son"; analogously, "the honor of the image refers to the archetype" (Belting 1994, 153). The mystery of Trinitarian unity was the rationale for honoring the divine image as a mere sign, conduit, or link of its prototype (rather than an end referent in itself). In the end, the iconoclast's charges of idolatry were founded on a very different semiotic economy of likeness—one that denied the interchangeability of the image created by divine "nature" (Greek *phýsis*) and that by human "imitation" (*mīmēsis*).

The second topic, which follows from the first on holy personhood, concerns the material and sensible nature of the holy icon. The early Christian father Clement of Alexandria's arguments, for example, later supported the Byzantine iconoclast position that "the only true image was the virtuous and pious Christian, in whose soul God and the Holy Spirit resided" (Brubaker and Haldon 2011, 41); material images were unnecessary for achieving piety. For iconophiles, to the contrary, the fleshly human nature of Christ warranted the material perceptibility of God's image on earth. As philosopher of the Byzantine imaginary Marie-José Mondzain clearly puts it, "The icon sets the visible and the invisible into a relation with each other without any concessions to realism, yet without contempt for matter" (2005, 85). More precisely, it is the visual sense that serves as the preeminent medium of divine perception, or the icon's visibility as a manifestation of grace. Following Mondzain's argument further, the icon's visibility indicates less divine presence and more divine withdrawal or self-absence from the world.

Historically speaking, Egypt's Copts had been imperial subjects of foreign Byzantine rule for only a relatively brief period, from 451 (when Coptic Orthodoxy acquired its independent identity as Christologically Miaphysite) until 641 with the onset of Fatimid Muslim rule (when the Byzantine iconoclastic movement was gaining momentum). Currently, Coptic Orthodox regard their traditions as intimately related to those of the Chalcedonian Eastern Orthodox churches, clearly partaking in the same Byzantium-originated imaginary of divine representation. For every Coptic Orthodox church, monastery, and shrine, one can find icon portraits and relics that honor the memory of their patron saints, enabling visitors to visually access holy men and women through images. To take baraka (blessing) from these images, people might also kiss and swipe their fingers on their surfaces or grip onto their frames (figure 6). Other sensory acts of veneration include bowing and singing or leaving behind written notes and lit candles as tokens of thanksgiving or petition.

Centuries after Byzantium's fall, the Coptic Orthodox Church underwent its own internal wars of iconoclasm. During its nineteenth-century period of widespread modernization, Pope Cyril IV, known as "the Reformer," built new schools and seminaries, renovated the Patriarchate Cathedral in Azbakiya, and introduced one of the first private Arabic printing presses in the Arab world. Cyril IV is additionally known for accusing his own flock of idolatry, prohibiting the display of icons in churches and destroying many images in Cairo and Asyut in public burnings (Meinardus 2002, 70). To this day, as a result of such lessons on the dangers of excessive attachment to "false" icons, Copts do not venerate statue-images of saints, which they recognize to be "idols" (*al-asnam*). It is worth mentioning that the beginning of Cyril IV's reign corresponded with the Coptic Evangelical Church's beginnings in Egypt with the arrival and proselytizing activities of American Presbyterians under British colonial protection (Sharkey 2008). Although there is no evidence of a direct correlation between iconoclasm and Protestant missionization, one might entertain the possibility that Protestant discourses of idolatry had some bearing on semiotic ideologies of modern individualism writ large in colonial Egypt (see Keane 2007).

The fact that Coptic Protestants now welcome portrait images of Christ in their chapels coincides with Orthodox characterizations of their own iconography as "cultural" or "national" art. Established in 1908, the Coptic Museum continues to showcase once-sacred objects from antiquity as national treasures, and in 1954 the Higher Institute of Coptic Studies began to train icon-writers to preserve the history and culture of Coptic civilization. The most prominent of these pioneering artists was Isaac Fanous Youssef, regarded as the father of neo-Coptic iconography, who ended up studying with the master iconographer Leonid Ouspensky in exile from Russia in 1960s Paris. Interestingly enough, before his return from France to Egypt in 1967, the nationalist Fanous surprised Ouspensky by declaring, "I would never paint a Russian icon on the soil of Egypt" (quoted in René 2014, 274).[5]

Developing new styles of contemporary Orthodox iconography, Fanous explicitly drew on pharaonic funerary portraiture (in addition to modern cubism and impressionism) in his icons, which rapidly gained popularity among Egyptians, including the diaspora abroad. For his staggering achievements in secular worlds of art appreciation, he was also clear that he wished for his images to aid Copts in remembering the hagiographic details of the saints. His portrait icons consistently emphasize sources of light from within saints, and his narrative icons translate verbal parables of their earthly biographies into visual pictorial form. Fanous ultimately intended for his new visual styles to serve as didactic tools of spiritual communication.

Before concerns over cultural style, the Coptic Orthodox Church is vigilant about disseminating its teachings against idolatry. One diasporic church in Milwaukee, Wisconsin, for example, cautions on its website against the temptations of worshipping the image:

> Soon, Christians began to venerate the icon itself and to forget the event or person it portrays. An icon is meant to be a window into the spiritual world helping us to contemplate spiritual matters, lead us to a prayerful frame of mind, and remind us of events in the Bible, the life of Christ, and the saints. The icon is *not* to be an object of worship. Again, we must contemplate the scene within the icon and not bow before it. We kneel to Jesus Christ, not to pictures. We kiss these pictures as if kissing the Lord, His Mother, the Disciples who touched Him, and the Saints who precede us to eternal life.[6]

Reminiscent of Byzantine defenses of image veneration, the warning underscores the difference between the archetype and the icon as its mere sign. The frequent metaphor of the "window" invokes the icon's value as a passageway and vehicle of movement toward someone other than itself. If Coptic Evangelicals are embroiled in debates about the proper use of icons as "art" (or objects of beauty in themselves), Coptic Orthodox are intent on maintaining the ritual value of icons as integral to remembering holy personhood. Lessons about false imagination from different sides are proof that the practical terms of iconoclasm are still up for correction and debate.

ANTHROPOLOGICAL THRESHOLDS OF THE ICON

Imagined as a window into the spiritual world, the holy icon is a "threshold" between the earthly and heavenly realms. As a passageway between the human being on earth and the saint in heaven, it serves as a go-between and limen to the extent that it represents its prototypical intermediary. The icon, in other words, intercedes only as much as its saintly referent is imagined to be an image of the divine. One necessary precondition for image veneration is the social recognition of the saint as "holy" or "divine": the human being (Greek *anthropos*) as a threshold of extraordinary power himself or herself. What is thus empirically central to the material imaginaries of holy persons is interactive perceptions of their miraculous activity and transformative powers in the world. For ethnographers, the task at hand is to track the histories and ritual traditions in which people interact with holy persons and perceive their activity as otherworldly and extraordinary.

Throughout the Eastern Mediterranean's interwoven histories of cult traditions, the bodies and graves of Muslim, Christian, and Jewish saints have attracted pilgrims seeking intercession (Meri 2002; Taylor 1999; Ghosh 1993). For these three monotheistic faiths, human capacities to act on behalf of God have consistently introduced anxieties around potential acts of idolatry. What are the proper limits surrounding the representation of holy persons, whether prophets, saints, wonder-workers, companions, friends, guarantors, or guardians? Which teachings and practices reflect the divine aspects of human mediation? For Egypt's Sunni Muslim majority, while anthropomorphic figurations of holiness are forbidden, visual signs evoking divine qualities such as bright light or calligraphic representations are commonly used to represent divine messengers and their names and virtues. Internally waged within the Islamic tradition, puritanical-minded Salafis and Sufi adherents continue to negotiate the legitimacy of saint veneration (Cornell 1998; Salomon 2017) and their material aesthetic implications. Aniconic teachings in Islamic thought are for the most part concerned with preventing *shirk*, or the idolatrous "association of other gods with God."[7]

Among contemporary Coptic Orthodox, Muslim suspicions of idolatry (around both Trinitarianism and sainthood) have in response produced strengthened vocabularies of monotheism. During my fieldwork in 2006 among lay youth taking courses in Coptic theology, I learned about the distinction between two categories of intercession. The first, called *al-shafaʿa al-kaffari* (intercession of expiation), refers to the singular act of Christ's death and resurrection or the full, perfect propitiation for sins. The second, called *al-shafaʿa al-tawassuli* (intercession of petition), refers to the secondary activity of human saints who, acting in Christ's image of intercession, also advocate on behalf of others. To be imagined as powerful and effective, saints must be felt and sensed as active in the lives of those who invoke their mediational authority.

Joining relics, holy icons are interactive foci of saintly presence. Standing in the place of the saint in heaven, the icon embodies the divine likeness of the otherworldly person. As such, it exercises supernatural agency in the material world and acts with extraordinary authority, performing miracles such as cures and healings, prophecies, exorcisms, visions, and visitations from beyond. By far the most popular saint in Egypt is the Virgin Mary, whose icons are carried during pilgrimages, festival days, and the feast day of her Assumption in August (Farag 2013, 261). Especially venerated by some Muslim devotees (particularly in Upper Egypt but also elsewhere), Marian icons and appearances provide sites of mixed pilgrimage, such as the blood-weeping Catholic portrait of the Mater Dolorosa in Wadi Natrun (Meinardus 1996) or the Virgin's apparitions in Zaytun, Shubra, and Giza (Heo 2013). The icon, in short, acts as a holy person on earth would act. Among faithful Copts, there are many popular accounts that describe the miraculous intercession of icons—Saint George jumping out of his image to defend a home against a thief, Saint Abanub the child martyr appearing to heal a bedridden woman—as well as miracle-icons that speak audibly, radiate hieratic light, or seep liquids such as oil or blood (Skalova and Gabra 2006).

In addition to the apostles and martyrs who died centuries ago, there are those special contemporaries who remain alive on earth, not yet dead. Unlike the heavenly dead, these prophets, wonder-workers, and mystics carry out their everyday lives in rural villages, churches, and monasteries, sought after for their powers of intercession. A handful of these miraculous actors are regarded as "holy men" or "holy women" but not as official saints of the Coptic Church: for instance, I have heard several times about the late Muqaddas[8] Aziz of Behbeh village from Beni Suef, who had attracted visitors looking for exorcisms and prophecies; ethnographer Valerie Hoffman describes Muqaddasa Elisabat of Sohag and her gifts of clairvoyance and spiritual vision (1995, 343–53); and most recently, the deaconess Mama Maggie Gobran of Cairo was a contender for the Nobel Peace Prize in 2012 for her charity work among slum children. Although these popular figures do not belong to the clerical hierarchy of Coptic Orthodoxy, they are few in number, and in fact the great majority of Coptic "living saints" are monks, nuns, priests, bishops, or popes. This is notably different from Sufi Muslim orders of sainthood, which are far more diffuse and decentralized.

Canonizing a saint in the Coptic Orthodox Church entails recognition of a given candidate's sanctity and heroic virtue. If someone is canonized, his or her name is remembered annually in the Holy Synaxarium and his or her icon-image is created and consecrated with the holy chrism to be used in shrines and churches. "Contemporary saints" (*al-qiddisin al-mu'asirin*), as opposed to the saints of antiquity, are those holy persons who have lived in relatively recent years, their deeds and virtues having been witnessed often by the still living. According to Coptic Church rules, a minimum of fifty years of miracles by a candidate must pass before he or she can be considered for canonization. However, there are many figures who are de facto saints (that is, "everybody knows he/she is a saint") despite the fact that they have not yet been canonized. The clearest example of this de facto popular canonization would be Pope Cyril VI, affectionately called "al-Baba Kyrillos," whose photo icons were to be found across homes and shrines long before his official entry into the Synaxarium in March 2014. There are numerous other holy contemporaries, though less well known, including Tamav Irini, the late abbess of the Convent of St. Mercurius; Abdel-Masih al-Makari of Manahra Minya; Abdel-Masih al-Habashi of central Ethiopia; Yustus al-Antuni of the Monastery of St. Anthony the Hermit on the Red Sea; and Father Bishoi Kamil of Sporting Alexandria.

In his seminal writings on the place of the holy in sixth- and seventh-century Mediterranean societies (preceding Byzantium's iconoclastic controversies), Peter Brown argues for the subversive value of the holy icon and the holy person. According to him, holy men and icons "both were, technically, unconsecrated objects. Not only was the holy man not ordained as a priest or a bishop; his appeal was precisely that he stood outside the vested hierarchy of the Byzantine church" (1973, 21). For the most part in modern Egyptian Christianity, by contrast, the rubric of holy contemporaries and their mass iconography is fully assimilated into the centralizing framework of Coptic Orthodox ecclesiastical power. The church's internal politics is further intimately linked to its external politics, its steep vertical clerical structure supported heavily by the authoritarian Egyptian state. The most visible evidence of this phenomenon is the widespread iconography of the late heads Pope Cyril VI and Pope Shenouda III, under whose reigns the Coptic clerical order was most consolidated. It is significant to note that much of their portrait imagery represents their status as both ruling popes and desert monastics who eschewed ordinary social life.

Featured in black ascetic garb, outside desert holes and abandoned windmills, they also signify the solitary status of the holy outsider.

Technically speaking, official icons are only those images that the Orthodox Church has consecrated with holy oil, in the Coptic case, or blessed with holy water in the churches of Byzantine derivation. Usually they are paintings, but in some cases they are print reproductions, like the Marian icon of Port Said and some images of Saint George with the dragon. When it comes to contemporary saints who await canonization, iconic photography is the key medium for disseminating their portrait presence. In the Monastery of St. Anthony the Hermit on the Red Sea, for example, there is a shrine dedicated to the late monk Yustus al-Antony, which includes enlarged photos of him from his life there. Although he has not yet been canonized, his unconsecrated images include icon paintings that are realist copies of a photo, rather than paintings fashioned in the abstract, simple neo-Coptic style of iconography (figure 7). In the larger Eastern Orthodox world outside Egypt, similar phenomena of a photo preceding the painting can be found. When in Thessaloniki, Greece, during August 2014, the contributors to this volume visited the grave of Elder Paisios at the Monastery of St. John the Theologian in Souroti. Also not yet canonized into sainthood, photo icons of this Greek Orthodox monk of Mount Athos were on sale in the shops (figure 8). Later on in downtown Thessaloniki's more urban alleys, lined with artisan stores and markets, our group stumbled upon an icon shop where paintings of Elder Paisios, in realist representations of his photos, were sold in anticipation of his canonization in 2015.

"A living icon" (Brown 1973, 12), the holy person is the anthropological threshold of divine origins, or "man made in the image of God." It is only at the point of death, when an earthly saint passes into heaven, that he or she can be made into a ritual object.[9] For contemporary saints, the period of fifty years after death ensures that a long enough time span has definitively passed after departure. Media technologies of visual representation also convey the ritual making of a saint's icon at the event of death: in Coptic director Magued Tawfik's hagiographic film *The Story of the Life of Marina the Martyr* (1993), for instance, the fourth-century Saint Marina's icon appears as a more stable fixation of her holy personhood after she is decapitated at the end of her tortures. As soon as a holy person dies, the ritual possibility of making him or her an icon is actualizable. Only after a person has died does it become morally legitimate to consecrate him or her as a permanent picture-icon. In the cult memory of all saints, the date of death is at once the date of commemoration. Thereby assimilated into the ritual cycle of annual feast days, a dead saint goes on living as a more fixed, regular image of collective memory.

REMEMBERING NAMES AND VIRTUES

The living quality of saints is often perceived through faces imagined in dreams and waking visions. Such imagined faces sometimes speak and intervene without their names being known. On one occasion, I was told that holy icons can also aid visionaries in locating the identity of such nameless faces. One Coptic Evangelical woman, who had been briefly exposed to Orthodoxy as a child in Sohag, described one dream of hers in which she envisioned herself holding in her arms a small young boy who prophesied the birth of her son. At that time an Evangelical Protestant, she was not very familiar with the saintly pantheon, having only known more widely disseminated portraits of popular figures such as the Virgin or Pope Cyril VI. Curious about the identity of the anonymous youth about whom she had dreamed, she went on a search for a name to match with his face and found his icon with his name in one of the bookstores of a neighboring Orthodox church: St. Menas the Wonderworker.

This woman's story fits into a common narrative type that upholds icons as visual tools for identifying the unknown. In the opening of another of Magued Tawfik's films, *The Story of the Life of St. Abanoub* (2003), a bedridden patient witnesses the luminous apparition of a cross-bearing child and later, after her miraculous recovery, locates his image in a church in Samanoud (Gharbiya, Delta). More well known is the story of the Marian icon of Port Said in which its owner, Samya Yusif Basilios, dreamed of three saints she did not know, only to find them revealed on the walls of her local Church of St. Bishoi. Icons thus serve as vehicles of increasing saintly literacy among the ignorant, that is, knowledge about intercessors and their biographical details, virtues, and powers. From a slightly different angle, they also reveal the sources of visionary encounter and bodily healing, authors not of word but of image. Getting to know holy figures requires social media of personal identity, which show what these saints look like to everyone—even within the intimate, private realm of dreams and apparitions.

Holy icons offer standardized depictions of the saints, which if anything else train believers in a shared sense of their appearances and thereby enable collective imaginaries. For any Copt raised in Sunday school and through regular pilgrimages, a familiar pictorial vocabulary of faces, names, and virtues renders the holy apostles, martyrs, ascetics, and miracle workers recognizable.

There is Saint Mark, the founding apostle of the Coptic Church, who is regularly depicted with a lion at his feet. And Saint Bishoi, the desert monk, who is portrayed either as carrying Christ on his shoulders or as washing Christ's feet. Or Bishop Ruways, the holy fool and ascetic, who is always shown flanked by his two camels. A personal portrait also often conveys the hallmark virtue of its prototype, tutoring viewers in the special capacities that characterize the identity of any given saint. Saint George the Martyr's act of spearing the dragon speaks to his physical skill and endurance for those looking for bodily strength to overcome obstacles. Or the Virgin Mary's tender embrace of the Christ child invokes her intercessory powers of compassion and mercy.

More than a delimited art object, the holy icon is thus an aggregate of various signs of personal identity. Faces, names, and pictures are all holy images, or likenesses of holy personhood, which signify the saint's identity. Simply put, the icon image enables viewers to remember a face and put it with a name and a biography filled with trademark virtues associated with the saint. One might experience an anonymous face in a miraculous dream or desire a particular type of divine aid, and it is the icon that directs people to the saint's personal identity. In keeping with a rich anthropological literature on names and naming practices (Geertz 1973; vom Bruck and Bodenhorn 2006), the social status of a person (living or dead) is created and represented through acts of address and kin-making. For an icon-object to be considered a proper subject of personhood, it must be treated according to the conventions of identity and order that encompass it. As Michael Herzfeld has illuminated in his work on the aesthetics of icons in Orthodox Crete, for instance, practices of referring to icons and their multiple copies are homologous to larger organizational principles of segmentation and solidarity (Herzfeld 1990). The identity of the saintly image, in these ways, stabilizes through social acts of interacting with it.

What is striking about the Coptic cases of dreamers, who use icons to identify unknown faces, is how their dream-visions appear to correspond to images they claim to have never seen before. Felt by the dreamers as arriving from radically elsewhere, the saints in heaven reveal their selves through the liminal space of dreams (Mittermaier 2011) and their icons on earth (Stewart 2012). The saintly imagination, in other words, is vested in a particular kind of virtual interaction that indexes the human-divine boundary once again. This threshold of visuality pinpoints the very special sociality of saints, active yet ultimately peripheral toward the world.

Here, Peter Brown's persuasive discussion of the living icon reminds us about the extraordinary social lives of holy men and women. Returning to living icons from late ancient hagiography, he describes ascetics praying alone on top of pillars or in holes, concealed out of sight. In sharp contrast to the ruling emperor and his imperial image at the center of all political activity, these intercessors were sought after at the edges of desert wilderness, withdrawn from the masses. Their spiritual lineage derived from their monastic schema that claimed "indirect consecration from the past," not through the bishop but rather through the garments conferred by the angels on Saint John the Baptist (Brown 1973, 21). Ironically, the result of their "asocial" personality is that they end up becoming very public images of holiness engaging various interpersonal realms of desire, need, exchange, and fulfillment.

Solitaries, cave dwellers, hermits, prophets, and anchorites are very much alive and active in the current imaginary of Copts. In Coptic Orthodox teachings on sainthood, the spiritual hierarchy of holy men and women is, from lowest to highest: (1) monastic (*rahib*), (2) solitary or hermit (*mutawahhid*), (3) anchorite (*sa'ih*), and (4) divine seer (*nazr Allah*). These different statuses of isolation from everyday society correspond to progressive stages of divine-human interaction. These special figures thus occupy a particular threshold of virtuous communication and access. Whereas priests are married, high-ranking bishops are celibate. Those monks who opt for eremetic life (as opposed to cenobitic communal life) are more likely to have miraculous abilities, like flying for the anchorite or clairvoyance for the divine seer. Remembered as a powerful mystic who could see into the past and future, Pope Cyril VI lived in an abandoned windmill on the high ledges of Muqattam Mountain. Recently canonized in 2014, his nicknames "al-Mutawahhid" (The Hermit) and "Ragul al-Salat" (Man of Prayer) capture his reclusive status as an intercessor with intimate ties to heaven. Even during his lifetime, crowds of people had visited his windmill shrine in search of his blessings and interventions.

While on earth, Coptic saints are known to hide their divine attributes from others in order to avoid idolatry. Yet another danger of false imagination is the making of the "living icon" into an idol, or the misrecognition of the human person as the divine archetype. To uphold the ethical bounds of image veneration, saints interact with public witnesses in strange, self-alienating ways. For example, Abuna Abdel-Masih al-Manahri of Minya would feign insanity, wearing dirty rags and flagrantly cursing his visitors who passed him. Erasing his own identity, he yelled out to people who asked who he was (often after witnessing a miracle he had performed), "I don't know my name!" This resort to "holy foolery" conforms somewhat predictably with a more generalizable Orthodox convention, arguably of Byzantine origins, of deflecting social attention and praise (see also Kormina and Shtyrkov 2012; Ivanov 2006). A less flamboyant example of self-erasure is Abuna "Bishoi" Kamil of Alexandria, who is remembered especially for his outstanding virtues of humility and forbearance in everyday life. Also known to hide his ability to converse with heavenly saints face-to-face, he would deliberately lie to others and pretend that they must have mistaken him for another with the name Bishoi.

Witnessing saints is thus an interactive activity that is temporally sensitive to the moral possibility of idolization. If names and naming confer social legitimacy and personhood, then it is important to name the holy person in the right way at the right time. Miraculous acts of intercession must be performed during a saint's lifetime in relative secret, only to be credited later posthumously. If not, excessive attention to the saint's abilities might tempt the saint into "vainglory" (*magd al-batil*). For this reason, Coptic saint Abdel-Masih al-Manahri had refused to be addressed by his name, and the saint Abuna Bishoi Kamil used popular confusion with names to dissimulate his extraordinary capacities to see beyond. Names spoken at the proper time are thus necessary to suspend cult glory until after saints are dead, so as to be preserved foremost as "human" images of divine power.

Names, virtues, and faces are all the preeminent signs that distribute the identity and attributes of saints. As we have seen, they do not always coincide, and in fact it is the appearance of one without the other that necessitates the quest for the icon image. This quest for saintly identity is oriented toward discovering what names to utter, what lives to recount and invoke, and what visual experiences to anticipate. Envisioning heavenly persons develops the anthropological potential for people to imagine saints interceding at the threshold of worlds.

ANGIE HEO is Assistant Professor at the University of Chicago Divinity School.

NOTES

1. Stanzas #25–26 of the "Glorification Hymn to St. Dimyana the Martyr" can also be found on the internet: http://st-takla.org/Lyrics-Spiritual-Songs/08-Coptic-Taraneem-Kalemat_Meem-Noun/Madee7-Al-Shaheeda-Dimiana.html.

2. During a trip to the old city of Dubrovnik, Croatia, for example, I noticed that Orthodox shopkeepers were very aware that their Marian icons differed from those of the Catholic majority (representing over 80 percent of the population). By contrast, Coptic Catholics (Uniate Catholics with a patriarchate established in the late eighteenth

century) have a minimal presence in Christian Egypt compared with their counterpart Coptic Orthodox. Most likely, Catholic images of the Virgin produced by the mass print industry in Italy were brought to Egypt via missionaries in the nineteenth and twentieth centuries (René 2014; Burckhardt 1967).

3. Coptic Christians make up 6–12 percent of Muslim-majority Egypt. Of this minority demographic, over 95 percent are Orthodox with smaller percentages of Coptic Protestants and Coptic Catholics. Although Protestants are small in number, they are disproportionately influential in economic and societal activity.

4. It is significant to note that, compared with the patriarch Nikephoros of Constantinople under Byzantine Christendom, John of Damascus enjoyed relatively more freedom to write boldly against his iconoclastic opponents under the protection of Dar al-Islam, which was "tolerant of a Christian theologian who defended the church's use of icons" (Pelikan 1990, 37).

5. In an interview with Marie-Gabrielle de Boncourt and Bernadette Sadek in 1999, Fanous elaborated on the aesthetic differences between Russian and Coptic iconography: "Russian and Byzantine iconographers study Greek legacy. In the Greek traditional style, there are details, and that is the imitation of nature that is put forward, while we, the Egyptians, we use abstraction to express our vision of eternity, of immortality.'" For more, see the transcript of this interview titled "A l'ecoute du maître," last accessed May 18, 2015, http://eocf.free.fr/text_fanous.htm.

6. See the section on "Coptic Iconography" on the website of St. Mary and St. Antonious Coptic Orthodox Church of Milwaukee, last accessed May 18, 2015, http://wiscopts.net/spiritual-library/72.

7. In recent years, world events, including the Taliban's destruction of Bamiyan Buddhas in Afghanistan in 2009 and the cartoon controversies in Denmark in 2005 and 2006, and then again in France in 2015, have galvanized scholarly stereotypes of Islam as iconoclastic and aniconic in its essence. As art historian Finnbar Barry Flood observes, these hasty conclusions fail to problematize the vocabulary of iconoclasm in Islam in the ways that the abundant literature on Byzantine Christian controversies has done (2002).

8. The Arabic title "Muqaddas" or "Muqaddasa" refers to a Christian who has made pilgrimage to Jerusalem (*al-Quds*).

9. Peter Brown draws on Delehaye's *Les saints Stylites* (1923) to illustrate beautifully the translation of the living icon into a ritual icon: "At his death, he instantly became an icon: 'for by the archbishop's orders the plank was stood upright—the body [of Daniel the Stylite, died 493] had been fixed to it so that it could not fall—and thus, like an icon, the holy man was displayed to all from every side'" (1973, 12).

REFERENCES

Films

The Story of the Life of Marina the Martyr. 1993. Directed by Magued Tawfik. Cairo: Sharja Intaj. DVD.
The Story of the Life of St. Abanoub. 2003. Directed by Magued Tawfik. Cairo: Sharja Intaj. DVD.

Books and Articles

Badawy, Alexander. 1978. *Coptic Art and Archaeology: The Art of the Christian Egyptians from the Late Antique to the Middle Ages.* Cambridge: MIT Press.

Belting, Hans. 1994. *Likeness and Presence: A History of the Image before the Era of Art.* Translated by Edmund Jephcott. Chicago: University of Chicago Press.

Bolman, Elizabeth, ed. 2002. *Monastic Visions: Wall Paintings in the Monastery of St. Antony at the Red Sea.* New Haven: Yale University Press.

Brown, Peter. 1973. "A Dark-Age Crisis: Aspects of the Iconoclastic Controversy." *English Historical Review* 88:1–33.

———. 1981. *The Cult of the Saints: Its Rise and Function in Latin Christianity.* Chicago: University of Chicago Press.

Brubaker, Leslie, and John Haldon. 2011. *Byzantium in the Iconoclast Era c. 680-850: A History.* Cambridge: Cambridge University Press.

Burckhardt, Titus. 1967. *Sacred Art in East and West.* Translated by Lord Northbourne. Bedfont, Middlesex: Perennial Books.

Cornell, Vincent J. 1998. *Realm of the Saint: Power and Authority in Moroccan Sufism.* Austin: University of Texas Press.

Elsner, Jas. 1988. "Image and Iconoclasm in Byzantium." *Art History* 11 (4): 471–91.

Farag, Lois M., ed. 2013. *The Coptic Christian Heritage: History, Faith and Culture.* New York: Routledge.

Finnestad, Ragnhild Bjerre. 1996. "Images as Messengers of Coptic Identity: An Example from Contemporary Egypt." *Scripta Instituti Donneriani Aboensis* 16:91–110.

Flood, Finbarr Barry. 2002. "Between Cult and Culture: Bamiyan, Islamic Iconoclasm, and the Museum." *Art Bulletin* 84 (4): 641–59.

Florovsky, Georges. 1972. *Collected Works.* Vol. 1. Belmont, MA: Nordland.

Geertz, Clifford. 1973. "Person, Time and Conduct in Bali." In *The Interpretation of Cultures: Selected Essays,* 360–411. New York: Basic Books.

Ghosh, Amitav. 1993. *An Antique Land: History in the Guise of a Traveler's Tale.* New York: Knopf.

Grabar, André. 1957. *L'iconoclasme byzantin: Le dossier archéologique.* Paris: Collège de France.

Heo, Angie. 2013. "The Virgin between Christianity and Islam: Sainthood, Media, and Modernity in Egypt." *Journal of the American Academy of Religion* 81 (4): 1117–38.

Herzfeld, Michael. 1990. "Icons and Identity: Religious Orthodoxy and Social Practice in Rural Crete." *Anthropological Quarterly* 63:109–21.

Hoffman, Valerie J. 1995. *Sufism, Mystics, and Saints in Modern Egypt.* Columbia: University of South Carolina Press.

Ivanov, Sergey A. 2006. *Holy Fools in Byzantium and Beyond.* Oxford: Oxford University Press.

Keane, Webb. 2007. *Christian Moderns: Freedom and Fetish in the Mission Encounter.* Berkeley: University of California Press.

Kitzinger, Ernst. 1958. *Byzantine Art in the Period between Justinian and Iconoclasm.* Berichte zum XI Internationalen Byzantinisten-Kongress, vol. 4. Munich: C. H. Beck.

Kormina, Jeanne, and Sergei Shtyrkov. 2012. "St. Xenia as a Patron Saint of Female Social Suffering: An Essay in Anthropological Hagiography." In *New Moralities and Religions in Post-Soviet Russia,* edited by Jarrett Zigon, 168–90. New York: Berghahn.

Lossky, Vladimir. 1974. *In the Image and Likeness of God*. Crestwood, NY: St. Vladimir's Seminary Press.
Luehrmann, Sonja. 2010. "A Dual Quarrel of Images on the Middle Volga: Icon Veneration in the Face of Protestant and Pagan Critique." In *Eastern Christians in Anthropological Perspective*, edited by Chris Hann and Hermann Goltz, 56–78. Berkeley: University of California Press.
Meinardus, Otto F. A. 1996. "The Virgin Mary as Mediatrix between Christians and Muslims in the Middle East." *Marian Studies* 47:88–101.
———. 2002. *Two Thousand Years of Coptic Christianity*. Cairo: American University of Cairo Press.
Meri, Josef W. 2002. *The Cult of Saints among Muslims and Jews in Medieval Syria*. Oxford: Oxford University Press.
Miskin, Matta al-. 1952. *Hayat al-Salat al-Urthuduksiya*. Wadi Al-Natrun: Dayr Abu Maqar Press.
Mittermaier, Amira. 2011. *Dreams That Matter: Egyptian Landscapes of the Imagination*. Berkeley: University of California Press.
Mondzain, Marie-José. 2005. *Image, Icon, Economy: The Byzantine Origins of the Contemporary Imaginary*. Stanford: Stanford University Press.
Ouspensky, Leonid. 1999. "The Meaning and Language of Icons." In *The Meaning of Icons*, by L. Ouspensky and V. Lossky, 23–50. Crestwood, NY: St. Vladimir's Seminary Press.
Peirce, C. S. 1992. *The Essential Peirce: Selected Philosophical Writings*. Vol. 1. Edited by N. Houser and C. Kloesel. Bloomington: Indiana University Press.
Pelikan, Jaroslav. 1990. *Imago Dei: The Byzantine Apologia for Icons*. New Haven: Yale University Press.
René, Monica. 2014. "Contemporary Coptic Art." In *Coptic Civilization: Two Thousand Years of Christianity in Egypt*, edited by Gawdat Gabra, 273–84. Cairo: American University in Cairo Press.
Salomon, Noah. 2017. *"The People of Sudan Love You, Oh. Messenger of God": An Ethnography of the Islamic State*. Princeton: Princeton University Press.
Sedra, Paul. 2011. *From Mission to Modernity: Evangelicals, Reformers, and Education in Nineteenth Century Egypt*. London: I. B. Tauris.
Sharkey, Heather J. 2008. *American Evangelicals in Egypt: Missionary Encounters in an Age of Empire*. Princeton: Princeton University Press.
Skalova, Zuzana, and Gawdat Gabra. 2006. *Icons of the Nile Valley*. Cairo: Egyptian International Publishing-Longman.
Stewart, Charles. 2012. *Dreaming and Historical Consciousness in Island Greece*. Cambridge, MA: Harvard University Press.
Taylor, Christopher Schurman. 1999. *In the Vicinity of the Righteous: Ziyara and the Veneration of Muslim Saints in Late Medieval Egypt*. Leiden: Brill.
Török, László. 2005. *Transfigurations of Hellenism: Aspects of Late Antique Art in Egypt, A.D. 250–700*. Leiden: Brill.
vom Bruck, Gabrielle, and Barbara Bodenhorn. 2006. *The Anthropology of Names and Naming*. Cambridge: Cambridge University Press.
Wessel, Klaus. 1965. *Coptic Art*. New York: McGraw-Hill.

SYRIAC AS A *LINGUA SACRA*

Speaking the Language of Christ in India

VLAD NAUMESCU

Orthodox christians are strongly aware that language is a privileged means for accessing the divine. They also know that some languages are better than others since they embody the spirit of ancient traditions, lending an aura of authenticity to their words of prayer. This is how Saint Thomas Christians in South India see Syriac, the liturgical language of Syriac Christianity emerging in the first century AD and continuing up until this day in churches of both West Syrian and East Syrian rites. Part of this large family of churches, Syrian Christians in India (Suryanikkal) claim their roots in the conversion of a few Hindu families by the apostle Thomas and in Syrian colonists arriving a few centuries later. While fully integrated in Indian culture and society, they maintained over centuries close connections with the Middle East for religious and commercial purposes, for which Syriac was the lingua franca. The patriarchs of Antioch or Iraq sent their messengers and metropolitans to the Malabar Coast to check on their flock, while Syrian Christians in return sent their aspiring bishops to be acknowledged by the patriarchs. In Kerala, Syriac was used in parallel with vernacular Malayalam (also written with Syriac script between the sixteenth and nineteenth centuries) for liturgical poetry, literature, and religious instruction and was taught by a Syriac teacher or *malpan*. Senior priests respected for their scholarship and linguistic skills, the *malpans* had their own residential "schools" similar to the Indian *gurukula* system, where pupils lived and studied with their master or guru. Knowledge transmission was based on family lineages and patronage networks in a tightly knit community of kin and church.

The use of Syriac decreased significantly with the nineteenth-century church reforms and the introduction of print and formal education, which led to a complete shift toward Malayalam. The liturgical language, however, still preserves many Syriac words and phrases, such as *Barekhmor* (Bless, O Lord!), *sleeba* (cross), *madbaha* (altar), and Qurbana (Divine Liturgy); in addition, all the church services and canonical prayers gathered in *Sh'himo Namaskaram* have kept their Syriac names. In this sense, despite the restricted literacy of Saint Thomas Christians, liturgical practice continues to provide a crucial space for the cultivation of a Syrian Christian identity. The language itself resonates with the people as part of a liturgical aesthetics meant to bring God closer to them in very tangible ways. A dialect of Aramaic, Syriac is for them concrete evidence of the continuity of their tradition since the beginning of Christianity and of its immunity to change. As one Sunday school teacher remarked, "Some teachers feel that learning a sacred language is necessary to establish proximity with God. Students are convinced that it is a matter of privilege to master Syriac, 'the language of Jesus,' to enjoy the liturgy, and this would make the prayer more powerful." They do so by learning by heart the words of prayers and songs transliterated into Malayalam script, trying to grasp the rhythm and tonality of Syriac and learning to recite correctly. In a religious tradition that claims its origins in the times of the apostles, the function of language is less to be understood for its denotative content than valued for its pure, familiar form. Linguistic sacredness makes Syriac integral to the mysteries of faith while preserving the cultural heritage and identity of these ancient Christians.

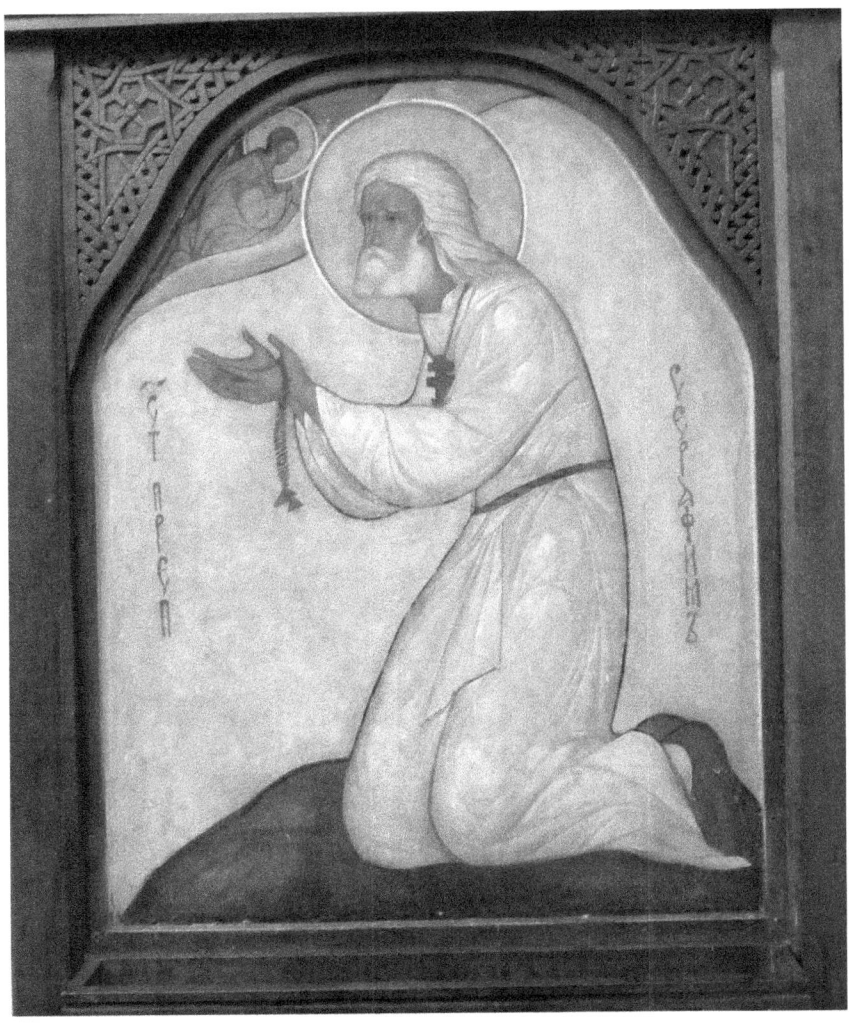

FIGURE 1. Saint Seraphim of Sarov praying on a stone. A twentieth-century icon by the monk Grigorii (Kroug, 1908–69), a Russian émigré who became an iconographer in France. Photograph courtesy of the Orthodox parish of Montgeron, France.

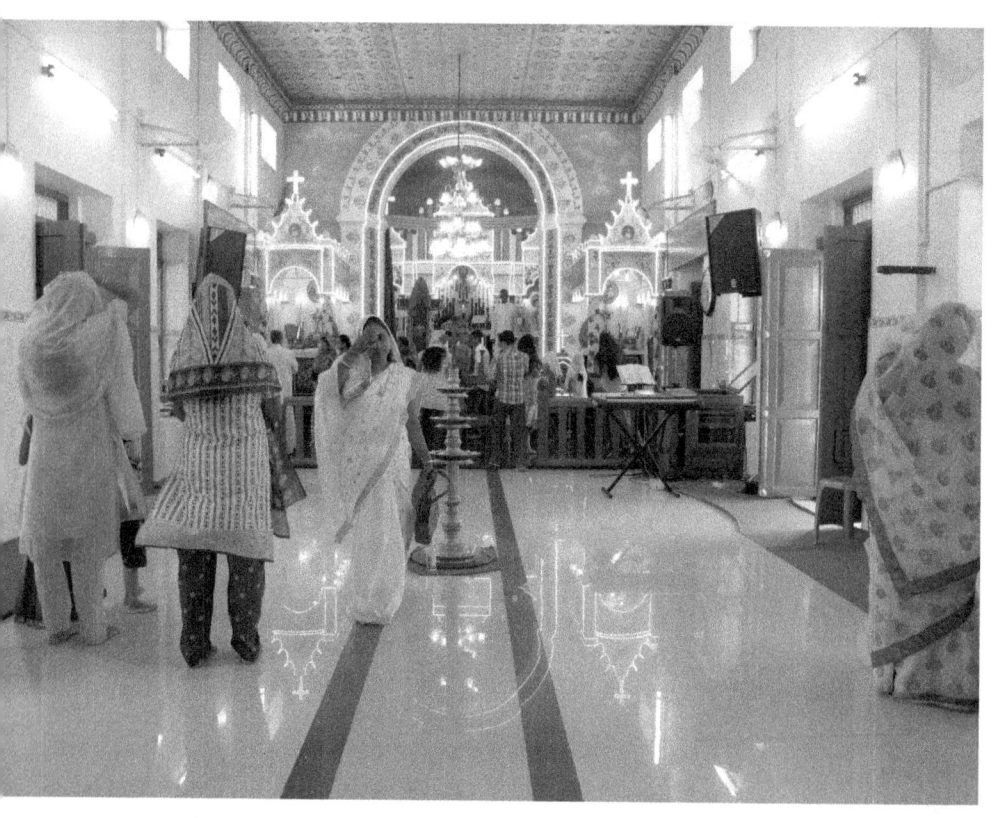

FIGURE 2. Anointing oneself with oil from the traditional lamp (*nilavilakku*) after the Sunday liturgy. St. Thomas Jacobite Church, Keezhillam, India, 2013. Photograph by Vlad Naumescu.

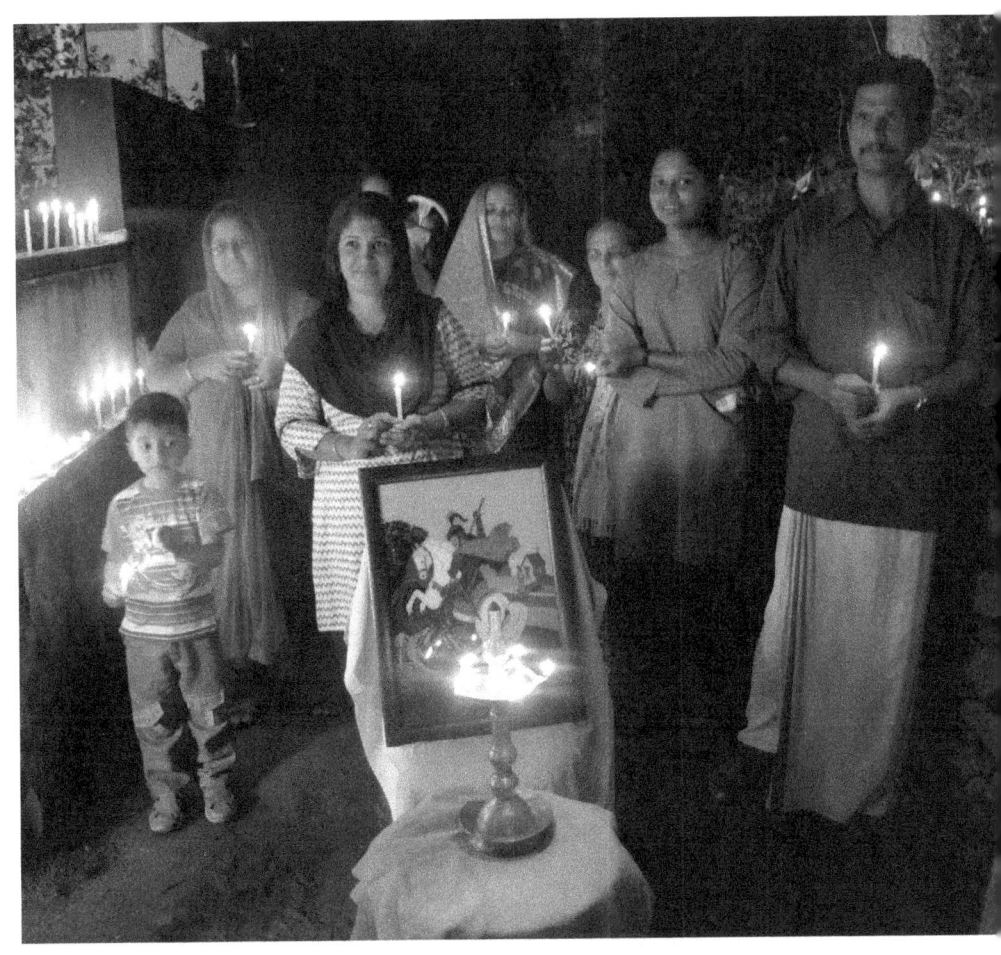

FIGURE 3. Family gathered in front of the house for the annual Puthuppally *perunnal* (feast). St. George Orthodox Church, Puthuppally, India, 2013. Photograph by Vlad Naumescu.

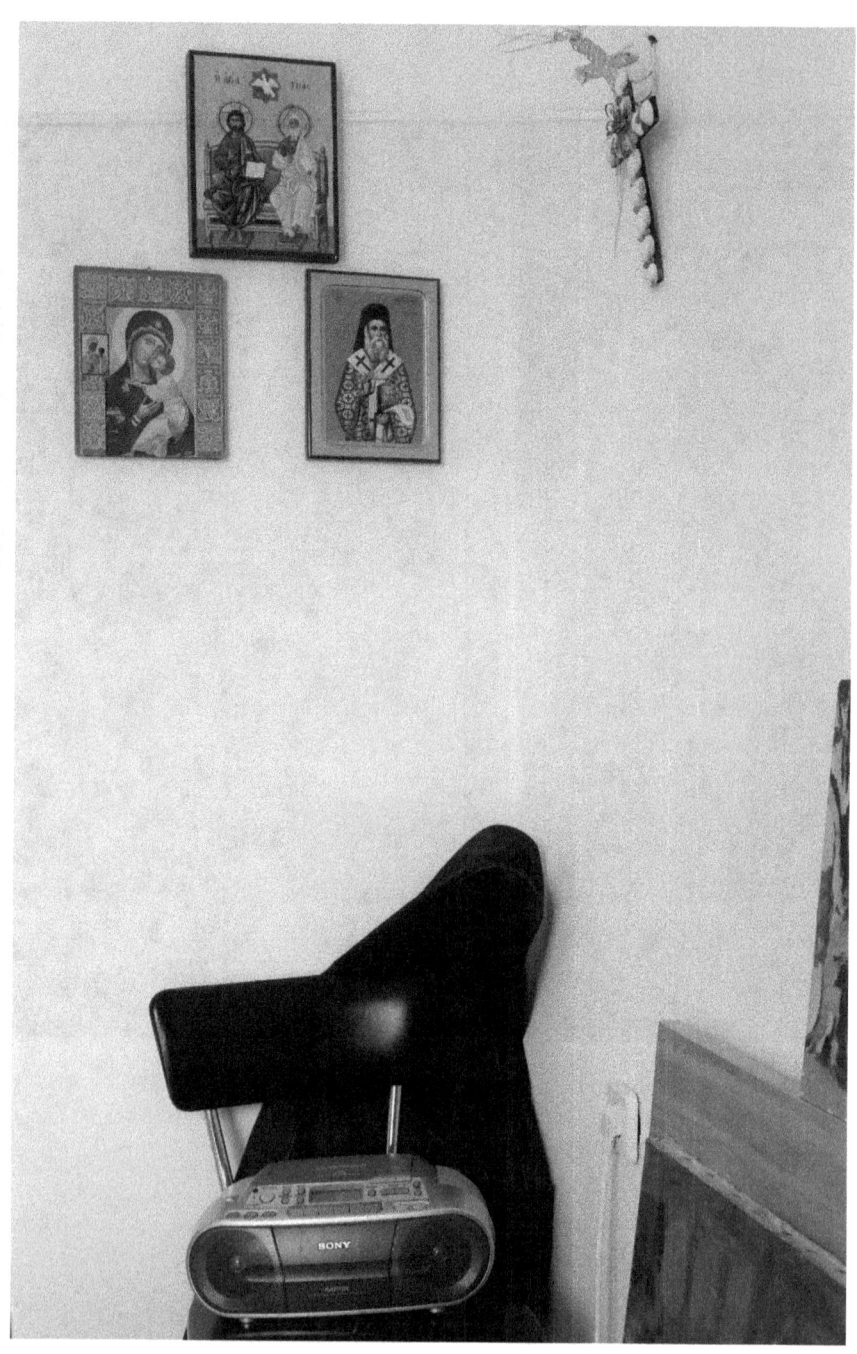

FIGURE 4. A household icon corner with portable radio/CD player for listening to recorded chant and broadcast services. Mesimeri village near Thessaloniki, Greece, 2014. Photograph by Jeffers Engelhardt.

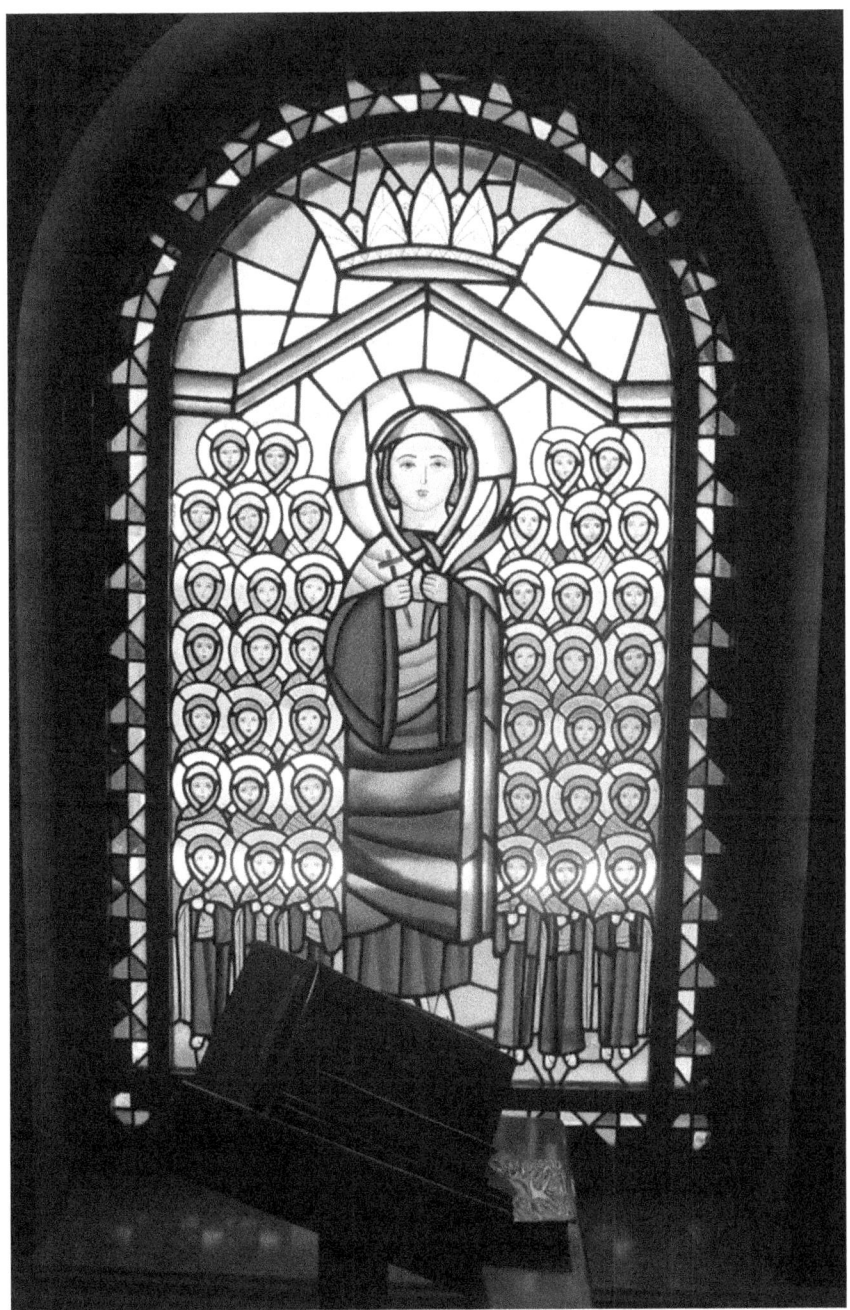

FIGURE 5. A stained-glass icon of Saint Dimyana and the Forty Virgins in the Convent of Saint Dimyana in Bilqas, Mansura, Egypt. Photograph by Angie Heo.

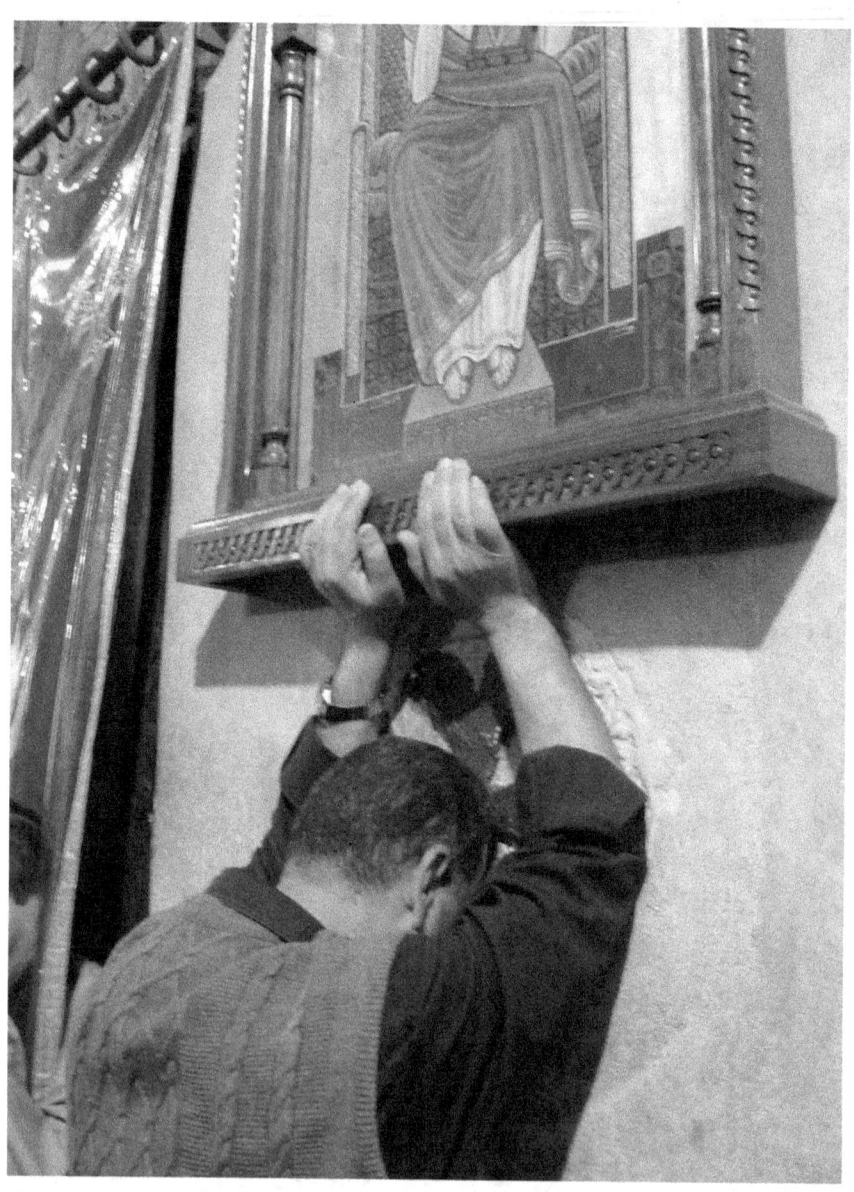

FIGURE 6. Gripping onto an icon while praying in the Church of the Virgin in Zaytun, Egypt, 2007. Photograph by Angie Heo.

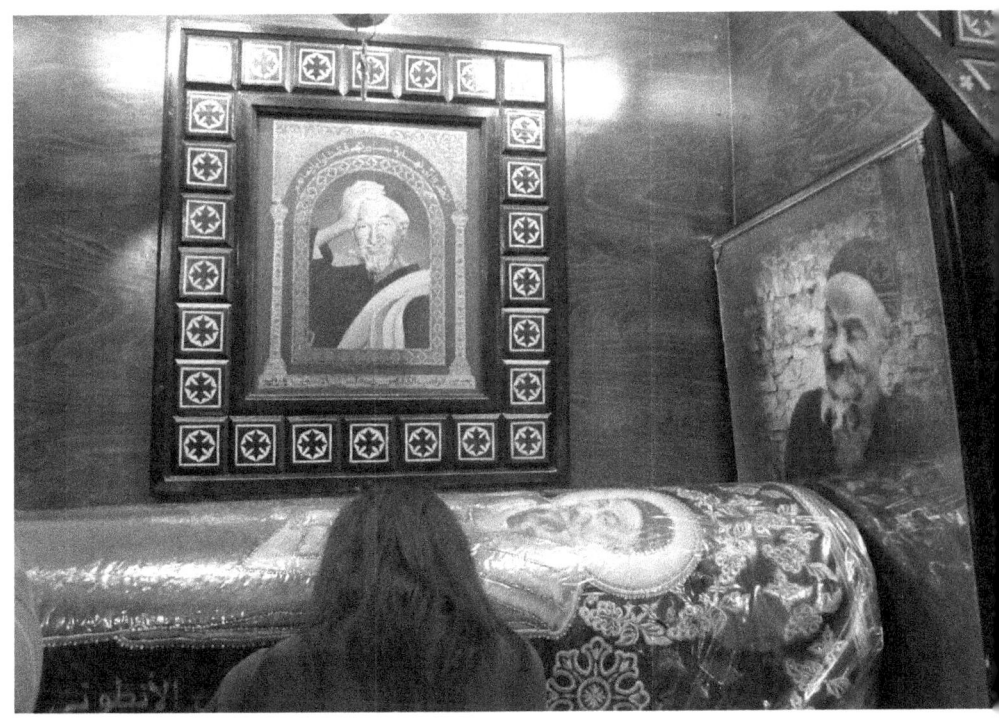

FIGURE 7. Shrine of Yustus al-Antuni in the Monastery of St. Anthony the Hermit on the Red Sea, Egypt, 2014. Photograph by Angie Heo.

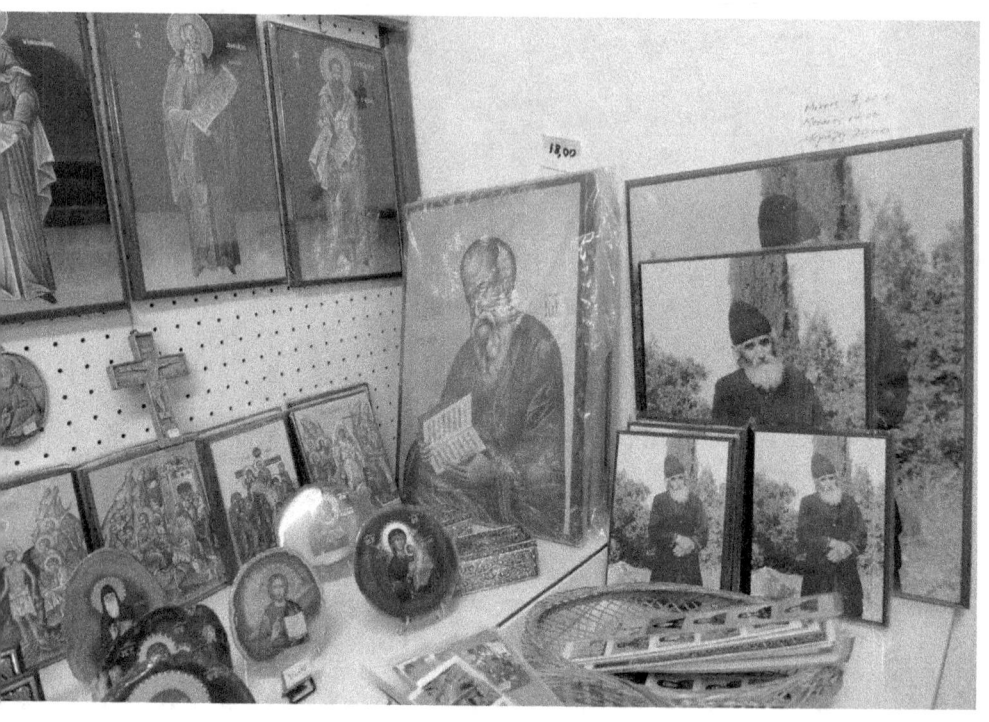

FIGURE 8. Photo-icons of Elder Paisios in the Monastery of St. John the Theologian in Souroti, Thessaloniki, 2014. These icons were for sale before the elder was officially canonized. Photograph by Angie Heo.

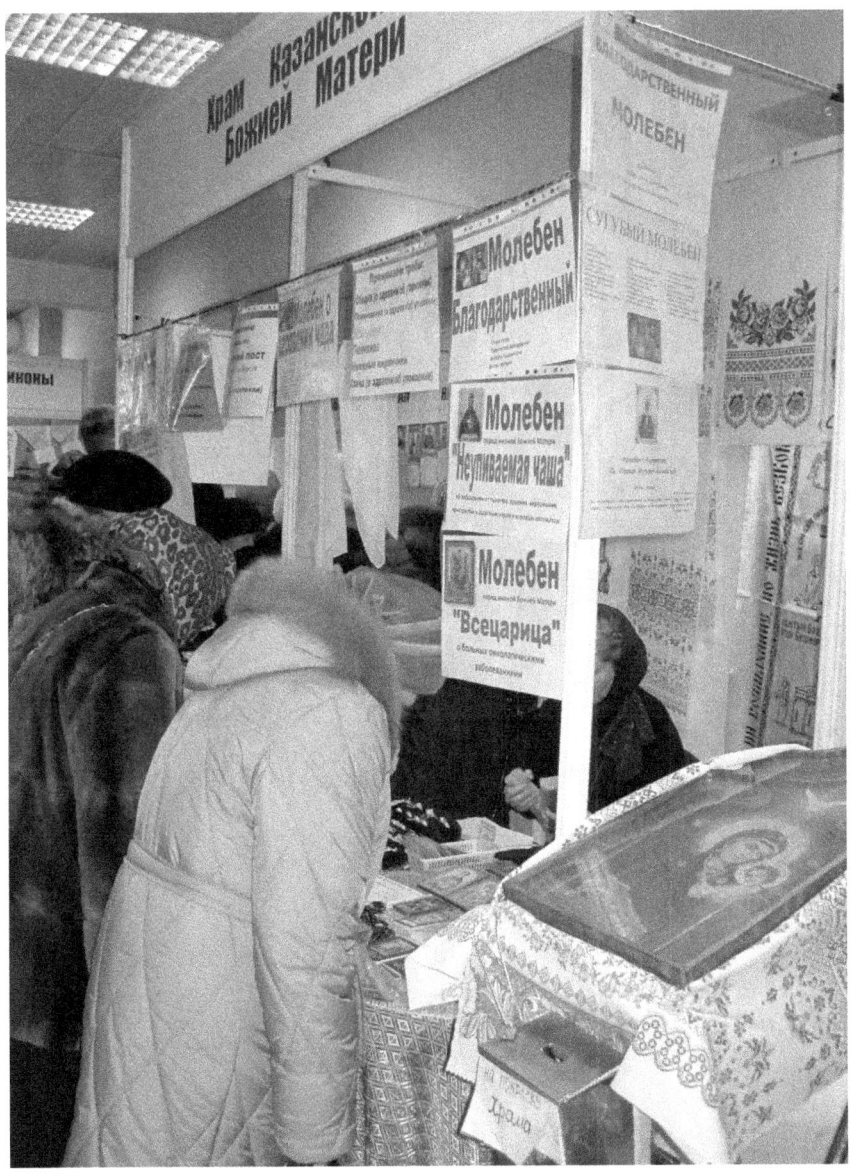

FIGURE 9. Prayers for various needs for sale at the Kazan Orthodox Fair. Clients at this stand pay a fee and write down names to be commemorated during prayers in front of specific icons, including the icons of Mary "The Cup That Cannot be Emptied" (for those afflicted with alcoholism or addiction) and "Queen of All" (for cancer patients). Kazan, Russia, 2012. Photograph by Sonja Luehrmann.

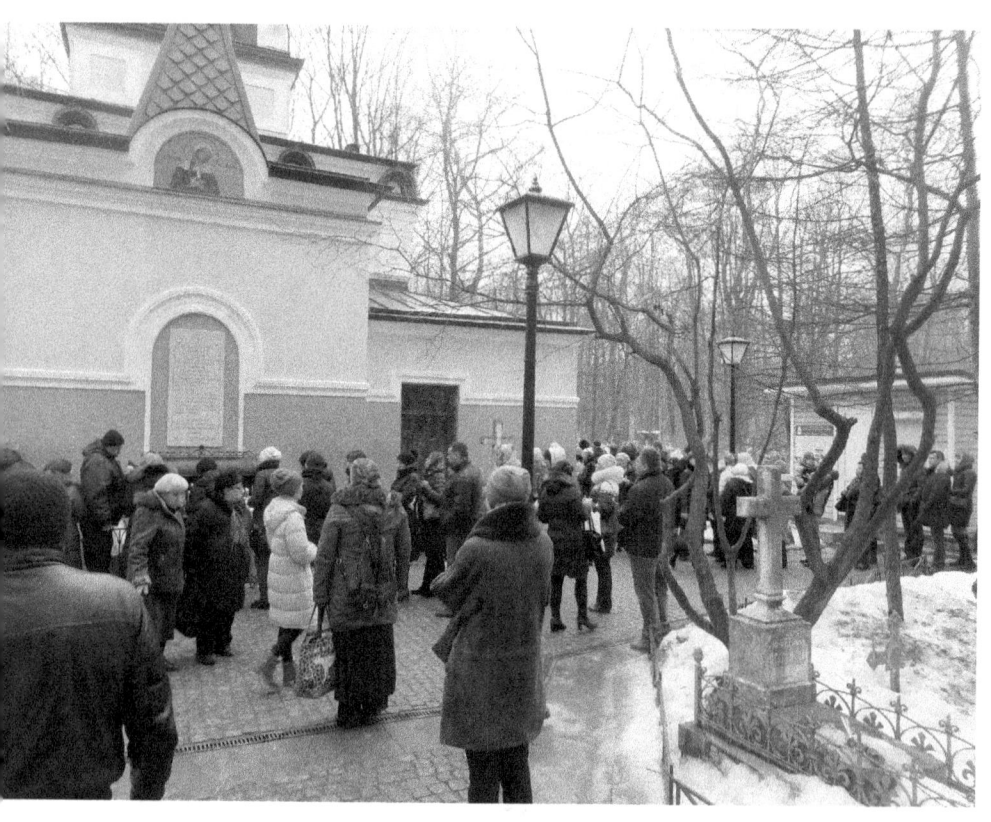

FIGURE 10. Individual pilgrims at Smolenskoe cemetery at the Chapel of Saint Xenia, Saint Petersburg, 2015. Pilgrims try to touch the chapel wall or leave a note when praying. Photograph by Jeanne Kormina.

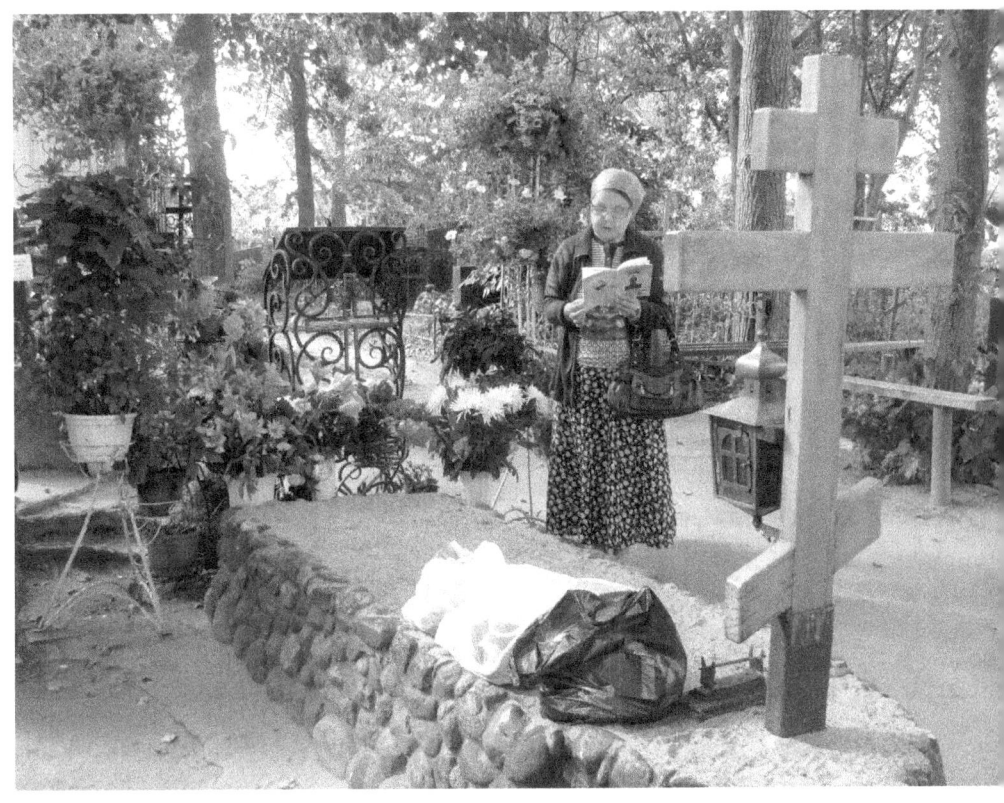

FIGURE 11. A pilgrim reads a noncanonical akathistos to the noncanonized saint Father Nikolai (Gurianov) at his venerated grave. Pskov region, Russia, 2016. Photograph by Jeanne Kormina.

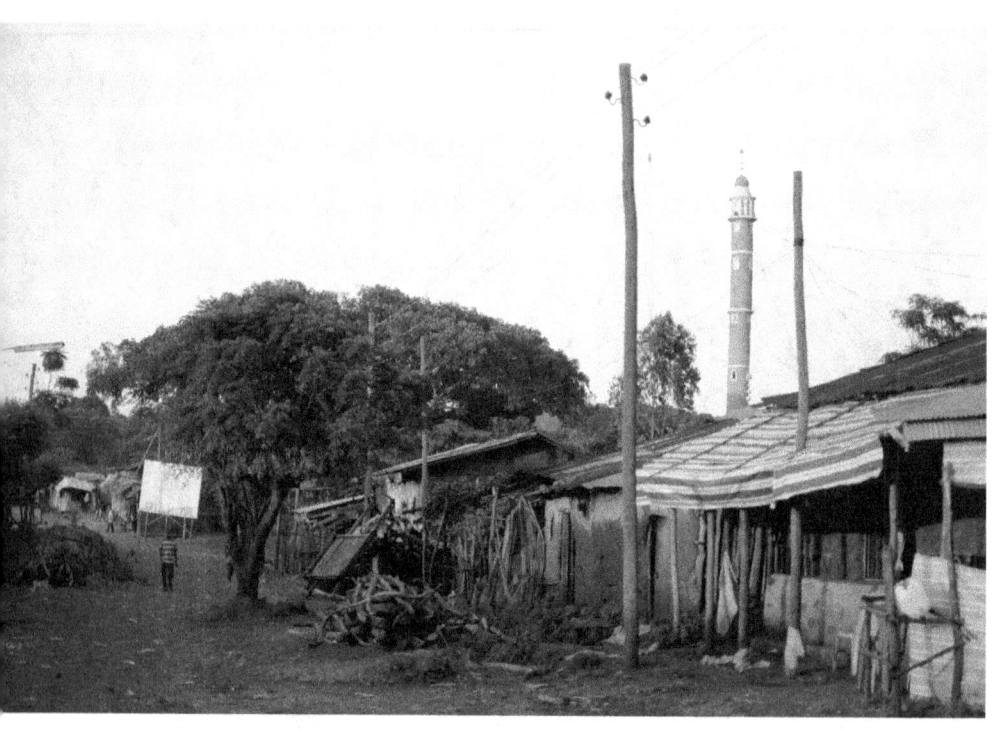

FIGURE 12. Minaret of the Zege mosque visible above the village. Zege, Ethiopia, 2013. Photograph by Tom Boylston.

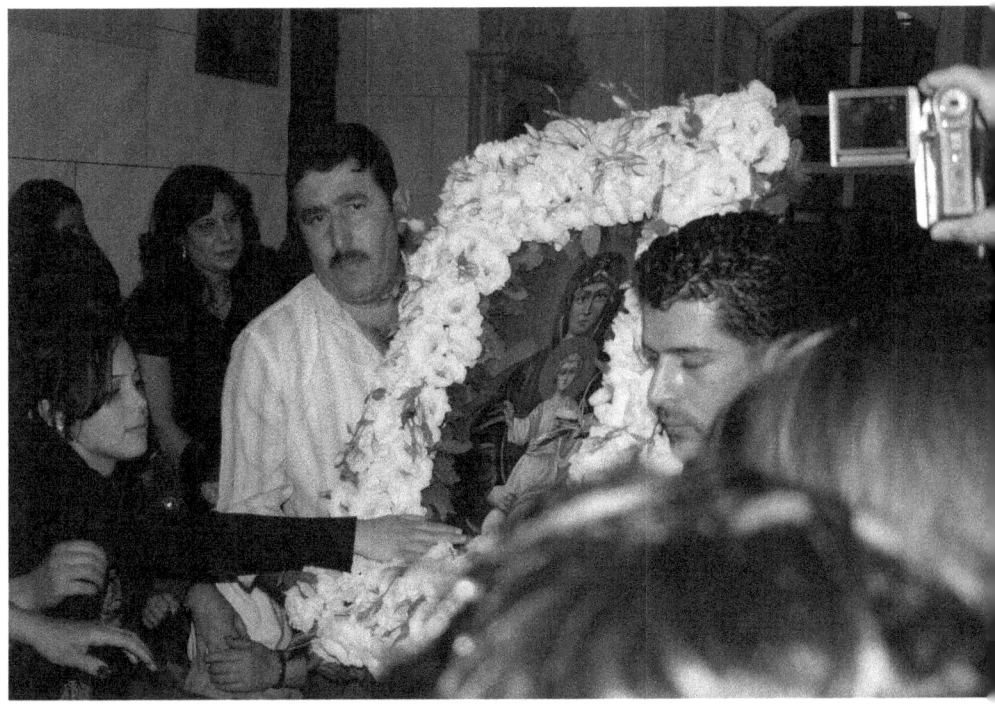

FIGURE 13. Orthodox Christians on the Celebration of Mary's Nativity on September 8 at the famous Greek Orthodox monastery of Our Lady in Saydnaya, Syria, 2009. Touching the icon is a way of accessing divine grace, common in many Orthodox countries. Photograph by Andreas Bandak.

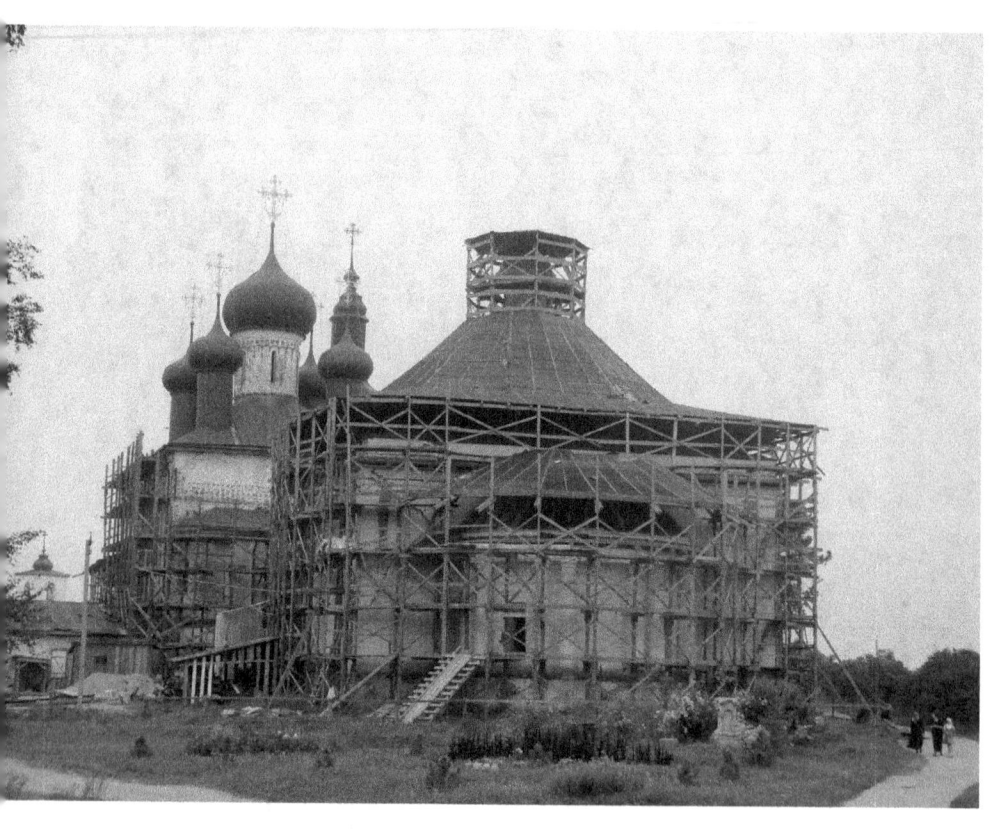

FIGURE 14. The Goritskii convent under reconstruction. Russia, 2010. Photograph by Daria Dubovka.

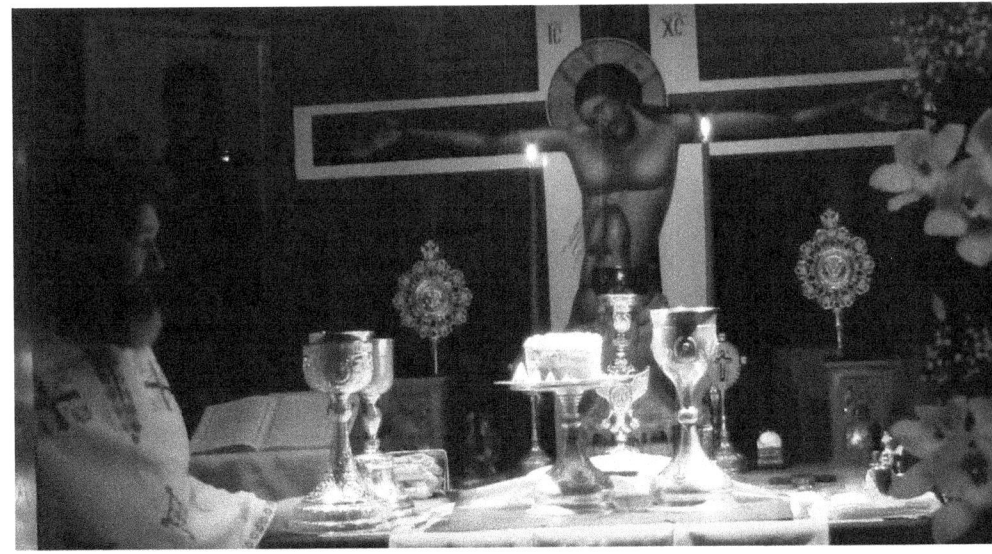

FIGURE 15. View of the Holy Eucharist through the open iconostasis doors at Father Mihail's church in Cluj, Romania, 2016. The open sanctuary expresses the idea of active participation and the way in which frequent communion helps transfer the drama of redemption from the altar to the faithful bodies. Photograph by Septimiu Rusu.

4 AUTHORIZING

The Paradoxes of Praying by the Book

SONJA LUEHRMANN

ALONGSIDE ICONS, MOST ORTHODOX CHRISTIAN FAMILIES own one or more prayer books. Often kept on the same shelf as the sacred images, the most obvious use for these books is to be taken up from the shelf and read aloud from while facing the icons. In Russian, one refers to "reading a prayer" rather than to reciting it. This expression comes from a shift in the meaning of the verb *chitat'* from Slavonic "recite, say out loud" to modern Russian "read," analogous to the semantic shift between Anglo-Saxon *raedan* and modern English "read" (Howe 1993). The persistence of the old meaning in the religious field reflects the close association between Russian Orthodox practice and the Old Church Slavonic language. It also shows a popular understanding that praying means to faithfully reproduce texts that are recorded in books, no matter if this happens by literally reading or by recalling a memorized text. For those who pray regularly, reciting from a prayer book is part of a complex process of actualizing pre-given elements in an act of correct worship, comparable to the generative process of using grammatical structures to create a new text. When trying to perform a prayer text correctly, worshippers engage in complex negotiations between their own skills and aesthetic preferences, the authority they ascribe to particular aspects of Orthodox tradition, and practical problems, such as how to make time for prayer in a busy day and maintain focus over a prolonged period of time.

At the same time, like other sacred things collected on icon shelves, prayer books have many uses that go beyond their ostensible purpose. The small books bound in cloth or leather may be given as gifts at baptism or by a more pious acquaintance but then rarely if ever opened. Because of the cross imprinted on these books' covers and the fact that they are sold in church shops, people may treat them more as an icon to be displayed on the shelf while using only a few stock prayers from memory or reading them from a digital device. Just as icons can serve as media of divine presence independent of their visual style or artistic accomplishment, prayer books can be signs of a household or an individual belonging to an Orthodox tradition without necessarily being used to verbalize prayer. Like icons and chants, their presence helps to create a canonical environment in which acts of prayer are anchored to the church as an institution (see also the chapters by Engelhardt and Boylston, this volume). In combination, the words of prayer and their material basis provide ways of forging connections between communal practice at church and individual devotions. This enables innovation in prayer at the same time as it remains anchored in tradition.

The effort of focusing on archaic and sometimes repetitive language and the silent presence of a closed book on a shelf show two characteristics of written texts that help changing generations of believers actualize a tradition whose essence is, they claim, unchanging: written or printed words have a material manifestation that remains constant over time, sometimes even across generations. One of the functions of writing is to make the transmission of texts somewhat independent of contact between concrete individuals, making the words immune from the changes that occur with person-to-person teaching (Goody 1986; Ong 1982; Urban 2001). Individuals perform prayer texts through acts of reading or recitation that depend on the skills and interests of particular human beings in their own time and location (Boyarin 1993). The insistence on authoritative texts, the actual variability of performance, and the way in which texts are sometimes overshadowed by a canonical environment are important parts of Orthodox Christian prayer. A closer look at how read prayer works and how new texts become part of accepted canons demonstrates the complex efforts that go into preserving right ways of doing things. In the interdependence between innovation and continual practice, there are surprising parallels between Orthodox prayer and forms that seem diametrically opposed at first glance, such as spontaneous evangelical prayer and charismatic praying in tongues.

GENERATIVE REPETITION

The anthropology of religion in general and of Christianity in particular offers few deep considerations of praying by the book. Although scholars interested in ritual language have long emphasized that creative innovation is enabled rather than hindered by the formal characteristics of ritual speech (Briggs 1988; Keane 1997), many have little to say about prayer books and the texts in them other than that they embody some form of social authority. Maurice Bloch's famous line "One cannot argue with a song" (1989, 37) describes a common attitude to read prayers as well. Part of the reason for this relative lack of attention to prescribed prayer texts may be that spontaneous, oral prayers are closer to the kinds of materials anthropologists like to record and analyze. Building on work on ritual and performance that focused on the processes of memory and transmission of ritual texts in the absence of writing (Hymes 1981; Vansina 1985), ethnographies of Christianity have paid much attention to the oral delivery of impromptu prayer and sermons (Harding 2000; Harkness 2014; Tomlinson 2014; Toren 2011). Glossolalia as the ultimate rejection of linguistic conventions in prayer has also prompted many to think of language in prayer as something on the border of human meaning-making (Csordas 1997; Engelke and Tomlinson 2006). When ethnographers turn their attention to religious traditions that value convention over spontaneity, it often seems easier to grasp the visual and material aspects of prayer (Dransart 2002; Mahieu 2010; Packert 2010) or the sonorous qualities of sacred languages (Graham 1987; Hirschkind 2006). An exception is the study of textual recitation and prayer in Islam, where ethnographers note that faithful repetition is not just an act of submitting to authority and reducing the scope of creativity, as Bloch argues. Rather, the habitual recitation of Quranic verses and prayer formulas can be an occasion for mental elaboration, pursuit of new skills, and witnessing to others through ritual performance (Haeri 2013; Gade 2004; Henkel 2005).

In order to form a more nuanced understanding of authoritative texts and their uses, one could think of the conventionalized media in Eastern Christian prayer—including prayer books, icons, and musical settings—as an answer to a dilemma faced by all religious traditions that consider divine beings to be in some way external to or transcending the sensory world. Anthropologist Tanya Luhrmann (2012, 47) discusses it as a problem of externalizing aspects of internal experience: "Whatever people do when they pray, they must learn to treat some inner mental phenomena as heard by an external presence, and other mental phenomena as not their own but as emanating from that presence." For the American evangelicals studied by Luhrmann, all experience during prayer is deeply personal and individual, and the problem is to distinguish between thoughts that belong to the person praying and those that represent the voice of God implanting ideas into his or her mind. In their effort to distinguish between internal and external causes of mental experience, Evangelical Protestants worry about the genuineness and immediacy of their experience of God more than about its conformity to church doctrine—for North American postdenominational Christians, the threat of "heresy fades into unimportance" (Luhrmann 2012, 84).

Orthodox Christian churches, whose liturgical texts and sermons drive home the need to be vigilant about remaining with the true faith (Luehrmann 2010), provide a different answer to the problem of externalizing mental experience. Though the God of Eastern Christianity is just as invisible and immaterial as that of evangelicals, worshippers are assured of the external origin of their experiences of the sacred through the sensory media that church tradition provides. The words in which an Orthodox Christian addresses God are literally not his or her own, neither in authorship nor in style, and those words that Orthodox liturgy puts into the mouth of God and God's agents are even further removed from ordinary conversation. The icons that worshippers are encouraged to look at while praying present images of a God-infused world that emphatically do not come from the individual's imagination but have been vetted by collective discernment (Heo, this volume; Luehrmann 2016). Ordinary laypeople will often say that texts of prayers and iconographic imagery were authored by saintly people whose spiritual advancement acts as a guide for the person striving for a similar experience. It could be said that the texts as well as the environments of Orthodox Christian prayer are meant to set limits to internal mental processes and model them after those of spiritual exemplars.

In order to attune the individual to this canonical environment, the use of set texts in prayer has to be more than an act of rote repetition. Orthodox prayer books are not instruction manuals to be read from cover to cover and followed step by step but look more like collections of poetry. Most prayer books for laypeople start with the most common sets of prayers for home use, the morning and evening prayers. Each of these takes about twenty to thirty minutes to recite in full, and neither is a continuous text but a collection of short individual prayers to be said in a particular order. Some texts come from the Bible and from the collective deliberations of the early church councils, such as the Lord's Prayer, various psalms, and the Nicene Creed. Other prayers are identified with an individual author—the prayer of Saint Makarius, for example, or the prayer of Saint Basil the Great. For the Orthodox Christian learning to pray well, the problem is not to recognize inner voices as actually coming from outside but rather to internalize voices that belong to others and model himself or herself after the attitudes of gratitude, contrition, or hope that are expressed by the saintly author.

The process of molding oneself to the interiority of a more spiritually advanced person through performing his or her speech is part of the Orthodox "morality of exemplars" (see Naumescu and Pop, this volume). Learning to do this involves more structure and repetition than the spontaneous chats with God encouraged by American evangelical churches, but it also requires variations and adjustments. A young man in his twenties who had left a Neo-Pentecostal church founded by American missionaries to work for the Orthodox diocese in a provincial Russian city explained that Orthodox prayer and liturgical practices were more repetitive and required more patience but that he felt that they "took him deeper" over time. A friend in Moscow used to comment on the same repetitiveness of the daily morning and evening prayers, struggling with boredom but valuing them as part of a "gospel way of life" passed on from generation to generation since the time of the apostles. Later, as a young mother, she started having difficulty saying daily prayers at all in the face of household responsibilities. Her parish priest agreed with her that in today's world, raising a family had become a spiritual exploit (Russian *podvig*) in its own right and told her not to worry about performing the prayers every day. This woman's prayer practice shrunk from reciting the half-hour-long morning and evening prayers daily when she was in her teens and early twenties to saying the Lord's Prayer and an invocation of the Holy Fathers with her children before meals and a prayer of thanksgiving afterward. What remains is the idea of prayer as an aspect of daily routines, a habitual part of life rather than a conversational comment on it.

The more seriously a believer tries to live out the daily cycle of prayers, the more it needs to be adjusted to changing life circumstances. In this way, praying by the book is a generative process, similar to using grammatical rules to construct new sentences (Bloom 1994). By using the texts provided by the prayer book but personalizing their performance with or without the blessing of a priest, believers can tailor their prayers to their own needs and abilities while acknowledging a common standard of correctness.

As the example of the young mother shows, one common way of personalizing the prayers is to abbreviate them or limit their recitation to special occasions. The frequency of abbreviation can be guessed from how often it is mentioned in advice literature since at least the nineteenth century. Opinions on the permissibility of abbreviating the prayers differ among authorities. The nineteenth-century bishop Ignatius (Brianchanninov, 1807–67) advised laypeople to say the prayers with focus and limit themselves to the amount of text that they could read before the mind started to wander: "Read the usual prayers, worrying not so much about the quantity of prayers, but about the quality, that is take care that it is done with attention and driven by attention, so that the heart is sanctified and revived by prayerful affection [*umilenie*] and consolation" (Ignatii 1998, 3). The charismatic urban priest Ioann Sergiev (1829–1908, canonized as Saint John of Kronstadt in 1990) by contrast admonished his followers to train themselves to focus on daily prayers from the beginning to the end, suggesting that they start all over again the moment they became distracted (Kizenko 2000). In his mid-twentieth-century lectures on pastoral theology held at the Theological Academy at St. Trinity-Sergius Lavra, Bishop Veniamin (Milov) warned priests in particular against the "danger of shortening the prayer rule," which he saw as a symptom of lack of faith in the saving powers of the church (Veniamin ([1948] 2002, 273). He quotes Saint John of Kronstadt's advice for how to prevent mind-wandering and purely mechanical reading: "When you carry out the prayer, especially following the book, do not hurry from word to word without feeling its truth, without putting it on your heart, but take up and always fulfill the work of feeling in your heart the truth of what you are saying" (quoted in Veniamin [1948] 2002, 277). Given that pre-revolutionary Russian laypeople were largely illiterate and unable to follow complex prayer rules, the idea that prayers should be performed with as much focus and completeness as possible was part of the reform tendencies of the nineteenth and early twentieth centuries, during which the lay piety of literate urbanites was modeled on standards that had formerly applied only to clergy and monastics. This trend continued through Soviet times among the smaller and more self-selected numbers of believers. The expectation and to some degree reality of prayer performance among lay faithful may have intensified, comparable to the emergence of more frequent confession and communion traced by Nadieszda Kizenko (2012).[1]

When abbreviating the prayers, many people reduce them to their most personal element: the commemoration of living and dead family members, friends, and benefactors for whom one requests health or eternal repose. This recitation of names has its fixed place in the morning prayers, and special blank "books of commemoration" (Russian *pomianniki*) are for sale in church shops to record one's personal list. In some traditional Orthodox communities, such as Old Believer villages or monasteries, *pomianniki* may be kept for several generations and constitute a record of the community across time (Kenworthy 2010; Naumescu 2013; Rogers 2009). In contemporary Russia, movements founded by Orthodox activists such as teetotalers (Russian *trezvenniki*), monarchists, and anti-abortion activists also create their own lists of names, using electronic means to distribute them to sympathetic clergy and laypeople across the country. Even for those who simply wish to commemorate family members, incorporating them into the daily prayers involves juggling between the prayer book and the list of names, in a miniature version of the shifts between four or more service books that are involved in any performance of the Divine Liturgy.

Recognizing the prompt to switch between prayer books and *pomianniki* is one of the most elementary generative skills a person must have in order to perform Orthodox prayers. In Russia, even people with relatively scant knowledge of Church Slavonic recognize the phrase *imia rek* (Slavonic "say the name") as a prompt to insert the baptismal name(s) of people being prayed for in lay intercessions as well as in liturgical texts for priests. Humorous anecdotes make fun of people who make the mistake of reading aloud this bit of stage instruction instead of replacing it with a name. While official prayer books clearly relegate lists of names to a secondary status within the prayer text, in practice the desire to intercede for family members often becomes the main purpose of private as well as public prayer. For example, during prayer services for particular needs (*moleben*), standing in line to write down the names of loved ones to be included in the final intercessions often takes precedence over joining the circle of worshippers standing with the priest. In prayers prayed at home, phrases from official prayer formulas can be used to bolster more intimate and local requests expressed in the praying person's own words. In this prayer for commemorating the dead I recorded in 2005 from an elderly Mari woman in a village in the Kirov region in northeastern Russia, this process of improvisation is also marked linguistically. Most of the prayer is spoken in Mari (one of the Finno-Ugric minority languages of the Volga region), but key phrases from prayer-book litanies use words borrowed from Russian or Church Slavonic. In the translation below, italics indicate places where the original uses Slavic terms.

> White Great God! Give us every day our drink and food.
> To the ancient ones give *rest*.
> Let everything be good.
> May there be harvest, may the cattle be plentiful for the family.
> Keep watch among us.
> God *forgive*.
> Rest their bones. May the *earth* be like *downs* to their *ashes*.
> Be so good as to *bless* everything. May it all be good.

> We have come again to *commemorate*.
> May God be so good as to *bless* us.
> Measure our *mind and spirit*. *Bless* us with *wellbeing, joy, success, peace and health*.
> Everything is good. Living well, we have come again to *commemorate*.
> Forgive Lord the sins of the handmaiden of God Klavdiia, those I have committed, those I have done, and those I have thought. Amen.
> Be so good as to *bless* us. *Bless* all relatives.
> All the desires of the Mari people fulfill.[2]

This is a prayer for the material and spiritual needs of living and dead relatives, spoken impromptu rather than read from a book and expressed in relatively informal language. However, the text is validated and structured by terms that resonate with prayer petitions in church, such as the imperatives "forgive" (Russianized Mari *prostitle*, from Russian *prosti*) and "bless" (*blagoslovitle*, from Russian *blagoslovi*). What makes this prayer especially uncanonical are the Mari phrasings that are influenced by that ethnic group's traditional rituals, which had been practiced in the village until the years of Klavdiia's youth. The name "White Great God" (Osh Kugu Iumo), for example, comes out of indigenous Mari cosmology, and Klavdiia goes on to address God with the Mari word "Iumo" rather than with the Slavonic "Gospodi" (Lord) that is used in official Mari-language translations of Orthodox prayers. The reference to earth being like "downs" comes from a Russian saying roughly equivalent to the English "May they rest in peace." With the exception of the influences from Finno-Ugric language and cosmology, the prayer is thus not so different from what might be said by Russian villagers who learned to pray without prayer books during the Soviet period but have been exposed to some key phrases from church services. In Klavdiia's prayer, such stock phrases include *um-razum* (Slavonic "mind and spirit"), the reference to herself as "handmaiden of God," and the formula for forgiveness of sins that recalls funerary services. Although she was not a regular churchgoer, she had absorbed these phrases over years of attendance at funerals and other occasional services and was able to draw on them in constructing her own prayer.

Whether performed spontaneously or from a prayer book, home prayers receive some of their performative force from the temporal openness of ritual formulas, which connect one set of petitions and concerns with those voiced in other times and places (Tomlinson 2014). At the same time, every individual performance is a negotiation between a textual template and the devotee's available time, ability to remember or read the archaic language, and degree of resonance with the concerns laid out by the saintly authors. The person praying also has to find his or her own footing within the contrasting stances of intercession for others and acts of praise, petition, and repentance for oneself that the texts themselves contain. Even people who are not religious virtuosi cannot help but personalize their prayer performance through these acts of adapting text to context.

DELEGATING PRAYER

Another way in which praying by the book differs from rote repetition is when speech roles are delegated or shared across several people, creating dynamic transitions between personal and corporate prayer. In the Gospels, Jesus speaks both of the virtues of secluded, individual prayer "in the inner room" (Matt. 6:6, ESV) and of the strength of multiple voices: "Again I say to you, that if two of you agree on earth about anything that they may ask, it shall be done for them by My Father in heaven" (Matt. 18:19). For evangelicals, collective prayer in public often raises issues of privacy—how much of one's innermost thoughts to reveal to others? Protestant converts around the world come up with forms of "collective-personal prayer," where several people pray aloud simultaneously so that no one can overhear what others are saying (Haynes 2017; see also Handman 2014 and Harkness, forthcoming). Confidential prayer hotlines and online requests are a technological solution to the same problem. For Pentecostals, praying in tongues combines the virtues of spontaneity with the privacy of an incomprehensible language. The Orthodox prayer book offers other answers to the problem of confidentiality in community: joint reading of generic texts to which each person attributes a different sense, and delegation of prayer to specific individuals who will perform them on behalf of known or unknown others. Within the family, it is often one of the older female members whose job it is to maintain relations with the household's heavenly guardians and to intercede for the rest of the family by attending church services or placing candles at monasteries or other sacred sites (Hirschon 1989; Kormina and Shtyrkov 2012).

When members of the household lack the time or confidence in their ability to pray over a particular concern, they will invite a priest or order prayers in a local church or a monastery. This means that the names of those in need of prayer will be included in a standardized prayer service (*moleben*) said for a particular concern, such as cancer, success in studies, or fertility. The details of the situation for which prayer is requested rarely become known to those who perform the prayer. This kind of standardized prayer based on lists of names is one of the main goods for sale in church kiosks as well as at Orthodox fairs that are held in many Russian cities throughout the year. Sometimes prayers for a variety of needs and concerns will be said in the presence of those who order them, as during a *moleben* in church. Sometimes the sponsors of the prayers are absent, as when someone pays a distant monastery for a forty-day-long commemoration of a loved one who suffers from alcoholism in front of an icon of the Mother of God "The Cup That Cannot be Emptied." In such cases, the sponsor is told the date when the prayers will start and is encouraged to join in during those days with some prayer effort of his or her own, such as reading a recommended prayer or akathistos hymn to the icon at home once a day. In the monastery, the prayer, hymn, and relevant Gospel passages will be inserted in the standard text of a prayer service read from the *trebnik* (Russian "book of needs," or book of occasional services). The *trebnik* is not usually owned by a lay household, but since the shorter prayers and hymns to popular icons are included in many lay prayer books, it is possible for sponsors to engage in their own synchronous actions.

Working with set texts for prayers thus allows delegation of prayerful duties as well as co-participation, even across distances. For many Orthodox laypeople, the predominant value seems to lie in the specialists' prayers: "He is a holy man; his prayer reaches God faster" is a common explanation, or "This person, whatever he asks God, God grants it." Through a combination of practice and charismatic gifts, priests and especially monastics become better at prayer, able to offset the shortcomings that seep into lay prayer through lack of time and daily distractions.

Although the market in prayers is driven by perceived value differentials between lay and clergy petitions, prayer by the book is not simply a good that is bought and sold. Rather, it is like a specialized service that may require some participation on the part of the client. The specialist's skill is complemented by the sincerity of the sponsor's amateur prayers, both of which are features that help speed up a prayer's way to God.

WHAT'S IN A NAME: THE POLITICS OF INTERCESSION

The lists of names that are used in intercession not only forge connections between private and corporate prayers but also, by bundling a prayer concern into a baptismal name, help to maintain confidentiality in public prayer. Upon entering a church or monastery, visitors will notice instructions for the right format in which to write "notes" (Russian *zapiski*), determining the order of names by clerical and lay status and gender and the right grammatical form in which to write them down. Since lists of names constitute the point of insertion of particular and temporal concerns into the generality of standardized prayer texts, they must be formatted properly. For example, all names must be written in the genitive case, because they will be inserted in the sentence "And still we pray for the health and forgiveness of sins of the servants of God [names]" or "And still we pray for the forgiveness and eternal rest of the servants of God [names]". Grammatically preformatted, the list of names can be read quickly by a priest with minimal conscious thought. Each note becomes part of a much longer litany of names of those about whom members of the community are concerned. Someone who enters the church and writes a note "for the health of Andrei, Olga, and Nataliia" may never recognize the moment when these names are read during the prayer service because there will likely be a flood of Andreis, Olgas, and Nataliias being commemorated. In this flood of names, the details of a prayer concern are also left open, merely hinted at by the nature of the service or through prefixes indicating the person's clerical or lay status, age group, or sometimes a short characterization such as "the sick Maksim" or "the traveler Valentina."

The names can serve as shorthand for the concrete circumstances that lead to the prayer requests by virtue of the most important formatting requirement: the use of baptismal names, all of which come from recognized Orthodox saints. In cases where someone gets baptized as an adult or parents of an infant have registered the birth under a name that is not in the register of saints, the baptismal name will be different, sometimes chosen for being close in sound, sometimes for being the saint commemorated on the birthday or day of baptism. For example, I have known an Èlina (a Tatar name) whose baptismal name was Elena and a Muza (a Soviet name referring to the muses of Greek mythology) whose baptismal name was Mariia but who still went by her secular name in her work as a Sunday school teacher. For some names, churches of Byzantine tradition use forms of names that are closer to the original Greek than those conventionally used in a particular country, such as Ioann for Ivan or Feodor for Fëdor in Russian or Mattias for Madis in Estonian. The baptismal name grants church membership and a special relationship with the name-giving saint. In intercessory prayer, it functions as a designator that God and the patron saint will recognize in the absence of any other information, comparable to a tax payer or patient identification number that gives access to a person's file.

Different from a personal identification number, however, the baptismal name is emphatically not unique to the individual but makes him or her part of a transtemporal community of Orthodox believers in which the living receive the protection of patrons who are dead but have a continued personalized existence in the community of the church (Hirschon 2010). "Christians pray for one another," explained the Orthodox priest Oleg Steniaev at a debate with Protestant clergy, noting that deceased saints could continue to intercede for the living because all were part of the church as a single community: "You may wonder: so how can Saint Nicholas or [Saint] Paul hear us? Are they ever-present? The thing is that we are in very close connection with them. We are in one body with them. That is the Church of Christ, which is one."[3] The capacity of baptismal names and saintly intercession to ensure the textual and metaphysical travels of petitions rests on the assumption that all or most of the people whom an Orthodox person prays for are baptized Orthodox Christians. Problems begin when one wishes to pray for someone who does not have an Orthodox saint's name because that person was either never baptized or is a member of another Christian church. That such people cannot be included in corporate prayers in church seems to be a general consensus in Russia. It is confirmed by signs in many church booths where candles are sold and prayers can be ordered: "The unbaptized, people of other faiths, unbelievers and suicides are not commemorated in the church." On occasions when I ordered prayers for Orthodox relatives in Russian churches, my foreign accent often provoked the question "Are they all baptized?"

Prayers at home or individual prayers in front of a venerated icon are a somewhat different matter, and strategies of how to include non-Orthodox loved ones vary. "One can pray for whomever one wants," said the young mother whose struggles with prayer time I discussed above, explaining that she had no problem praying for non-Orthodox friends in private. Commemorating those who have no name at all is more problematic, to the point that parents who wish to pray for a child who died before baptism or for an aborted fetus will sometimes dream a name or simply give one to the child, whose only regular use will be in private prayer (Lar'kina 2012; Luehrmann 2017). The lack of a name and a baptized identity bars these categories of departed from corporate prayers, as reflected in the lack of a funeral service for stillborn infants in the *trebnik* (Baum, Kishler, and Kishler 2010).

When it comes to people who have names but cannot be included in corporate prayers for other reasons, specialized saints may be called upon to present their cases to God. In churches throughout Russia, the Roman martyr Varus (Russian Uar) is becoming known as a patron of those who died without baptism or who renounced the church, and prayers to him are included in many prayer books "for times of trouble" or "for loved ones." There is also a special prayer on behalf of suicides, attributed to one of the famous elders of Optina Pustyn' Monastery, Lev Optinskii (1768–1841). It ends with the request "Do not count my prayer as sin. May Your holy will be done" (*Kak molit'sia* 2009, 12). The uncertainty about the permissibility of the prayer request is written into the text itself. By distributing such prayers for personal use by the faithful, the church recognizes the fact that in the aftermath of socialism or secularizing and pluralizing processes, many contemporary Orthodox believers will count people among their loved ones who do not fit the requirements for inclusion in corporate prayers. Prayer texts respond to historical changes and popular demand, but change always needs to be legitimated by an established authority within the Orthodox discursive tradition.

AKATHISTOI AND INNOVATION

In the domain of names and intercession, innovation happens through the legitimization of new prayer concerns. But there are also prayer genres that are more open to innovation than others. A particularly dynamic genre that is gaining in popularity in several Orthodox countries is the akathistos (Old Church Slavonic *akafist*), or hymn of praise to the Virgin Mary, a saint, or a feast day. As with the emerging forms of intercession, the flexibility of this genre is partly owed to its use outside of church liturgy. The Greek name refers to a hymn sung "without sitting down," and the original akathistos was a hymn to the Virgin Mary, composed in honor of the successful defense of Constantinople against a Persian attack in 626 (Goltz 1988). A handful of Greek hymns with similar schema and meter followed between the thirteenth century and the fall of Constantinople in 1453. Like modern akathistoi composed in other liturgical languages, they share the structure of the original hymn: twelve kontakions ending in the word "Alleluia" alternate with twelve *oikoi* containing a number of lines starting with "Rejoice" (Greek *khaire*, Slavonic *raduisia*) and ending in a refrain. In the original akathistos to the Virgin Mary, this is "Rejoice, unwedded bride" (Greek *Khaire nymphe anympheute*, Slavonic *Raduisia nevesto nenevestnaia*). Another poetic device used in the original Greek text of the akathistos that recurs in some but not all modern akathistoi is the acrostic—with the exception of the first kontakion, each stanza starts with a consecutive letter of the Greek alphabet.

Other than the structure, modern akathistoi are often considered to fall far short of Byzantine hymnology in poetic expression and originality. However, the genre gained popularity at a time when there was higher literacy among laypeople and greater demand for opportunities to praise and address saints outside of church services. Starting in the nineteenth century, increasing numbers of laypeople wrote akathistoi. For example, the akathistos in honor of the Kazan icon of the Theotokos was written by a professor of Kazan Theological Academy in 1868 (Shevzov 2007); the akathistos for the Holy Martyrs Faith, Hope, and Charity and their mother, Sophia, was written in 1892 by Leonid Ivanovich Denisov, a graduate of Moscow University and "the author of many books and brochures of religious-moral content" (Popov [1903] 2013, 348–49). Writing akathistoi was a relatively unregulated practice because they were not, strictly speaking, liturgical texts. With the exception of the akathistos to the Virgin Mary, which is performed during matins on the fifth Saturday of Lent, other akathistoi have no place in the Typikon and are either printed for home use or performed after the Divine Liturgy or as stand-alone evening services at the discretion of the rector of a church.

In the Russian empire, it was the role of the Holy Synod, the highest instance of church governance, to correct akathistoi and approve them for printing. After the Bolshevik revolution of 1917, few new Slavonic akathistoi could be officially approved, but a large number of them were written and circulated as typescripts or handwritten copies (Liudogovskii and Pliakin 2013, 587). The same was the case with new service texts, which were written for newly canonized saints or newly arising liturgical occasions, such as the collective prayer of confession before communion, which was used in many churches in response to the dearth of priests who could hear individual confessions (Kizenko 2012).

Starting in 1989, a liturgical commission under the auspices of the Holy Synod started to edit and standardize these texts; since 2011 there is a separate commission on akathistoi, reflecting the specifics and importance of this genre. According to commission member Father Feodor Liudogovskii (personal communication, June 2014), members mainly find texts for consideration on the internet, but sometimes dioceses also write with requests for approval of a new text. Since neither the commission nor the Holy Synod have the time and personnel to work through the huge number of new akathistoi, many hymns continue to exist in a gray zone between popular literature and liturgical text. The blessing of a local bishop; approval from a Ukrainian, Belorussian, or Serbian liturgical commission; or the remark "translated from the Greek" often replaces the imprint "Approved for publication by the Editorial Council of the Moscow Patriarchate," which is officially required for all literature distributed in church shops since 2011.

Although some of the new texts have unconventional addressees (for example, Tsar Ivan the Terrible or the Immaculate Conception of the Virgin Mary, which is part of Catholic, not Orthodox, dogma) or vary the required length and structure, the Russian commission has not come across any akathistoi that have completely abandoned the variation between *oikos* and kontakion or that were intentionally composed in modern Russian. Even if the author's command of Old Church Slavonic is weak, the use of Slavonic endings and commonly used words from services and prayer litanies demonstrates the intention to write in the liturgical language (Liudogovskii and Pliakin 2013, 598; Liudogovskii, personal communication). Even in this most dynamic of contemporary prayer forms, innovation happens through intentionally following existing models.

Akathistoi are thus a good example of the combination of deference to traditional authority and relatively decentralized mechanisms of innovation that are part of how contemporary Orthodox Christians engage the prayers of their church. At the same time, the popularity of akathistoi also shows that accessible prayer texts do matter to lay believers, despite stereotypes of Orthodox Christians who are content to merely cross themselves in response to half-understood petitions. In the opinion of two priests who are members of the commission on akathistoi of the Russian Holy Synod, among the reasons for the popularity of akathistoi are the proximity of the Slavonic language used in them to modern Russian, the easy and cheap availability of akathistoi to particular saints in a variety of church and secular shops, and the possibility of "visual intake of the text" while following along with the service (Liudogovskii and Pliakin 2013, 594). Different from other services, which would require a complicated combination of liturgical books to fully follow, it is easy to purchase an akathistos booklet and read along. In many congregations that regularly sing akathistoi to a local icon or a saint venerated for a particular need, regulars arriving for the service retrieve booklets from their bags or purses, while newcomers can buy one in the church shop. The priest usually reads the kontakia and narrative parts of the *oikoi*, and members of the congregation join with the choir in singing the *khairisma*, or successions of lines starting with "rejoice."

Additionally, the popularity of akathistoi shows that people form prayerful attachments to particular saints or icons and seek ways to address them independent of the days prescribed by the church calendar. As Feodor Liudogovskii and Maksim Pliakin (2013, 595) explain, the canon or official service text for a saint is often taken as something to be performed only on the appointed saint's day and only at church. Akathistoi, however, are portable temporally as well as spatially and provide an accepted way to address a saint any time, alone or in a group, in a church or outside. Although its lengthy repetitive structure can make an akathistos unwieldy to perform, outside of the church setting it is often possible to vary the length and completeness of a reading. On the bus to the starting point of a walking pilgrimage in the Kirov region, an elderly woman who had just recited the prayers before Holy Communion and the prayer to the Holy Spirit "for starting out on an undertaking" took out a slim booklet with the akathistos to Saint Nicholas (a protector of travelers but also a helper in a variety of situations of illness or loss). "I always read this on Thursdays, took the blessing [from a priest] for this," she explained to her companion. "And I read it whenever it feels right to my soul [*kogda mne po dushe*]," said the other. Together in a whisper they started the akathistos but skipped a number of stanzas toward the end to get to the final prayers, which ask the saint to protect the devotee in this life and intercede with God for her soul in the afterlife. What precise misfortunes or punishments each was trying to avert by reciting this prayer remained as confidential as the concerns of an individual in a church full of people praying in tongues or speaking their petitions simultaneously. At the same time, the printed text enabled the two women to embody the pilgrimage ethos of doing something together rather than separately and to inform other pilgrims of an important prayer to say for many occasions.

CONCLUSION: READING ONE'S PRAYERS

During the same pilgrimage, one could see the effect of an extraordinary time on people's abilities to say their prayers: every morning and (especially) evening, pilgrims separated out in small groups to read the daily prayers. One reason for the groupings was that not everyone had brought a prayer book (presumably because they did not say prayers at home). Those without books joined others who had one, often people with whom they had come on the pilgrimage. Within the groups, the oldest person or the one most literate in Church Slavonic read the words aloud, sometimes in a speaking voice, sometimes in a version of the chant used in church reading. In groups that had a male member, the reading task fell to the man, just as in a group where an ordained member of the clergy is present, he will usually be the person reading the prayers.

The small groups in which prayer was read out loud illustrated some features of Orthodox Christian prayer: "read" or recited prayer is both a private and a collective affair, something one does for and with others but as inconspicuously as possible. The text matters both as a sound that is produced and carries semantic meaning to God or the saints and also as an object of focus and aid in concentration. The length of the prescribed texts and their habitual sameness make the performance of prayers a special feat of faith that is part of the efforts of a pilgrimage or a time of crisis but that relatively few people maintain on a day-to-day basis. And finally, part of correctly performing the prayer text is to defer to others with greater claim to expertise for reason of ordained status, gender, or age. Thick prayer books as well as thin akathistos booklets are media that can take prayer routines outside of their usual settings, as shown by the woman who continued her routine praise of Saint Nicholas during the extraordinary time of pilgrimage. Though in some ways reading from the prayer book could not be more different from glossolalia, the foreign and yet familiar words of repetitive texts seem to accomplish similar tasks as automatic "speaking in tongues": they shut out everyday worries and conscious thought through a focus on sound itself (Marshall 2009), and they can be shortened but also extended almost indefinitely through repetition. Like much ritual language, they mediate strangeness while maintaining a sense of the distance to be crossed (Keane 1997; Seligman et al. 2008). Both praying in tongues and praying by the book also invoke communities that can be joined through learning: a group reciting evening prayers together is an invitation to bystanders to do the same, both on pilgrimage and at home (see Henkel 2005), while a group engaged in charismatic prayer is an invitation to neophytes to acquire "the gifts of the Holy Spirit" and join in or start their own group. If charismatic forms of prayer are often considered a perfect way to create community under the individualizing and flexible tendencies of (post)modern religiosity (Csordas 1997), praying by the book offers similar features of shift to automatic thinking, marking sacred time, and the simultaneous possibility of communal experience *and* private withdrawal. At the same time, it forces the person praying to encounter the words of other people who have prayed and thought before, connecting each prayer event to a transtemporal community that goes beyond those gathered together at a given place and time.

SONJA LUEHRMANN is Associate Professor of Anthropology at Simon Fraser University in Vancouver, Canada. She is author of *Secularism Soviet Style: Teaching Atheism and Religion in a Volga Republic* (IUP) and *Religion in Secular Archives: Soviet Atheism and Historical Knowledge*.

NOTES

1. The link between literacy and book learning and heightened expectations of the correct performance of prayer texts is not unique to Orthodoxy but has parallels among Muslims in Turkey and India. See Henkel 2005 and research-in-progress by Parvis Ghassem-Fachandi.
2. I thank Svetlana Semenova-Avramova for help in transcribing the prayer.
3. I am grateful to the missionary department of the Orthodox Diocese of Ioshkar-Ola and Marii El for making available the transcript of this debate, which was held in the early 2000s.

REFERENCES

Baum, Michael, Andrew Kishler, and Patricia Kishler. 2010. "For Words at a Loss: The Church's Response to Miscarriage and Stillbirth Needs More Work." *Touchstone Magazine* 23 (January/February). Last accessed July 15, 2014. Retrieved from http://www.touchstonemag.com/archives/article.php?id=23-01-018-f.

Bloch, Maurice. 1989. "Symbols, Song, Dance and Features of Articulation." In *Ritual, History and Power: Selected Papers in Anthropology*, 19–45. London: Athlone.

Bloom, Paul. 1994. "Generativity within Language and Other Cognitive Domains." *Cognition* 51 (2): 177–89.

Boyarin, Jonathan, ed. 1993. *The Ethnography of Reading*. Berkeley: University of California Press.

Briggs, Charles. 1988. *Competence in Performance: The Creativity of Tradition in Mexican Verbal Art*. Philadelphia: University of Pennsylvania Press.

Csordas, Thomas. 1997. *Language, Charisma, and Creativity: The Ritual Life of a Religious Movement*. Berkeley: University of California Press.

Dransart, Penelope. 2002. "Concepts of Spiritual Nourishment in the Andes and Europe: Rosaries in Cross-Cultural Contexts." *Journal of the Royal Anthropological Institute* 8 (1): 1–21.

Engelke, Matthew, and Matt Tomlinson, eds. *The Limits of Meaning: Case Studies in the Anthropology of Christianity*. New York: Berghahn Books.

Gade, Anna. 2004. *Perfection Makes Practice: Learning, Emotion, and the Recited Qur'ān in Indonesia*. Honolulu: University of Hawai'i Press.

Goltz, Hermann. 1988. *Akathistos: Hymnen der Ostkirche*. Leipzig: St. Benno.

Goody, Jack. 1986. *The Logic of Writing and the Organisation of Society*. Cambridge: Cambridge University Press.

Graham, William. 1987. *Beyond the Written Word: Oral Aspects of Scripture in the History of Religion*. Cambridge: Cambridge University Press.

Haeri, Niloofar. 2013. "The Private Performance of *Salat* Prayers: Repetition, Time, and Meaning." *Anthropological Quarterly* 86 (1): 5–34.

Handman, Courtney. 2014. *Critical Christianity: Translation and Denominational Conflict in Papua New Guinea*. Berkeley: University of California Press.

Harding, Susan. 2000. *The Book of Jerry Falwell: Fundamentalist Language and Politics*. Princeton: Princeton University Press.

Harkness, Nicholas. 2014. *Songs of Seoul: An Ethnography of Voice and Voicing in Christian South Korea*. Berkeley: University of California Press.

———. Forthcoming. "Glossolalia and Cacophony in South Korea: Cultural Semiosis at the Limits of Language." *American Ethnologist*.

Haynes, Naomi. 2017. "Learning to Pray the Pentecostal Way: Language and Personhood on the Zambian Copperbelt." *Religion* 47 (1): 35–50.

Henkel, Heiko. 2005. "Between Belief and Unbelief Lies the Performance of Salāt: Meaning and Efficacy of a Muslim Ritual." *Journal of the Royal Anthropological Institute* 11 (3): 487–507.

Hirschkind, Charles. 2006. *The Ethical Soundscape: Cassette Sermons and Islamic Counterpublics*. New York: Columbia University Press.

Hirschon, Renée. 1989. *Heirs of the Greek Catastrophe: The Social Life of Asia Minor Refugees in Piraeus*. Oxford: Clarendon.

———. 2010. "Indigenous Persons and Imported Individuals: Changing Paradigms of Personal Identity in Contemporary Greece." In *Eastern Christians in Anthropological Perspective*, edited by Chris Hann and Hermann Goltz, 289–310. Berkeley: University of California Press.

Howe, Nicholas. 1993. "The Cultural Construction of Reading in Anglo-Saxon England." In *The Ethnography of Reading*, edited by Jonathan Boyarin, 58–79. Berkeley: University of California Press.

Hymes, Dell. 1981. *In Vain I Tried to Tell You: Essays in Native American Ethnopoetics*. Philadelphia: University of Pennsylvania Press.

Ignatii (Brianchaninov). 1998. *O molitve*. Moscow: Sestrichestvo vo imia Velikoi Kniagini Elizavety.

Kak molit'sia o samoubiitsakh? Kanon o samovol'ne zhivot svoi konchavshikh. 2009. Moscow: Neugasimaia lampada.

Keane, Webb. 1997. "Religious Language." *Annual Review of Anthropology* 26 (1): 47–71.

Kenworthy, Scott. 2010. *The Heart of Russia: Trinity-Sergius, Monasticism, and Society after 1825*. New York: Oxford University Press.

Kizenko, Nadieszda. 2000. *A Prodigal Saint: Father John of Kronstadt and the Russian People*. University Park: Penn State University Press.

———. 2012. "Sacramental Confession in Russia and Ukraine." In *State Secularism and Lived Religion in Soviet Russia and Ukraine*, edited by Catherine Wanner, 190–217. New York: Oxford University Press.

Kormina, Jeanne, and Sergei Shtyrkov. 2012. "St. Xenia as a Patron Saint of Female Social Suffering: An Essay in Anthropological Hagiography." In *New Moralities and Religions in Post-Soviet Russia*, edited by Jarrett Zigon, 168–90. New York: Berghahn.

Lar'kina, Ol'ga. 2012. *Kogda ty byla vo mne tochkoi, dochka: Rasskazy zhenshchin, sovershivshikh abort*. Riazan': Zerna.

Liudogovskii, Feodor, and Maksim Pliakin. 2013. "Zhanr akafista v XXI veke." In *Pravoslavnye russkie akafisty*, by A. V. Popov, 586–636. Moscow: Izdatel'stvo Moskovskoi Patriarkhii.

Luehrmann, Sonja. 2010. "A Dual Quarrel of Images on the Middle Volga: Icon Veneration in the Face of Protestant and Pagan Critique." In *Eastern Christians in Anthropological Perspective*, edited by Chris Hann and Hermann Goltz, 56–78. Berkeley: University of California Press.

———. 2016. "Iconographic Historicism: Being Contemporary and Orthodox at the Same Time." *Material Religion* 12 (2): 237–40.
———. 2017. "Innocence and Demographic Crisis: Transposing Post-abortion Syndrome into a Russian Orthodox Key." In *A Fragmented Landscape: Abortion Governance and Protest Logics in Postwar Europe*, edited by Silvia de Zordo, Joanna Mishtal, and Lorena Anton, 103–22. New York: Berghahn.
Luhrmann, Tanya. 2012. *When God Talks Back: Understanding the American Evangelical Relationship with God*. New York: Vintage.
Mahieu, Stéphanie. 2010. "Icons and/or Statues? The Greek Catholic Divine Liturgy in Hungary and Romania, between Renewal and Purification." In *Eastern Christians in Anthropological Perspective*, edited by Chris Hann and Hermann Goltz, 79–100. Berkeley: University of California Press.
Marshall, Ruth. 2009. *Political Spiritualities: The Pentecostal Revolution in Nigeria*. Chicago: University of Chicago Press.
Naumescu, Vlad. 2013. "Old Believers' Passion Play: The Meaning of Doubt in an Orthodox Ritualist Movement." In *Ethnographies of Doubt: Faith and Uncertainty in Contemporary Societies*, edited by Mathijs Pelkmans, 85–117. London: Tauris.
Ong, Walter J. 1982. *Orality and Literacy: The Technologizing of the Word*. London: Methuen.
Packert, Cynthia. 2010. *The Art of Loving Krishna: Ornamentation and Devotion*. Bloomington: Indiana University Press.
Popov, Aleksei Vasil'evich. (1903) 2013. *Pravoslavnye russkie akafisty*. Moscow: Izdatel'stvo Moskovskoi Patriarkhii.
Rogers, Douglas. 2009. *The Old Faith and the Russian Land: A Historical Ethnography of Ethics in the Urals*. Ithaca: Cornell University Press.
Seligman, Adam, Robert P. Weller, Michael Puett, and Bennett Simon. 2008. *Ritual and Its Consequences: An Essay on the Limits of Sincerity*. New York: Oxford University Press.
Shevzov, Vera. 2007. "Scripting the Gaze: Liturgy, Homilies, and the Kazan Icon of the Mother of God in Late Imperial Russia." In *Sacred Stories: Religion and Spirituality in Modern Russia*, edited by Mark Steinberg and Heather Coleman, 61–92. Bloomington: Indiana University Press.
Tomlinson, Matt. 2014. *Ritual Textuality: Pattern and Motion in Performance*. New York: Oxford University Press.
Toren, Christina. 2011. "The Stuff of Imagination: What We Can Learn from Fijian Children's Ideas about Their Lives as Adults." *Social Analysis* 55 (1): 23–47.
Urban, Greg. 2001. *Metaculture: How Culture Moves through the World*. Minneapolis: University of Minnesota Press.
Vansina, Jan. 1985. *Oral Tradition as History*. Madison: University of Wisconsin Press.
Veniamin (Milov). (1948) 2002. *Pastyrskoe bogoslovie s asketikoi*. Moscow: Izdatel'stvo Moskovskogo podvor'ia Sviato-Troitskoi Sergievoi Lavry.

PART II
WORLDS

5 INHABITING ORTHODOX RUSSIA: RELIGIOUS NOMADISM AND THE PUZZLE OF BELONGING

JEANNE KORMINA

According to a survey conducted in November 2013 by the Levada-Center (a Russian nongovernmental polling organization), while 68 percent of respondents across Russia identified themselves as religious and Orthodox, 62 percent of those Orthodox Christians claimed they had never taken communion.

There are many ways to interpret this data. Church representatives would criticize the majority, who are not churchgoers, for not being true Christians and for merely roaming *around* the church instead of being *in* the church. Some analysts suggest that Orthodoxy in Russia is understood by many as a sort of official state religion, which helps people identify themselves with the Russian nation or Russian ethnicity but which, in fact, no longer has anything to do with lived religion, as it does not provide people with potential opportunities to have religious experiences. However, as a social researcher I take this data as an intellectual challenge. Where, for example, are those who state that they are Orthodox Christians *and* believers? If we take their statement of belonging to the church seriously, we can formulate a research problem in the following way: How do these people understand the idea of belonging to a church, and, more important, how do they practice their belonging? Furthermore, if we believe that they are believers, we have a chance to learn more about the fabric of religious life of a mainstream Orthodox person whose religion is culturally dominant in a post-Soviet, postsecular, and postmodern setting.

How do the majority of Orthodox people who are not churchgoers live their religious lives, and what concepts and practices of belonging to religious communities do they develop? To which religious communities do they belong? This alternate regime of belonging is developing alongside traditional modes of religious life within the framework of local, and originally peasant, parish communities; I will call it the *nomadic* religious regime. Those who compose this majority prefer making pilgrimages to sacred sites or visiting urban Orthodox fairs (*iarmarki*)[1] to a regular religious life in their local parishes. Even those who do visit the church on a more or less regular basis tend to participate in nomadic practices too, either going on pilgrimages or venerating traveling holy objects such as the Belt of the Theotokos.[2]

Within the last two decades, many social researchers of religion use the "believing without belonging" dichotomy in their analyses of the forms taken by the secularization process. Sociologist Grace Davie introduced this dichotomy to scholarly debates and pointed to the divergence between an individual's faith and his or her participation in a particular ecclesial institution, either the Anglican Church in Great Britain (Davie, 1990, 1994) or the Catholic Church in Italy (Marchisio and Pisati, 1999). These scholars' arguments are based on results of quantitative surveys, a research technique that cannot grasp, and does not intend to, the meaning the informants ascribe to a particular aspect of their worldview. In the dialect of Orthodox Christians in Russia, the word *votserkovlenie* (literally "enchurching") means to become an Orthodox believer; there is no way to be a believer without belonging to the institution of the church, at least to some extent. However, there are many different ways to participate in the ecclesial institution and to articulate, in narratives and practices, that sense of belonging.

In my ethnography of belonging, I focus on the church's practices of *domesticating* those *religious nomads* who are roaming around the institution of the church rather than being within it. *Nomadic* concepts of inhabiting via travel and pilgrimage work as a way of building personal connections with both the land and the imagined "Orthodox nation." These concepts compete with the *parish* approach to inhabiting. The parish approach includes everyday routine efforts to build and maintain the local parish community in all its material practicalities, from restoration work and cleaning to singing in a church choir.[3] Regular investment of one's time is as highly appreciated as monetary donations, if not more. As a result of these efforts, mutual belonging develops between a person and the local church (and parish)—the believer belongs to the church and community just as they belong to him or her. The nomadic concept focuses on movement, leisure, entertainment, and adventure as a means of building a community of belief, whereas the parish concept stresses situatedness, work, responsibility, obedience, and community-building. What does their combination or interaction tell us about the way Orthodox communities are organized?

PILGRIMAGE AND MINIMAL RELIGION

Pilgrimage to a particular site "puts it on a map" (Christian 1981, 105)—that is, the site becomes visible and desirable for actual and potential travelers. By "map" I mean here an imagined and shared scheme that indicates significant places in a particular territory that everybody could and even should visit at least once. The importance and visibility of one of these places increase or decrease based on the activities of its promoters, as well as on the site's infrastructure and the potential of the place itself.

It is almost impossible to have a tour in any region or city of Russia without experiencing at least some light religious touches. Thus, in June 2014 my university organized a one-day trip for its administrative staff to the Konevetz Monastery, located on Konevetz Island in Ladoga Lake. The tour was operated by a secular tourist agency that advertises itself as one specializing in "intellectual travels." For the two hours of bus travel to the harbor, the guide told us a long history of the region in an absolutely secular way. However, when the highway ended and our bus started jolting over a rutted dirt road, she eagerly explained to us that anyone who approaches a sacred place such as the monastery is a kind of pilgrim, and every pilgrimage has a bit of suffering in it.

Nowadays, in fact, religious places seem to predominate as sites of interest in the domestic tourism market in Russia. This is not surprising, as churches and monasteries are in many cases the richest places culturally, from both aesthetic and historic standpoints. These characteristics make them "natural" points of interest, and their appearance on the maps of cultural travelers seems to be a logical consequence of post-Soviet and post-atheist developments, which are represented by a proliferation of religious markets with both "recycled" and brand-new cultural/religious constructions (Luehrmann 2005; Pelkmans 2009). Similarly, the territories that used to be blank spots on the map of cultural tourism during the Soviet era are now reclaiming their attractiveness with the help of religious symbols. Thus, the big industrial city of Ekaterinburg has recently become internationally known as the place where, in 1918, Bolsheviks murdered the last Russian emperor, Nicholas II, along with his family and servants. The Church on the Blood, built from 2000 to 2003 at the site of this tragic event, has become one of the most visited tourist destinations in the city.

The post-Soviet reinvention of religion has provided people with a new lens for looking at the cultural and historical landscape of the nation; this new perspective, alongside other developments, transforms this territory. Cultural heritage tourists typically do not participate in religious services or other pious practices, instead reserving for themselves the position of observers of "authentic" religious life when visiting monasteries and other religious places. Nonetheless, they claim, if asked, that they do belong to the Russian Orthodox Church, on a par with the more intentional pilgrims.

There are different kinds of explicitly religious pilgrimages in terms of, among other things, who organizes them, who participates, and how long a trip lasts.[4] Popular in contemporary Russia are weekend bus pilgrimages. Such a pilgrimage takes one to three days, starting Friday night and ending before Monday morning. Travelers, sometimes called *avtobusniki* (pilgrims who travel by bus; see Kormina 2010), can spend a night or two on a bus or sleep in a monastery's hostel. These trips are usually organized by local activists, who can be affiliated with a particular church parish or a diocesan office but as a rule don't have this kind of affiliation, or have it just nominally and operate independently. Literally anybody can organize such a trip. All they need do is rent a bus, decide about a sacred site or a set of sites they want to visit, and spread the word among potential participants.

In big cities, pilgrimage entrepreneurs advertise trips via their websites and announcements published in the Orthodox media and on leaflets distributed in churches, in church shops, and at Orthodox fairs, along with other places visited by potential clients. In smaller towns and villages this information is often spread via personal networks: an organizer invites his or her friends as well as participants of former trips, and these people are encouraged to invite friends and neighbors. In many cases, these kinds of activities are based in a local enterprise or state institution that employs enough people, women especially, to fill up a bus. In villages and small towns, centers of this sort can be located in hospitals; in bigger places, the initiative can spread from a library, museum, or academic institution where the pilgrimage activists work. In these cases, the pilgrimage trips continue the Soviet tradition of organized leisure time for workers, which trade unions used to be responsible for (regarding Soviet tourism, see Gorsuch 2011).

The organizers of these trips require, and search for, legitimacy, which may include using church announcement boards to advertise pilgrimages or having the pilgrimage blessed by a charismatic bishop or some other authorized person with religious charisma of either an institutional or noninstitutional kind (for example a *starets*, a kind of living saint; see more in Kormina 2013). Organizers can say in their advertisements and on their web pages that they have the blessing of the official representative of the church (a local bishop) for this particular pilgrimage or, if this is a long-term project, for their activities in the pilgrimage market in general. To give a blessing (*blagoslovenie*) means "to allow" and "to command" at the same time. In the Orthodox vocabulary, the concept of blessing is closely connected with the idea of strict obedience as a way of living a proper religious life, which may in turn lead to salvation (Dubokva, this volume). Ideally, the believer who receives a blessing for doing something has to carry out his or her plans even if the circumstances have changed and there is no sense in doing it anymore. Hence, to receive a blessing for doing something means to reduce both one's own participation in decision-making and responsibility for the results. On another level, in small towns and villages the organizers of pilgrimage trips tend to ask for a blessing from a local priest for every trip. This way they perform an act of responsibility for him and for the church he represents and at the same time, again, they make their pilgrimage initiatives more legitimate. Very few priests would refuse to give their blessing for these trips, as such a refusal could lead to conflict with religious activists, who might instead simply ask some other priest for this blessing-as-permission or go on the pilgrimage with no blessing at all.

The dominant ideology of pilgrimage in Russian religious life before its crucial transformations in the 1990s had been a reciprocal exchange between a believer and the sacred (see, for example, Green 2010). According to available ethnographic data, a typical reason for taking a pilgrimage to a local or more distant shrine, of regional or national significance, was a silent personal vow. A person promised to make this trip in gratitude for God's help for the pilgrim or for his or her close kin (especially children) to, for example, be healed from serious illness or survive a war. This agreement was kept in secret from everybody; neither church nor priest was involved in it. As I have written elsewhere (Kormina 2004, 29–30), this old practice of a personal agreement with God has apparently vanished from the modern version of Orthodox religious life.

Why then do people go on pilgrimages today? Is it simply a cheap variant of tourism and entertainment? Do they wish to consume culture and history in this way, just as many did during Soviet times when traveling to secular sacred sites? Or maybe they view the pilgrimage itself as a transformative practice and travel to new or restored holy sites in hopes of experiencing the *presence* of the sacred (see Engelke 2007; Orsi 2008; Meyer 2014)? According to observations made during my long-term fieldwork among Orthodox pilgrims throughout Russia, all these possibilities proved true. This chapter will focus on how experiencing the presence of the sacred can be not only a driving force for nomadic pilgrims but also a draw for domesticating them as parishioners.

It seems obvious that the religious life of any believer is built around his or her desire to feel the presence of the sacred. In other words, a minimum definition of religion could be formulated today as a personal but shared "experience of the presence of the sacred." Especially prominent in contemporary evangelical movements, this sensualistic shift in religious lives is also characteristic of Orthodox religious cultures. An essential feature of this experience is that it has to be shared with co-believers. In other words, while experience of the sacred, as with any personal body experience, is felt individually, it still needs to be proved by others who belong to the shared understanding as to which sites, people, and natural phenomena are of the same group, unstable as the borders of such a group may be. Similarly, the sacred is predicated on shared knowledge.

Obviously, the most reliable way to have this desired religious experience is as a parishioner within a local religious community, where believers can experience divine presence by participating in church rituals, in particular Holy Communion. The communal and nomadic regimes of religiosity vary in the ways in which believers localize the sacred, in how they legitimize it, and in how access to the sacred is organized. Within the communal, parish-based religious regime, the bureaucratic institution (a church) distributes and controls the sacred; this control is legitimized by means of appealing to tradition, in particular historical continuity, either real or imagined. The sacred in this case is embodied in holy objects, church rituals, and religious professionals, namely clergy. On the other hand, pilgrims localize religious charisma in holy material things, such as the grave of an elder or a stone imprinted with God's footprint, objects that, according to their imagination, can serve as a kind of container of charisma outside the church walls and without the blessing (and control) of religious professionals. Believers, in narratives about sacred objects and in the practice of dealing with these objects, insist that those objects have their own agency, entirely independent of human will. Thus can icons cry and bleed, stream myrrh and clean themselves of soot and stains (*obnovliat'sia*, literally "renew themselves").

The church tries to domesticate the uncontrolled sacred by establishing churches, chapels, or monasteries at those places where the divine revealed itself in some way; by so doing, the church brings the newly revealed "containers of charisma" within the church walls, just as it probably always has (see, for example, Shevzov 1999). In this way the church canonizes some folk saints, taking their bodies from the graveyards and into the monasteries, as recently happened to Matrona of Moscow. Canonized around the turn of the twenty-first century, she has been attracting many pilgrims to the Pokrovskii Monastery in

Moscow and has become a holy representative of the Russian Orthodox Church throughout the world. Although she did not bring people *into* the church, she manages to bring them closer to it, as those who come tend to venerate the icon but still not participate in a church service.

Paradoxically, this fixing of the sacred within a particular ecclesiastic framework helps to further develop the nomadic practice of religious trips. An important part of a typical pilgrimage program is a Divine Liturgy at the church located at or near the pilgrimage destination. Hence the weekend pilgrimage programs are timed to coincide with a Sunday liturgy. This does not necessarily mean that every pilgrim takes part in the Eucharist; according to my observations, many take the position of observers rather than participants and limit themselves to lighting candles in front of favorite icons and buying inexpensive books and icons in the church shop. Often a pilgrimage provides the opportunity for confession with an unknown priest whom the believer will never see again. For many people this is a welcome relief and can allow for a more sincere confession and, by extension, a more sincere experience of faith. Some pilgrims participate in the liturgy for the first time in their life, while other nonchurchgoers do so after a long period of not participating in the Eucharist. And for others a pilgrimage can become an enlightening or missionary project that gives them the opportunity to learn more and to experience their faith more deeply.

"INSTEAD OF GOING SOMEWHERE ELSE, GO TO YOUR OWN CHURCH!" DOMESTICATING RELIGIOUS NOMADS

Nadezhda, whom I met in the early 2010s during my fieldwork in the Sverdlovsk region of the Urals, is one of those post-Soviet Orthodox people whose religious conversion and later catechization was carried out during pilgrimage tours and other activities outside of the church. In the late Soviet period she worked as a director of the village house of culture and was elected as a deputy in the District Council of the People's Deputies. With these administrative resources, in the beginning of the 1990s she was enthusiastically involved in restoring her local church. She was proud that, due to her efforts, the church building in her village was the first in the district to be returned to the Orthodox Church. For Nadezhda, however, the restoration work was connected with the preservation of the collective cultural heritage rather than with her own religious search. In her sixties and a mother of four when I met her, she had begun occasionally visiting churches and sacred places in the mid-1990s. In her case, a program of pilgrimages included participation in the Eucharist at a particularly holy place, such as a monastery or a special church. Every Sunday morning, rather than going to her local village church she went instead to one of the churches of her choice, either as a participant of a bus pilgrimage or on her own, together with her husband who drove her there.

Her nomadic way of living Orthodoxy was interrupted by a new priest, Father Aleksii, at that time in his mid-thirties, who was appointed to her village church in the spring of 2012. Since his appointment, Father Aleksii started building a parish community in the village. Although the church had opened more than twenty years before his appointment, parish life was not well developed there, as previous priests were apathetic about pastoral work and had lived in Kamensk-Ural'skii, a district center an hour's drive from the village. Father Aleksii did not move to the village either, but he was very active in doing missionary and social work and started building a parish community there in order, as he explained to me, "to unite these people." Very soon he learned that a group of people in the village traveled to various sacred places, either together or separately, by joining pilgrimage trips organized by individual activists or agencies in the larger neighboring village, in the district center of Kamensk-Ural'skii, or in the city of Ekaterinburg. Nadezhda was one of those who often participated in these trips and sometimes organized them herself.

In his program of building the parish community, Father Aleksii made special efforts to restrict the religious mobility of his flock. He insisted that they needed to receive his blessing for these trips and advised (or ordered) people to go on pilgrimage no more than twice a year. "I know many people for whom it became a kind of a habit—they need to run somewhere," he said, "and they spend a lot of money there, they pay for church services, and so on. . . . This is not all to the good; there is a place, a house which is yours [the local church], and you have to support it." Father Aleksii criticized pilgrims for their economic behavior as they bought candles, services, and so on somewhere else instead of investing in their local church and community. His critique about roaming around to different churches and monasteries was not purely pragmatic, however, but also involved ethics and religion: "They [who travel too much] entertain demons, you know. They boost their vanity; they are looking for something that is simpler [to accept], or better, or holier. They go on pilgrimage to tell everybody that they did it, that they had a marvelous priest to whom they confessed as never before in their lives. They would say that the water in the spring there was different from the water in this local spring, that the holy bread there was sweeter, and so on and so forth." Father Aleksii also pointed to the staged authenticity (MacCannell 1973) at the sacred (or so-called sacred) places: "Within the day or two they spend in these monasteries they don't have a chance to see the real routine of these places; all they see there is an advertisement, and the show performed for them."

Father Aleksii's remarks, however, do not mean that he was skeptical about the sacred itself or about the possibility of approaching the sacred at pilgrimage sites. He was certain that a believer could lose consciousness when venerating a holy object such as a miracle-working icon, but he also thought that contact with very powerful containers of charisma should occur only occasionally. Pilgrimage, from his point of view, should be a rare feast rather than a routine of religious life. The everyday life of a believer should be concentrated on serving the local parish church.

Nadezhda accepted his arguments and stopped going on pilgrimages, at least for a while. Her decision, she explained, was the result of personal difficulties that were caused by her pilgrimages. When she organized these trips, she said, she did not know the thoughts or intentions of the people who joined the group, and as a result she suffered, as organizer and believer, from "the devil's attacks" (*vrag napadaet*) in the form of illness and problems at work and in personal relations. In other words, organizing a pilgrimage was itself a religious deed that had negative ramifications in terms of damage to her personal and family life. Father Aleksii gave her his blessing to carry an old icon through the village church instead of going on a pilgrimage. This localized form of pilgrimage could be considered a means of domesticating religious nomads.

The more experienced and sophisticated a believer, the more particular he or she becomes in building contacts with the sacred. A typical step in an Orthodox religious career is to decide to venerate a particular icon; this veneration provides the believer with constant communication with the sacred. Usually, this commitment to an icon arises as a result of a personal "abundant event,"[5] that is, when the sacred intervenes in the believer's world, in the form of a dream or apparition. It is important to remember that icons, according to believers, have agency and the ability to act and so, for example, can choose a particular believer as their special devotee. Thus, Nadezhda was chosen by the Tikhvin icon of the Mother of God.[6]

About ten years ago Nadezhda was driven by her husband to the nearby town of Kamensk-Ural'skii to receive communion there. She entered the church and began her usual religious routine of lighting candles and kissing icons when suddenly she was attacked by a woman who verbally assaulted her, shouting, "Why have you come to the church? You shouldn't be here" (*nechego tebe zdes' delat'*), and attempted to eject her from the church for no clear reason. "Have you touched the Tikhvin icon of the Mother of God?" asked a bystander, an elderly woman who turned out to be a kind of leader in that church. Nadezhda explained to her that she had simply venerated (*prikladyvalas'*) the icon. "How did you do this?" the woman asked. Nadezhda replied that she had kissed the icon, touched it with her forehead, and lit a candle before it, just as she usually did with holy icons. She behaved properly, she explained, and did not touch it with her hands or anything like that. The woman explained that the angry parishioner had been behaving unconventionally in the church lately, but Nadezhda later interpreted her attack as a sign from God.

That night Nadezhda saw this same icon in a dream. It was beautiful and as big as a church. Nadezhda heard a voice, which she later interpreted as an angel's voice. The voice said: "Pray to this icon. Venerate [*prikladyvaisia*] it. Carry this icon [wear a small replica of this icon around your neck, together with a neck cross], and it will help you in all your needs." "And what do you think?" she continued, when we were having tea in the churchyard with some other parishioners one sunny day in July. Recently, Father Aleksii had given her his blessing to carry the old, heavy Tikhvin icon of the Mother of God around their church on a daily basis.

In her story of her profound relationship with a particular icon, Nadezhda tried to explain that it was the icon itself, or the divine powers behind it, that chose Nadezhda for this special relationship. This divine wish was transmitted via the hostile woman in the church. As the elderly woman hinted, the angry parishioner had recently been behaving as if she were possessed by demons (see Worobec 2001; Panchenko and Shtyrkov 2001). According to widespread opinion, demons reveal themselves in the presence of holy things by speaking in nonhuman voices and by causing the individuals they possess to commit blasphemy and sacrilege. In Nadezhda's story, this occurred when the supposedly possessed woman informed her, in a perverse way, that this particular icon was destined for her. Or, in other words, Nadezhda's personal religious deed and her way to salvation became the dedicated veneration of this icon. The second sign came to her in a compelling dream. She identified the voice she heard as the voice of an angel from God. These two voices came from the unseen world, and she was attuned to hear them and to understand the messages they transmitted (Engelhardt, this volume).

In the Orthodox religious tradition, in Russia and elsewhere, icons used to miraculously appear to claim particular sites as special. There are plenty of stories of this sort, including within the biography of the above-mentioned

Theotokos of Tikhvin. According to legend, an icon appeared hovering over a lake in the town of Tikhvin in the late fourteenth century. The people who encountered these holy objects in dreams or visions became the icons' mediators, who addressed the local community. An icon could, via these mediators, insist on building a new chapel for itself in a village of its choice, or it could reveal itself in a dream and ask to be discovered where it had been forgotten in a monastery attic (see, for example, Shevzov 1999). A visionary would report a dream to a local community and its authorities, who, after establishing special veneration of this icon, would benefit from its holy protection as well as from the stream of pilgrims it would attract.

In Nadezhda's case, on the contrary, an icon came to her in order to establish an intimate personal connection with her alone. The icon in her dream did not have a message for the community, her fellow villagers, or her fellow believers. Rather, the icon provided Nadezhda with the feeling of belonging to the Orthodox Church as an imagined community of believers. She could wear a small replica of this icon on her necklace alongside her cross and pray to it at home or celebrate it on this icon's feast day. She could carry it with her wherever she went. As a matter of fact, her "contract" with the icon did not necessarily include her hard work venerating an old Theotokos of Tikhvin icon in her local village church. She added this part due to her local priest's advice.

Since then, Nadezhda has taken her daily pilgrimage around her village church. Each day at noon she goes to the church, takes the heavy old Theotokos of Tikhvin icon from where it hangs on the wall, and circles around the church 150 times. The initiative to do precisely 150 circles a day came to her mind after her pilgrimage with a group from Ekaterinburg to the famous convent of the Holy Trinity in Diveevo. When carrying the icon, she prayed the Orthodox version of Hail Mary, "Theotokos and Virgin, Rejoice," one prayer per round, just as the Diveevo people had taught her and the other pilgrims to do when following the Mother of God path (the Holy Canal) around the convent.

"I feel the same, the same grace [*blagodat'*] and sense [*oshchushchenie*], when carrying the icon around the church 150 times, as if I've been doing the Holy Canal path," Nadezhda confessed, when we were sipping tea in the churchyard. In her everyday devotional rounds she imitates the practice every pilgrim does at the holy Diveevo convent. To help the pilgrims to experience the presence of the sacred, the nuns and staff of Diveevo support an etiological narrative of the "Diveevo obedience." As the legend goes, one day Saint Seraphim of Sarov, who served as a spiritual guide for the convent,[7] saw the Mother of God walking around the boundaries of the monastery. He understood that this vision had been given not only as a sign of her protection but also to indicate that the very path she walked would be a blessing for those who followed in her steps, praying. In 1830 Saint Seraphim asked Diveevo's nuns to dig the Holy Canal, which would surround the elected place chosen by the Mother of God for the building of the convent. Advertising materials for pilgrims recall Saint Seraphim's saying that "he who walks along the Holy Canal praying 'O Theotokos the Virgin, Rejoice. . .' 150 times, for him this place will be Athos, Jerusalem, and Kiev."[8]

This place is advertised among the Orthodox people as the Fourth Appanage ("allotted portion") of the Mother of God on Earth, a place where one has special opportunity to feel her presence. There is no need to make long pilgrimages to the very holy places of Athos or Kyiv[9] to fully experience this presence; it can be experienced as the result of proper efforts, through physical suffering and multiple repetition of the same short prayer. In this older mode of domestication on a national level, pilgrimage is more about work than adventure.

In Nadezhda's twenty-first-century parish, the imitation of a particular body practice of veneration developed in Diveevo provided her with the experience of direct contact with the sacred by doing 150 devotional circles with a heavy icon in her hands. The same prayer and the same bodily practice (walking) made this imitation meaningful for Nadezhda and helped her to locate her devotional activities at her parish church. What began as religious nomadism became embedded in a local context and, thus, domesticated, at least for a while.

Obviously, Nadezhda's religious career is not typical for the majority of religious seekers who identify as Orthodox but keep their distance from regular church life. Instead of *roaming* around the church chaotically as *avtobusniki* do, she is following her own trajectory, led by her personal religious calling. However, the difference between her and other religious seekers is not so crucial; Nadezhda, a kind of religious virtuosa, is probably more attuned than the majority, but nonetheless all of them play in the same key. All manner of contemporary Orthodox believers search for personal and direct contact with the divine and demonstrate a readiness for self-development, centering on cultivating religious bodies and disciplining the senses.

ATTUNING THE RELIGIOUS BODY: DISCIPLINING THE SENSES

For an average, minimalistic Orthodox believer, religious competence to a great extent is measured by mastering the technologies of dealing with sacred things. These are material items that, according to shared knowledge, contain a kind of divine or supernatural *presence* (in Russian the term *blagodat'*, literally meaning "grace," refers to this presence). Communication with these things provides the believer with an opportunity to have a personal religious experience, as well as to have a kind of communion with other believers who share the same ideas and narratives about the "abundant events" that provide or confirm the divine presence. Bodily techniques of venerating sacred objects are acquired by newcomers to the church before they learn any prayer texts. Thus mothers bring their toddlers to the church or other sacred places to kiss holy icons or a cross or to bathe in a holy spring. Together with the habit of crossing oneself and some knowledge of how to pray, this habit of venerating holy objects constitutes the obligatory minimum religious repertoire of an Orthodox person.

The introduction of a newcomer to Orthodox Christian practice starts with the training of his or her senses. The scent of church incense, the light from the candles, the sounds of singing and praying, and the taste of holy bread and wine create the somber atmosphere of the place of faith. Yet, the tactile element of Orthodox sacred practice is even more prominent, as it does more than contribute to the atmosphere of the religious space: it provides direct and personal communication between a believer and the sacred (Engelke 2007). In other words, at the pilgrimage destinations, pilgrims may not experience the smells or acoustics of a church, but they would nevertheless have access to the sacred through the contagious effects of the material objects. Contagion (if you touch something sacred, the sacred comes to you and into you) gains its power because the prayers are materialized in an object or place and thus endure over distance and without the intervention of a priest.

One of the very first things every newcomer is taught is how to venerate holy icons properly, *prikladyvat'sia*. This word is used only in religious language and means "to have bodily contact with a holy thing in an act of veneration," especially an icon or relics. In practice this specifically means to kiss a sacred object, such as an icon, a box with holy relics, or a holy cross. An Orthodox manner of greeting a priest includes the kissing of his hand. Thus one can conclude that following these Orthodox protocols helps people to learn about the location of grace in the church and to behave accordingly. Moreover, acquiring this bodily practice introduces believers into a specific sensual regime of Orthodox Christianity and helps them to train their senses to be more attuned to the whole religious atmosphere the church provides.

The ritual of kissing a sacred item creates a special kind of relationship between a believer and a material object. This ritual makes people and objects comparable but unequal members of the same religious network. This kissing is simultaneously both intimate and public. Public notices posted in the church about appropriate behavior often include a prohibition against lipstick, in order to keep the icons clean. These hygienic precautions, however, predictably ignore the fact that many people kiss the same holy image or object; this practice, together with the ritual of distributing Holy Communion with the same spoon for the entire congregation, was one of the common science-based criticisms against the church by the Soviets. This literal and physical co-participation in church rituals creates a strong feeling in a believer of being a member of the same collective body, attested to by the senses.[10]

Acquiring the religious body techniques and bodily discipline is an important part of the process of becoming a churchgoer (see Naumescu, this volume). Learning this body language, together with the social dialect of Orthodox believers, is a crucial part of the process of "catechization," or rather self-education in the church. In the narratives of believers, the process of adjusting to church life is often represented as hard work, a kind of physical training, when one learns new and difficult bodily practices. The Russian Orthodox Church is especially strict in its demands about the appearance of believers, particularly in terms of requiring humble, feminine attire for women. In most churches in Russia, women are prohibited from wearing trousers, skirts must be long, and the head must be covered with a headscarf. In some other Orthodox countries, such as Greece, the dress code is less strict, if articulated at all. But in Russia, nearly every church has the dress code posted at the entrance, along with a box containing headscarves and long skirts for visitors to borrow. As modern women rarely use such garments in their everyday life, they must acquire particular body techniques to wear this female Orthodox uniform.

Most believers take the church dress code for granted, and although some find it inconvenient, they accept it as a part of the "tradition" that they embody through this fashion. How they are dressed helps strengthen their sense of belonging to the Orthodox religious community. Although in conversations the women hardly mentioned their specific struggle with skirts and scarves, their stories of becoming Orthodox were nonetheless cast in terms of disciplining their bodies. In particular, they usually stressed how difficult it was, when they had just begun their church life, to stand for the entirety of the long church service (*vystoiat' sluzhbu*). Usually, there is no seating in Orthodox churches, so parishioners must stand for one to several hours, with very minimal movement.

Conversion narratives typically mention the first time a believer manages to stand up till the end of the church service. Nadezhda told this kind of story about her husband:

He stayed [in the church] and told me: "I don't want to stay in the church any more. I feel hot coals under my feet. Let's go home." I said: "No, no, we have to stand through the whole service. . . . Let's say the prayer to the Mother of God [Hail Mary] and Our Father." At that time, they were the only two prayers I knew; I know more now, thank God. . . . We started praying and managed to stand to the end. When we went back home, he was in a sweat, and all his body was wet, so that he had to change all his clothes. He went to have a nap, while I was cooking. And he saw an angel in a dream, two angels, the white and the black. They were fighting; eventually the white hit the black and turned him into dark water. He came to him [to the husband], embraced him, and said: "I will be with you forever." From that time on, we have been standing during the church services up to the end.

To stand in the church until the end of the service is itself a religious deed, as it involves physical suffering and purifying.

For Nadezhda, and likely for her husband too, standing in the church until the end of the service is a disciplinary practice that serves to create the body of a good Orthodox believer. Through physical suffering a believer goes through his or her long conversion (*votserkovlenie*), and after the conversion is complete, the suffering ends. Once a believer has the body of a true Orthodox Christian, he or she would no longer have problems standing during a long church service.

However, Father Aleksii explains it a bit differently:

Yes, this is hard to stand, even for me if I am present at the service as a parishioner. In June, I visited the relics of Saint Aleksii of Moscow [his personal patron saint] at Epiphany Cathedral in Elokhovo [in Moscow]. Really, it was hard to stay through the service. And when is it easier? When you understand what is going on, when you can follow the church service. It is easier when you yourself, inside of you, with all your mind, participate. You are there, not here. And you just forget about your legs. But if you stay mindless, if you neither see, nor hear or understand, then everything draws your attention from the service easily—in a word, if you are not in, you feel it so hard.

Interestingly, both Father Aleksii's intellectualist approach to full conversion (understand and participate) and Nadezhda's sensualist approach take the believer's body and senses as indications of how attuned one is to the service.

While prayer can help the neophyte gain endurance, the proper behavior of a believer in church, at holy sites, and in private life is also a prerequisite for strong (*sil'naia*) prayer. According to Nadezhda, there are very few "people of prayer" (*molitvenniki*) in Russia, because to be this kind of person one has to start going to church in childhood. In theory, one can become a *molitvennik* at a later stage of life if one practices the Jesus Prayer (see the chapter by Pop in this volume). Yet, to gain this higher stage of spiritual life, first of all one has to "work on oneself" hard (*nad soboi rabotat'*), starting with strict observation of fasts, including not only seasonal fasts (of which there are four on the Orthodox calendar) but also weekly fast days, Wednesdays and Fridays. This is a higher stage in developing the religious self, which can be obtained only through further work in attuning the religious body.

CONCLUSION

The domestication of religious nomads is a very difficult task for the Russian Orthodox Church. The church advocates for a premodern conception of belonging, rooted in a parish-based organization of society; such a concept helps create a narrative of the continuity of religious tradition with the pre-Soviet peasant past but is hardly acceptable as a mode of life for the majority of contemporary believers. Their understanding of how to be correctly Orthodox is framed by a pattern of religious life that is self-centered rather than community-centered. In this pattern, religious identity is loosely connected, if at all, with local identity; after all, the icon that chooses you has no registration in a particular place and is present everywhere, including in every copy, from newspapers to museums, in old images as well as new.

However, the continuity argument is still quite strong and successful. It is shared by nearly everyone who goes through deep Orthodox conversion, or enchurching, which is a painful process of learning the body language of the Orthodox tradition through participating in long church services and in church processions or pilgrimages. This suffering, in tandem with this kind of nonintellectual knowledge, combines to create the religious self. In disciplining their enchurched bodies and senses, believers acquire religion as tradition, precious in its continuity. Yet, while mastering the physical elements of religious culture, believers develop their own strategies of approaching and consuming the sacred. They acquire specific rhythms and styles of communication with the sacred, within the framework of existing broad conventions.

Nomadic religiosity does not require any local legitimization; by definition, it is not rooted in the local religious tradition, materiality, and social structure. Indeed, does local religion exist in contemporary Russia as it existed in the prerevolutionary past or in premodern segments of society (such as the peasantry) of this and other countries (Christian 1981)? Probably not. Likewise, strong parish identity is problematic. While not impossible, it is exceptional. For a mainstream religious person, regular participation in parish life is an ideal but not really acceptable in practice. Most such people prefer to enjoy "proper" parish life in the mode of interactive performance, reserving for themselves the role of perceptive observer rather than active participant, even if they have enough bodily knowledge to fully participate.

Training the religious body and developing a religious self are part of the process of inhabiting the religious world. Contemporary believers are constantly engaged in creative searching—for a better parish to attend, a more powerful spiritual father to confess to, a more sacred holy site to visit, and a stronger prayer to recite. The Russian population's general lack of trust in institutions, including the church, allows this seeking tendency to proliferate. As a result, churches, monasteries, and other sacred sites become mere stations in the personal journey of a believer. These stations have unique religious acoustics, where the sounds of prayer can become louder. In many cases these acoustics amplify the presence of the sacred due to elaborate religious aesthetics, both visual and aural. The aesthetics of the major holy sites attract various kinds of visitors, especially pilgrims like Nadezhda, who come from churches with no choir and few or only newly made icons.

The bishop removed Father Aleksii from his parish soon after we met. After that, Nadezhda quit her pilgrimage around the church in favor of distant religious travel. At the same time, she joined a small circle of religious activists in the parish to serve there as a reader. She comes to the church every day to read, according to the church calendar, an akathistos to a saint and goes on a pilgrimage with her Orthodox friends from other parishes only once or twice a year, just as Father Aleksii had strongly recommended.

JEANNE KORMINA is Professor of Social Anthropology and Religious Studies at the Higher School of Economics, Saint Petersburg. She is author of *Sending Off Army Recruits in Post-Reform Russia: An Ethnographic Analysis* and coeditor of *Dreams of the Mother of God* and *The Invention of Religion in Post-Soviet Space*.

NOTES

1. The Orthodox fairs in Russia have become a very visible phenomenon within the last decade or so. They simultaneously follow the patterns of industry fairs and officially organized local community feasts. Sellers at these fairs include parishes, monasteries, or enterprises (publishing houses, icon workshops, etc.).

2. In the fall of 2011, a piece of the Cincture (the Holy Belt) of the Theotokos was brought to Russia from the Vatopedi Monastery on Mount Athos to allow Russian Orthodox pilgrims to revere it in different cities. It attracted hundreds of thousands, including representatives of the state. A piece of the same holy object kept permanently in St. Petersburg's Kazan Cathedral, on the other hand, hardly draws the attention of believers at all. The advertisement of the holy item as an object of pilgrimage coming from the especially holy place of Athos greatly enhanced its attraction.

3. Needless to say, these mundane routines are understood as religious deeds. To do the volunteer work for the church, one has to get a blessing from a priest or an invitation from the divine—from the Holy Trinity, for instance, as happened to Nadezhda:

> It was just before the Feast of the Holy Trinity, [and] I was back home from the hospital after I gave birth to a child. I had a flare-up of kidney stones, and while lying in bed, I heard a voice. It said: "Go to the church to clean it up for the feast." I asked my neighbor, a girl, to help me get to the church, and I took a bucket and a mop and went to the church. I was saying a prayer all the time on my way and while I was cleaning. How could I manage it without a prayer? And suddenly I felt a push—this was the kidney stone passing—and I felt such relief. I said my thanks to God and came back home.

4. For a survey of scholarship in the field of pilgrimage, see Badone 2014; in the field of Russian Orthodox pilgrimage, see Rock 2015.

5. Robert Orsi (2007) suggests the useful concept of the abundant event. Orsi writes that such events have five characteristics: (1) they present themselves as sui generis: people experience these events as singular, even if they are recognizable within cultural conventions; (2) they are real to those who experience them; (3) they arise at the intersection of the conscious and the unconscious; (4) they arise at the intersection of past/present/future, and at the moment of such an event one has a new experience of the past while at the same time the horizon of the future is also fundamentally altered; (5) they are intersubjective (and this intersubjectivity may include, for instance, the dead or saints).

6. The Tikhvin Mother of God, or Theotokos of Tikhvin, is traditionally one of the most venerated icons in Russia. It was said to have miraculously fled Byzantium before the arrival of the Ottomans, taking up residence in the Russian north and reportedly saving the town of Tikhvin from Swedish invaders in the seventeenth century (Kaiser 2011, 129). In 1941 the icon was taken by the German troops from Tikhvin Assumption Monastery, where it had been kept since the fourteenth century. In 2004 it was returned to Tikhvin, in a solemn event organized with strong support from the secular state authorities; the event provided the icon with a great deal of inadvertent advertising. Due to folk etymologization of its name (*tikhii* means shy, calm, still), in the folk religious tradition the icon used to purportedly be an effective means of calming a crying baby or a person with a mental disorder or of stopping a fire.

7. Saint Seraphim of Sarov is now one of the most venerated saints in the Russian Orthodox Church. He was canonized in 1903 with enthusiastic support by Emperor Nicholas II in his "efforts to find a usable national myth" and "to resacralize the authocracy" (Green 2010, 75; Freeze 1996).

8. See http://eparhia.karelia.ru/diveevo.htm, last accessed October 30, 2016.

9. According to Orthodox tradition, the Theotokos has four "allotted portions" or territories under her special holy protection. The first (chronologically) is Iveria (Geor-

gia), the second is Mount Athos, the third is Kyievo-Pechers'k Lavra in Kyiv (Kiev), and the last is Diveevo.

10. In regard to secular questions of hygiene during communion, a typical response has been given by the famous Orthodox theologian and publicist Andrei Kuraev: "I am a deacon. After all parishioners have taken Communion, I have to drink all that is left in the Chalice. Then, I have to wash the Chalice, and even this water I cannot pour out—I have to drink it. From the hygienic point of view, all infections of my parishioners are mine. But I have to assure you that in 15 years of service I have never had an infectious disease" (Kuraev 2006).

REFERENCES

Badone, Ellen. 2014. "Conventional and Unconventional Pilgrimages: Conceptualizing Sacred Travel in the Twenty-First Century." In *Redefining Pilgrimage: New Perspectives on Historical and Contemporary Pilgrimages*, edited by Anton M. Pazos, 7–31. Farnham, UK: Ashgate.

Christian, William A., Jr. 1981. *Local Religion in Sixteenth-Century Spain*. Princeton: Princeton University Press.

Davie, Grace. 1990. "Believing without Belonging: Is This the Future of Religion in Britain?" *Social Compass* 37 (4): 455–69.

———. 1994. *Religion in Britain since 1945: Believing without Belonging*. Oxford: Blackwell.

Engelke, Mathew. 2007. *A Problem of Presence: Beyond Scripture in an African Church*. Berkeley: University of California Press.

Freeze, Gregory L. 1996. "Subversive Piety: Religion and the Political Crisis in Late Imperial Russia." *Journal of Modern History* 68 (2): 316–23.

Gorsuch, Anne E. 2011. *All This Is Your World: Soviet Tourism at Home and Abroad after Stalin*. Oxford: Oxford University Press.

Green, Robert H. 2010. *Bodies Like Bright Stars: Saints and Relics in Orthodox Russia*. DeKalb: Northern Illinois University Press.

Kaiser, Daniel H. 2011. "Icons and Private Devotion among Eighteenth-Century Moscow Townsfolk." *Journal of Social History* 45 (1): 125–47.

Kormina, Jeanne. 2004. "Pilgrims, Priest and Local Religion in Contemporary Russia: Contested Religious Discourses." *Folklore* 28:25–40.

———. 2010. "Avtobusniki: Russian Orthodox Pilgrims' Longing for Authenticity." In *Eastern Christians in Anthropological Perspective*, edited by Chris Hann and Hermann Goltz, 267–86. Berkeley: University of California Press.

———. 2013. "Russian Saint under Construction: Portraits and Icons of Starets Nikolay." *Archives de sciences sociales des religions* 162:55–74.

Kuraev, Andrei. 2006. *Tserkov' v mire liudei* [The church in the people's world]. Moscow: Sretenskii Monastyr'.

Luehrmann, Sonja. 2005. "Recycling Cultural Construction: Desecularisation in Postsoviet Mari El." *Religion, State and Society* 33 (1): 35–56.

Marchisio, Robert, and Maurizio Pisati. 1999. "Belonging without Believing: Catholics in Contemporary Italy." *Journal of Modern Italian Studies* 4 (2): 236–55.

Meyer, Birgit. 2014. "Mediation and the Genesis of Presence," with a response and comments by Hans Belting, Pamela Klassen, Chris Pinney, and Monigue Scheer. *Religion and Society: Advances in Research* 5:205–54.

MacCannell, Dean. 1973. "Staged Authenticity: Arrangements of Social Space in Tourist Settings." *American Journal of Sociology* 79 (3): 589–603.

Orsi, Robert. 2007. "When 2 + 2 = 5." *American Scholar*, March 1.

———. 2008. "Abundant History: Marian Apparitions as Alternative Modernity." *Historically Speaking* 9 (7): 12–16.

Panchenko, Alexander, and Sergey Shtyrkov. 2001. "Chuzhoi golos: Iz materialov o russkom klikushestve." *Kanun* 6:316–36.

Pelkmans, Mathijs. 2009. "Introduction: Post-Soviet Space and the Unexpected Turns of Religious Life." In *Conversion after Socialism: Disruptions, Modernisms, and the Technologies of Faith*, edited by M. Pelkmans, 1–16. New York: Berghahn.

Rock, Stella. 2015. "Touching the Holy: Orthodox Christian Pilgrimage within Russia." In *International Perspectives on Pilgrimage Studies: Itineraries, Gaps and Obstacles*, edited by J. Eade and D. Albera, 47–68. London: Routledge.

Shevzov, Vera. 1999. "Icons, Laity, and Authority in the Russian Orthodox Church, 1861–1917." *Russian Review* 58:26–48.

Worobec, Christine. 2001. *Possessed: Women, Witches, and Demons in Imperial Russia*. DeKalb: Northern Illinois University Press.

BARAKA: MIXING MUSLIMS, CHRISTIANS, AND JEWS

ANGIE HEO

ACROSS THE ARAB MEDITERRANEAN WORLD, Muslims, Christians, and Jews have long shared a terrain of prophets, wonder-workers, and holy intercessors. Every December, Jews and Muslims celebrate the festival of the Moroccan rabbi Abu Hasira in the Nile delta city of Damanhur. When Christians and Muslims convene every August in the Delta village of Mit Damsis, it is Saint George the Martyr to whom they make their appeals for exorcisms and healings.

These special saints, dead or living, are known to carry baraka, an Arabic term common across traditions that registers a family of concepts in English: blessing, holiness, charisma, divine power, potent force. To take baraka from the saints who left their holy traces in Egypt, pilgrims travel to the places where their bodies once were. Baraka is treated like an interpersonal substance, not unlike the Melanesian magic of *mana*, which has inspired many classic anthropological theories of religion (Firth 1940; Hocart 1914; Mauss [1902] 1972; compare Mazzarella 2017). Fluid and tactile, baraka is conveyed via media like water, oil, dust, air, electricity. Wellsprings and caves where the Virgin Mary and Christ child stopped to rest from their flight from Israel offer sites for accessing the physical remains of their presence.

In the city of Musturud on Cairo's gritty industrial perimeter, the feast of the Virgin attracts thousands of Muslims and Christians to the ancient well of "sweet water" and the underground grotto where the Holy Family drank and slept. Wound around the church like a fluid ribbon, queues of people waiting inside guardrails, men on one side and women on the other, inch up to take baraka. At the well, teenage volunteers fill and tie up plastic bags with holy water from the spring's spigots. Tossing the handheld bags into the sweaty queues, they help speed up the pilgrimage process so that the conduits of blessing keep moving.

On these summer evenings beyond the church's grotto and well, the streets are packed with food stalls, tattoo stations, souvenir shops, and even an enormous Ferris wheel with blinking lights. This is the familiar scene of a *moulid*, a Muslim term that refers to the birthday celebrations of prophets and saints. In recent history, *moulids* and their "perils of joy" (Schielke 2012) have raised concern among clerics and reformists as venues for immoral entertainment, like belly dancing or magic tricks. For the police, street festivals are a potential site for public disturbance and disorder. The idea that latent sectarian tensions might erupt at any moment looms large in the backdrop. But Musturud's festival of the Virgin is different from other saintly celebrations—when Jews are in their synagogues, Christians in their churches, and Muslims in their mosques.

Mixing Muslims and Christians together, the Virgin's festival in Musturud spills over into the open streets. Perhaps this excessive quality is also part of baraka's design. With its promise to extend the holy saint's presence, baraka moves across religious borders and boundaries as an offering for even the unbelieving to be touched.

REFERENCES

Firth, Raymond. 1940. "The Analysis of Mana: An Empirical Approach." *Journal of the Polynesian Society* 49:483–510.
Hocart, A. M. 1914. "Mana." *Man* 14:97–101.
Mazzarella, William. 2017. *The Mana of Mass Society*. Chicago: University of Chicago Press.
Mauss, Marcel. (1902) 1972. *A General Theory of Magic*. Translated by Robert Brain. London: Routledge.
Schielke, Samuli. 2012. *The Perils of Joy: Contesting Mulid Festivals in Contemporary Egypt*. New York: Syracuse University Press.

6 SHARING SPACE

On the Publicity of Prayer, between an Ethiopian Village and the Rest of the World

TOM BOYLSTON

THE ZEGE PENINSULA, where I have conducted fieldwork since 2008, was Christianized in the fourteenth century by the itinerant Saint Betre Maryam—some nine centuries after the conversion of King Ezana of the Axumite Empire by Syrian missionaries. The peninsula is majority Orthodox with an established Muslim minority living in the market village of Afaf. The demographic division across Ethiopia is more even: roughly 44 percent Orthodox Christian, 34 percent Muslim, and 19 percent Protestant, according to the 2007 census. But it is Orthodox Christianity that has dominated religious narratives of Ethiopia, largely because of its close association with the Ethiopian imperial state and with the northern highland areas where that state first emerged.

This Orthodox dominance and its association with the Amhara and Tigrayan ethnic groups is now being challenged on various fronts, and religious equality has been enshrined in the constitution since the early 1990s (Haustein and Østebø 2013; Samson 2015). This follows from the disestablishment of the Orthodox Church under the socialist Derg regime (1974–91)—a move that was met with a revival of grassroots devotional practice among Orthodox Christians and a general and public reaffirmation of kinds of Orthodox belonging that had once been taken for granted (Clapham 1988; Bonacci 2000).

The Ethiopian Orthodox Tewahedo Church is one of the non-Chalcedonian or "Oriental" Orthodox churches. These churches, including the Coptic and Armenian, split from the greater church for mainly Christological reasons that have come to be associated with the doctrine of Monophysitism: that Christ was of one nature, both divine and human, rather than two natures in one (note that both sides agreed that Christ was fully divine and fully human and that the dispute centered over the question of "natures" or *phýsis*; Ayala 1981). Monophysitism has become a derogatory (and orientalist) term designating the Oriental churches as somehow uncivilized or at least unsophisticated, and "Miaphysitism" is now preferred, though it has much the same semantic meaning. But I have been told privately by some theologically engaged Christians in Addis Ababa that the Christological differences among Chalcedonian Orthodox, non-Chalcedonian, and even Roman Catholic churches are relatively insignificant.

Ethiopian Orthodox Christianity has developed a quite distinctive set of traditions and practices, among which the high emphasis on fasting and the use of consecrated *tabots* in churches, derived from Hebraic tradition and representing the biblical ark of the covenant, are often noted (Ephraim 2013, 50; Antohin 2014). The twentieth century has seen developments in the use of vernacular language for parts of the liturgy—for example, the Gospels tend to be read in contemporary Amharic or other languages in common use, while the Eucharistic *anaphora* and other chants remain in classical Ge'ez (Aymro and Motovu 1970). There have also been important contacts between the Ethiopian Orthodox Church and the Caribbean, starting from the Ethiopianist movements of the early twentieth century and resulting in the establishment of churches in Jamaica, Trinidad, and Guyana, as well as in the UK and United States (Brahana 2000). This chapter takes up the question of how developments in media technology played into the religious politics of the post-imperial era in one particular part of the traditional (but not exclusive) heartlands of Ethiopian Orthodoxy.

PUBLIC PRAYER

For Orthodox Christians in Zege, prayer, in the narrow sense (*s'elot*), is largely a matter for specialists. Priests perform prayers for the liturgy, for funerals, and for baptisms, each requiring specialized training. The prayers are often in Ge'ez, the classical language that predates vernacular Amharic, and are prescribed for each occasion (an improvisational, free-form mode of prayer-poetry, *k'iné*, exists, but this is even more specialized than other prayer skills). The idea of an individual on hands and knees, praying to God or Mary in his or her own home, is not unknown, but it just isn't something people do or talk about all that much. After all, that's what priests are there for. When a person prays in the churchyard during a service by prostrating himself or herself on the ground, this is referred to as *sigdet*, "obeisance" or "surrender." It is the bodily show of deference, rather than the uttering of words, that is highlighted.[1] The result is that prayer is largely a public matter, and communication with God is achieved not through individual speech acts but through public networks of petition and deference, all the more so now that prayers surrounding the liturgy are broadcast over electric loudspeakers.

This is not to say that the laity are disengaged from religious practice, only that prayer in the narrow sense is only part of a diffuse range of religious activities that Orthodox Christians practice in conjunction with priests, saints, and each other. Most prominent of these is fasting (Ephraim 1995; Boylston 2013). All Orthodox Christians in Zege avoid meat on Wednesdays and Fridays and during Lent and Advent, while many, including clergy, keep much stricter regimes. For more specific religious petitions, the usual form is a vow (*silet*) made to a saint; if one's request is granted, the petitioner will hold a memorial feast (*zikkir*) on the saint's annual day, thus including his or her neighbors in the exchange (Boylston 2013). The use of holy water—usually blessed by priests' prayers—is another extremely common way by which people can engage with divine power in material form (Hermann, forthcoming).

It seems incorrect to separate spoken prayer from these broader practices that articulate with it. Spoken prayer (in institutionally specified forms) is essential for the practice of the holy sacraments, but at the broader social level it is not a privileged form of religious engagement. "Prayer," broadly construed, is intersubjective and embodied through collective and individual fasting, through public gestures of collective submission, and through hearing the prayers of the priests. These practices alike constitute worshipful, communicative forms of engagement with the divine, and there is no clear empirical reason to separate linguistic forms of prayer from these others. At the very least, we should not assume an a priori distinction.

The public, shared quality of prayer (broad sense) is intrinsically related to the importance of the medium of prayer—bodies, food, loudspeakers—because the medium is what allows the prayer to be shared.[2] This sharing does not just link a person to God but also draws others into the relationship in more or less active roles. But this public and broadly mediated nature of prayer also turns prayer into a political concern (Hirschkind and Larkin 2008). The first half of this chapter traces the development of Christian-Muslim relations in the past seven years in Zege through changes in the way these believers occupy space through a combination of architecture and media technology. The second part investigates how media technology changes the relationships between person, prayer, and public and private space among Christians themselves. In each case, I will argue, developments in media seriously alter both the experience of space and the ways in which social and political relations across that space can be formed through prayer, understood as a public and social endeavor. But these changes are not entirely determined by technological developments. Rather, I argue, a distinctively Orthodox focus on the importance of the public medium shapes the ways in which people take up the new possibilities that technology offers.

CHRISTIANS AND MUSLIMS (IN LOCAL, NATIONAL, AND DIGITAL SPACE)

The Zege Peninsula, about ten miles by boat from the regional capital Bahir Dar, is known for its monasteries, the first of which was founded in the fourteenth century. The peninsula itself is almost entirely Orthodox Christian, but the small market town that abuts it, Afaf, has a well-established Muslim minority. The pattern of Christians inhabiting the countryside and Muslims mainly living in towns conforms to a broad normative association of Christians with farming and Muslims with trade. But the dominant narrative of the area has long been as an Orthodox heartland, a land of monasteries, whose Muslim population was depicted as largely incidental.

In this aspect, Zege mirrors the prevalent narrative of Ethiopia as an Orthodox Christian nation. The key symbols of this narrative are familiar: the rock-hewn churches of Lalibela; the myth of Prester John, the lost medieval Christian king in the East; the references to Ethiopia in the Psalms and in Acts. But this story is largely one of the Ethiopian state, not of the entirety of its peoples (Clapham 2002; Triulzi 2002). And since Orthodox Christianity was disestablished as a state religion with the fall of Haile Selassie in 1974, the narrative has become increasingly difficult to sustain. Religions are now constitutionally equal, Protestantism is gaining rapid ground in Orthodox homelands, and Ethiopia's large and long-established Muslim population is mounting renewed claims to public recognition (Haustein and Østebø 2013; Abbink 2011, 2014; Samson 2015).

While relations between Orthodoxy and Islam are in a moment of increasing tension, there is also a well-established and much-touted tradition of mutual tolerance and cooperation. In Afaf, as in much of Ethiopia, Christians and Muslims do not share meat (some have told me, significantly, that this is because different prayers are said during the slaughter). However, they will always make sure to serve some non-meat dishes at feasts so as to be able to host their neighbors. Personal relations among Christians and Muslims in town have generally been cordial and cooperative, accompanied by mutual recognition of the meat separation as proper on both sides.

In 2008, when I began fieldwork, there were occasional signs of unacknowledged tension. Most surrounded the small mosque that lay in the center of town. It had a powerful loudspeaker and would broadcast the call to prayer at a volume that would often wake the whole town in the small hours of the night. I would occasionally hear Christian friends complain of tiredness, but there was never any open acknowledgment of a problem: ethics of neighborly respect for religious activity, combined with an aversion to provoking conflict, meant that nobody wished to speak out. Most actively denied that anything was wrong. That this was not entirely true became clear when, about a year into my fieldwork, somebody stole the mosque's amplifier.

The traditional rural-urban divide between Christians and Muslims is significant here. At this time there were seven churches in Zege to one small mosque, and most had amplifiers of their own. But all were situated outside of town, as is usual, to maintain proper separation between worldly and sacred space. For those living in town, the churches just weren't very loud, if they could be heard at all. Nonetheless, aside from the theft of the amplifier, things were peaceful when I left the field in 2009.

Village religious politics would become much more fraught over the next few years until my most recent visit in December 2014. The most obvious flashpoint was the reconstruction of the mosque, from a nondescript mud house to a vast painted concrete structure with a minaret tower that dwarfs any other building in the area. In a town of one-story houses of mud and straw with corrugated iron roofs, the new mosque stands out.

From a Muslim perspective, this was an assertion of legitimate and longstanding presence; many had clearly felt unrecognized and unrepresented for some time. The mosque was one of many similar construction projects across the country, as Ethiopian Muslims are seeking to assert their equal status in the federal era. It was not clear to locals where the money had come from, but many suspected that donations were coming from the Middle East as well as from Ethiopian Muslim associations. Chatting to Christians, on the other hand, I heard two sorts of responses. In public they once again downplayed any kind of tension, saying that there was "no problem." But privately I heard complaints that the construction was inappropriate in a place of such historic Christian importance and that local officials had been bribed.

At the same time, local Christian organizations moved to counter the mosque construction and so reestablish their claims to primacy on the peninsula. Raising money from their own national connections, they built two new churches in the peninsula: Medhane Alem, in the forest near Afaf, and Rufael, near the northern shore of the peninsula on the site of a previous church that had been dismantled during the Italian occupation in the 1930s, its stones used to make a military camp whose remains are still visible. Neither of these churches has anything like the visual presence of the mosque. They are low, single-story buildings situated in the forest, not like the much larger and more elaborate structures now found in towns. This is in line with established practice: churches have not traditionally been built to dominate space; they are supposed to be sheltered, in line with their traditional role as monastic refuges and places of separation from the world. The monasteries of Zege are known for their murals, the treasures they house, their histories, and the power of their holy water, not for their architectural majesty. By comparison, Orthodox churches in cities have become much more visually imposing in the last century, and in the last two years the facade of Saint George's church in Bahir Dar has been renovated to include a vast and eye-catching bas-relief of George and the dragon. These developments seem to derive initially from the influence of European architectural styles and lately in the need to produce structures that match the Islamic occupation of space (Boylston 2014).

The new churches in Zege do more than compete for visual presence. For one thing, they emphasize the Christian argument that the peninsula is Orthodox: there are now nine churches rather than seven to the one mosque. But perhaps more important, the Orthodox demonstrated that they could call on their own support networks in the form of Christian associations (*mahber*) that are backing church construction across the country. These associations promote church building but also provide funds for the training of church students (future priests and religious scholars) in an age of great concern that their numbers are diminishing. So Zege now hosts a number of boys who are entering church training, with new robes and books to work with and some support for food. Building the churches includes making investments in the future of the church as a whole and so combats perceived threats to Orthodoxy's preeminence.

The most significant change in the experience of religious relations in Zege between 2008 and 2015 has been the heightened awareness that the local churches and mosque are intimately tied to a highly politicized struggle of national and international proportions. Both the mosque regeneration and the new churches were realized by calling upon large-scale support networks, whose financial backing had direct and tangible effects in Afaf town and on the peninsula. The presence of the new buildings, and the political wrangles that surround them, gives evidence of the broader interests behind them. The churches and the mosque are understood to stand for something much bigger that lies just out of sight: on one axis, God, but on another the great organizational networks of those who share the faith. People feel these developments acutely because they entail massive transformations in the experience of sensory space, due to both the visual and tangible presence of religious buildings and the greatly enhanced sonic range of the apparatus of prayer.

Another key development that has changed local Christian and Muslim conceptions of their interrelationships has been the spread of polemical discourse through public media (Abbink 2011). As Samson Bezabeh (2015) shows, sermons from both Christian and Muslim speakers, which circulate on CDs and video, draw heavily on international discourses of religious conflict, invoking a clash of global forces of Christianity, Islam, and secular modernity. These circulations may not reflect the subtler realities of coexistence and cooperation on the ground, but they are powerful enough to gain a reality of their own and begin to produce the conflict they describe. It seems at the moment that the speedy development of media technology for circulating religious material has intensified a sense of conflict rather than cooperation.

The rapid growth of Facebook use among young people in Zege has provided a striking instance of this phenomenon, particularly potent because of the way that Facebook allows users to share images and slogans at the press of a button. In 2008 nobody in Zege had a Facebook profile (or much use for the internet at all); by 2010 I had a couple dozen "friends" from Zege, and the number has continued to grow. When I returned to the field, I happened to ask my research assistant about a mutual friend, Mulat. My assistant told me that they didn't really talk any more—Mulat had moved to Bahir Dar, and now "he only posts about Islam." I did not remember Mulat having discussed Islam much at all when I had known him, but through Facebook there was suddenly a steady stream of prayers, exhortations, and macros (images with text edited in) that he could simply "share" and so declare his agreement with them. This meant the possibility of developing a new kind of public identity, and one that some of his Christian friends found irksome—although they were doing much the same thing with the sharing of Christian images and slogans, and perhaps more so. Most of Mulat's posts were fairly innocuous statements like "I am a Sufi and I love my prophet," written on a football shirt, or a picture of the Qur'an that said "We love Al-Quran," along with pictures of cute children dressed in Muslim garb and performing prostrations.

The most recent and shocking example of Christian outrage at the time of writing has been the response to the Islamic State releasing a video purporting to show the beheading and shooting of some thirty Ethiopian Orthodox Christians in Libya (widely reported April 19 and 20, 2015). Images from the video, some extremely graphic, have been shared by many of my Zege friends on Facebook (which, of course, is exactly the purpose of releasing such videos) alongside expressions of outrage and prayers for the victims (for example, "To die in the name of the cross is an honor" and "They will know my faith by the cross around my neck," each accompanied with a gruesome picture of a beheaded man). My friends now feel personally, viscerally affected by world political events in a way that was not evident before and galvanized to affirm their Christian loyalty, though they often do so not in their own words but in those provided along with the images that are circulating. In another example of a polarizing event that could never have happened in the pre-Facebook era, one of my friends shared a photoshopped image of a giant Caucasian woman defecating on the Mecca Kaaba. It is hard to think of a more inflammatory gesture, but I do not think the person who shared the image harbors any significant anti-Islamic feelings beyond a certain reactionary Facebook tribalism. He would certainly never show such an image to anybody face to face or make any other similarly outrageous statement. But on Facebook it was easy, something you could click on as a joke and end up causing extreme anger, which of course it did. An on-screen shouting match predictably broke out, though I do not know of any further ramifications.

A number of things are happening here. First, Facebook blurs lines between what is public and what is among friends and even changes what it means to say something publicly, resulting in statements that one would never make face to face. Second, the ability to circulate posts made by others makes it much easier to repeat a discourse originating elsewhere. This means both that users feel connected into a much wider debate—they know that the things they post come from a wider group of people who share some interest—and that they may publicly make statements that they would not in other circumstances have even formulated.

The online response to the Libya killings did not just take the form of Christian-Muslim opposition, however. Many of the image macros and statements that people were sharing appealed instead to a common national identity, contrasting the Ethiopian tradition of interreligious cooperation with the foreign organization of extremist Islam. Some people responded to all of these events simply with prayers and petitions to Mary to protect the country (see also Dulin 2016).

Add to this the public connections that Facebook enables with those outside the country. Selam, a woman in her early twenties who has been working as a maid in Saudi Arabia for the last two years, posts a steady stream of macros containing either prayers or laments about missing Ethiopia. In the week of the Libya and South Africa killings, she posted even more prayers, some in very topical forms. In one example, a photo of a man being burned in front of South African police officers is superimposed with an Amharic prayer that reads:

> My heart bleeds
> And my eyes cry
> When my brother burns
> While the police laugh.
> To whom shall I say it?
> Who will hear me?
> Best if I talk to
> Omnipotent God:
> Creator, please
> Say enough of
> My brothers' blood
> And my sisters' tears.
> Please, if not by our faults
> Then by your mercy
> Guide us, Amen.[3]

Selam had shared this from another friend, and forty people have commented beneath at the time of writing, most simply saying "Amen amen amen" or adding macros with further prayers and images.

The combination of righteous anger, mutual support, and public prayer (along with a fair amount of spurious gossip) that met the Libyan and South African episodes epitomizes much of the circulation of image macros on Facebook among young people in Zege. It is not all anger and conflict; pictures of icons and prayer slogans are equally easy to share, and quite popular. We can think of these as existing in a tradition of public prayer—short, stylized declarations of fidelity, just in newly mediated form. And while nobody would mistake a digitally shared photo of a picture of Mary for a spiritually empowered icon, that is no reason for such photos not to act as personal reminders and public indicators of deference and allegiance.

The growth of Facebook and the construction of the Afaf mosque happened at around the same time. For people in Zege, especially the young, these two factors combined to produce a vastly increased sense of being part of translocal religious-political factions. This developing sense has clear material foundations: the building of the mosque and churches, but also the networks of money that funded them and the improving internet infrastructure that allowed people from Zege to access the internet, first in the regional capital nearby and then from their phones in Zege. This does not mean that developing media technology always increases factional conflict. It does show, however, that changes in the media of public prayer have significant effects on how people experience their religious allegiances, connections, and claims to shared space. Public prayer, I have argued, has always involved a division of labor and the formation of public allegiances under the divine aegis through shared media of prayer. And while these changes in the mediation of prayer, whether through buildings, loudspeakers, or the internet, are enabling rapid transformations in the fabric of that allegiance, they are doing so within a recognizably Orthodox idiom.

MEDIA AND THE EXPERIENCE OF SPACE

The circulation of Facebook prayers gave an indication of new possibilities afforded by media technologies and the consciousness of new kinds of connection that they may provide. But Facebook emerged at a time when mass media technologies had already begun to have significant effects on the contours of religious practice in Zege, since electricity came to Afaf town a decade ago. We have already seen an indication of this in the theft of the mosque's amplifier, and I now turn my attention to the broader ramifications of the electrified religious soundscape, produced by loudspeakers but also by radio and, especially, the circulation of recorded preaching and religious music on CD and Video CD. In particular, we will see how these technologies are leading to a refiguring of the religious experience of space.

Loudspeakers have been used to broadcast the call to prayer in the Muslim world since at least the 1950s and have been regarded with ambivalence and controversy, by Muslims and non-Muslims alike, for just as long (Khan 2011; Weiner 2013). In Ethiopia, churches and mosques now use loudspeakers as a matter of course. While debates within Islam revolved around the propriety of mediating the voice in prayer and so stripping it of its sacred status (Khan 2011, 576), Orthodox Christians have been concerned about the projection of the sacred liturgy beyond the walls of the church, where it is heard by Christians who have not fasted and are not in the proper reflective state. One theologian in Addis Ababa told me that, while he saw the value of loudspeakers in the city, he was concerned about the consequences of hearing the holy liturgy while sitting outside the church, perhaps in a café, not having fasted, perhaps while quarrelling. The projection of the liturgy over distance was causing problems for him precisely because the grounds of church services are supposed to be restricted, attended only by those in proper bodily and affective states.

However, if the liturgy is closely restricted, Ethiopian Orthodox Christians have always found other means of prayerful engagement when unable to attend church. Classic examples include taking holy water and fasting, but media technology is opening up new avenues for making nonchurch spaces religiously vibrant. This is especially important for junior women, who are often kept from going to church by housekeeping duties, and especially true of the servant women who work in Afaf's bars, most of whom hail from poorer and more rural areas than Zege.

One of the more significant restrictions on serving women, as they see it, is their inability to attend church on anything like a regular basis. One classic way for servants to engage with their religion is to fast, and they can arrange with their soul fathers (*yenefs abbat*) to observe extra fasts in lieu of going to church. Extra fasting is also a common recourse for women who are kept from going to church by health or purity issues (Hannig 2013). What media make possible is for servant women, via recorded hymns, to make their spaces of work into temporary religious zones.

The availability of Amharic hymns in digital formats adds a whole new dimension to domestic religious life, especially in the bars. It allows serving women, and others, too, to use their employers' stereo systems to play religious music from the moment they wake and start work until the first customers arrive. These spaces recall the "Christocentric everyday" described by Jeffers Engelhardt (this volume), although usually focused on Mary or the saints rather than on Christ. The place of business becomes a devotional space—though once business starts and people are drinking and eating, this is no longer appropriate. I once heard a friend's wife scold him for singing religious songs while eating; the logic of separation of religious activity from feasting and drinking extends beyond the church walls.

The vernacular Amharic hymns are of recent, post-1991 composition but use only traditional instruments. However, unlike the traditional classical Ge'ez hymns of the church, they are often performed by women (Shelemay 2012) and are in a language everyone can understand. They are slow, devotional songs of reflection and penitence, particularly suitable for the morning, before one has breakfasted or done other worldly things. The slow, irregular drumbeat and sparse traditional instrumentation set the hymns clearly apart from any other kind of music. This is not music you can dance to, although the singers in the accompanying video perform a slow swaying of upturned hands—video versions of the songs are as easily available as audio, copied and distributed by vendors near churches in Bahir Dar.

It is not just servants and not just women who listen to hymns in the morning. Anyone with the requisite technology can do so, but it is especially important for the servants given the restrictions on their movement and the nature of the space they inhabit. As they cook the day's food and clean the premises, they can assert a form of control over their surroundings and develop their devotional lives in ways that would not otherwise be possible. When I ask women why they listen to the hymns, they almost always answer quite simply that it makes them happy to do so.

If fasting has always enabled people to engage in devotion no matter where they were—in the space of their bodies, as it were—recorded hymns allow for the creation of new kinds of devotional spaces in homes and places of business, which for servants are the same thing. They also enable new partitions of time, in which each day starts in a religious mode until breakfast is eaten, and this time is clearly differentiated from the rest of the day and its worldly affairs. Since hymns are usually played loud enough to be audible beyond the building's walls, these listening practices begin to shape the shared soundscape of the town, especially in the early mornings. In cities, it has become common to hear hymns played in cafés during the day (an action under the control of the waitresses), especially during fasting times, further pushing devotional sound into the public, shared sphere.

There are other ways of bringing religiosity into the home, many based around print. While icons do not have quite the same prominence as in other Orthodox traditions, and most icons are to be found inside the church, many people at least hang a religious picture or two on their walls. The most common are an image of Gabriel saving the three boys from the fires of Nebuchadnezzar and printed posters from Greece or Russia of Christ or of the Virgin and child that many people hang across corners of the house (where demons are known to hide), perhaps shrouded with a lacy veil. (While icons exist in Ethiopian Orthodox practice, their use is not so common among laypeople as in other Orthodox traditions.) These domestic images are not consecrated and so are not technically icons, but I do know of cases of them being used for personal prayer. Prayer books are also becoming more common, available cheaply from the same vendors who sell the recorded hymns. Especially in cities, large parts of the congregation may now be found reading in the churchyard during the liturgy. But prayer books also facilitate prayer in the home. In Afaf, too, a man called Temesgen told me about how he liked to start each day reading a section of the Widasé Maryam, the Praises of Mary, before breakfast. With printed posters and books as with audio recordings, mass reproduction allows people to bring a certain Orthodox sensibility into the home, at least as a way to begin the day, which is important for those whose work lives make churchgoing difficult.

The significance of aural media and religious soundscapes for creating spaces of ethical formation and deliberation has been widely discussed (Hirschkind 2006; Schulz 2008; Oosterbahn 2008; Engelhardt, this volume). Part of this is due to transportability of media technologies, which "move practices and experiences related to the aural perception of spiritual presence into new arenas of daily life, beyond the immediate sphere of ritual action to which these aural forms of spiritual experience used to be restricted" (Schulz 2008, 175). But just as much has to do with the capacity of sound to cross boundaries in ways that more solid modes of mediation do not (although large buildings may have similar effects, to the extent that they dominate lines of sight, as in the case of the Afaf mosque).

A soundscape, as Martijn Oosterbahn (2008) shows, is a shared living space inhabited by multiple overlapping noise sources. Sound is integral to creating ethically charged environments, but, because of its quality of being shared whether we like it or not, a soundscape always has political and territorial dimensions at the same time.

THE AUTHORITY QUESTION

So what of the prayers of priests? If Facebook and recorded hymns open up new sites for religious engagement, will these new channels circumvent and undercut established religious authority, as Dale Eickelman and Jon Anderson (2003) argue? It seems that the reverse is true: increased engagement by Orthodox Christians in the public sphere entails a reaffirmation of the importance of the priesthood and the institutional church. The reasons for this have much to do with Ethiopian Orthodox and Muslim "theologies of mediation" (Eisenlohr 2012) and received notions of the public nature of prayer.

For one thing, the new importance of church construction and the use of loudspeakers serve to amplify, quite literally, the voice of priests. The emphasis, evident all over Ethiopia, on larger and more numerous churches and mosques indicates a reaffirmation of the importance of traditional authority, bolstered by technologies of amplification and with enhanced projection over soundscapes and sightlines. We can also look to where ordinary people are putting their money. Both the evidence from Zege and my interviews with Orthodox donors in Addis Ababa show a clear emphasis on two fronts: building and rehabilitating churches and providing for the upkeep of church schools and trainee priests. Orthodox activists regard the continuation of the specialist priesthood as integral to the survival of the religion. The two newly built churches in Zege serve another purpose, beyond reestablishing a territorial claim: they are bases for church students, funded by the same revenue streams that built the churches. Architectural renovation goes along with the renewal of the specialist priesthood.

Images that circulate on Facebook, as well as many of the recorded sermons that have recently become popular, may stray far beyond the authorized doctrine of the Orthodox Church. There are still widespread debates about whether the new Amharic hymns are appropriate or whether they constitute deviations from tradition. To this extent, media enable diversions from centrally controlled Orthodoxy. However, Orthodox Christians are expressly and actively returning to the authority of the church and the priests as the public instantiation of Orthodox belonging. The apparent paradox, of increasingly heterodox ideas combined with increasingly vocal loyalty to Orthodox institutions, tells us that there is more at stake here than doctrinal questions of content. Prayer is public, and its media of instantiation, the allegiances it forms, and the institutional basis of its authority are all widely recognized as being integral to the action of communicating properly with God.

In the recent anthropology of religion and media, there is an overwhelming focus on the production of authority through claims to immediacy, in which factions compete to show that they possess the most direct and uninhibited channel to God (Eisenlohr 2011). Of course, the argument goes, these communications are always mediated, but the winners of the debate are those who can most successfully render their religious media invisible.

This is manifestly not what is happening in Zege, and in Orthodox Ethiopia generally. On the contrary, there is a general recognition that the media of religious communication are foundational and even required—hence the proliferation of ever-more imposing churches, the use of loudspeakers, the circulation of images, and especially the reaffirmation of the importance of priests. Orthodox Christians are affirming not unmediated contact with divinity but the properly public, and hence shared, political nature of prayer. After all, one of the key characteristics of a medium is that multiple people can see, hear, and interact with it at once.

These observations should make us hesitate to adopt too enthusiastically a "media constructivism" or determinism (Eisenlohr 2011) that would assume that advances in media technology are unilaterally driving religious and political change. Clearly, people are bringing to the party their own ideas and ideologies of what constitutes proper mediation. Media bring new affordances and new kinds of consciousness, but their usage is conditioned by preexisting values (which may nonetheless be constantly updated). And as Engelhardt (this volume) shows, new media for Orthodox Christians enter a "rich, reflexive discourse on the nature of religious mediation" that has long paid attention to the relations between bodies, senses, and the material techniques of communication.

We should also note that, to the extent that media technologies contribute to politicized interreligious conflict, or at least to discomfort, it is usually not just in the circulation of images but in the affective ways that media articulate with the occupation of lived space through churches, mosques, and loudspeakers. Equally, the effects of media are contingent on the material infrastructures and financial networks that underpin them (Boyer 2012; Larkin 2013). In the case of the new churches and mosque, these constructions may be taken as indexical evidence of the political-religious networks and interests that underlie them.

In his survey of approaches to religion and media, Patrick Eisenlohr (2012) advocates those frameworks that regard religion as always already mediated. There is a case for saying that Ethiopian Orthodox Christians have always known this. A corollary of this insight, as I hope to have shown, is the conviction that prayer is at heart a shared, public endeavor that translates effectively between local and long-distance materialities. Tales of the efficacy of prayer almost always possess the public dimension: a priest in Addis Ababa telling me how the prayers of the church brought victory to Ethiopia over Italian invaders at the 1896 Battle of Adwa, for example, or local ideas in Zege that the prayers of priests enact an ongoing covenant with God to protect the local environment and make sure that the rains fall.

The polemicization of Ethiopian religious discourse that some observers have described is real enough, and certainly exacerbated by the speed and visceral quality of digital media. But it is important to note how frequently the flashpoints that result in prayerful declarations of Orthodox, Islamic, or Ethiopian identity involve migrants. The victims of the Islamic State were reported to be on their way to Europe and the migrants in South Africa killed for traveling to seek work. Those sharing images and money are also frequently those who have gone abroad and are reaffirming old connections and new identities of memory. The more global consciousness of people in Zege is not just a result of media technology coming to them but of people from Zege going out into the world. That prayer is one of the primary idioms for thinking through these long-distance connections and memories makes sense when we think of the material scales at which public prayer operates: a combination of local materializations and long-distance connections that allow for shared participation among Christians, and then the notion, always there in the background, that God is witness to these prayers wherever they take place.

The interface between religion and politics exists in the spatial and material mediations of religious practice (Hirschkind and Larkin 2008). What is interesting about prayer is its dual audience: other people (local and long-distance) and God (in this case, often via saintly and angelic intermediaries). The divine audience can hear and see prayer wherever it emerges, but communication with the human audience is limited and defined by spatial mediations and the material limits of the available media. And without these media, it would be much more difficult for humans to imagine or engage with divinity in anything but the most extreme mystical sense (Debray 1991). So prayer integrates two axes of communication: geographical and (for want of a better term) spiritual. The spatial, material mediations that make God imaginable for humans, and allow them to understand God as responsive and engaged, are very frequently the same ones that allow us to imagine community. The mass mediation of prayer forces people to imagine anew the relationship between their territorial and their religious commitments.

TOM BOYLSTON is Lecturer in Social Anthropology at the University of Edinburgh.

NOTES

1. In Addis Ababa and other cities, the use of prayer books has become much more common, either for private prayer at home or for reading, silently or out loud, during church services.

2. We might note, with Webb Keane (1997, 2007), that speech itself is a material medium that enables sharing. But Keane's point is exactly that speech is a medium that gives the impression of immediacy, of being both "less material" and more intimate and private, than other forms.

3. Translation by author.

REFERENCES

(Ethiopian authors are listed by first name.)

Abbink, Jon. 2011. "Religion in Public Spaces: Emerging Muslim-Christian Polemics in Ethiopia." *African Affairs* 110 (439): 253–74.

———. 2014. "Religious Freedom and the Political Order: The Ethiopian 'Secular State' and the Containment of Muslim Identity Politics." *Journal of Eastern African Studies* 8 (3): 346–65.

Antohin, Alexandra. 2014. "Expressions of Sacred Promise: Ritual and Devotion in Ethiopian Orthodox Praxis." PhD diss., University College London.

Ayala Takla-Haymanot, Abba. 1981. *The Ethiopian Church and Its Christological Doctrine*. Addis Ababa: Graphic Printers.

Aymro Wondmagegnu and Joachim Motovu. 1970. *The Ethiopian Orthodox Church*. Addis Ababa: Ethiopian Orthodox Mission.

Bonacci, Giulia. 2000. *The Ethiopian Orthodox Church and the State, 1974–1991: Analysis of an Ambiguous Religious Policy*. London: Centre of Ethiopian Studies.

Boyer, Dominic. 2012. "From Media Anthropology to the Anthropology of Mediation." In *The SAGE Handbook of Social Anthropology*, edited by Richard Fardon et al., 383–92. London: SAGE.

Boylston, Tom. 2013. "Food, Life, and Material Religion in Ethiopian Orthodox Christianity." In *A Companion to the Anthropology of Religion*. edited by Michael Lambek and Janice Boddy, 257–73. Hoboken, NJ: Wiley-Blackwell.

———. 2014. "What Kind of Territory? On Public Religion and Space in Ethiopia." *The Immanent Frame*, August 26. http://blogs.ssrc.org/tif/2014/08/26/what-kind-of-territory-on-public-religion-and-space-in-ethiopia/.

Brahana Selassie. 2000. *Towards a Fuller Vision: My Life and the Ethiopian Orthodox Church*. London: Minerva Press.

Clapham, Christopher. 1988. *Transformation and Continuity in Revolutionary Ethiopia*. Cambridge: Cambridge University Press, 1988.

———. 2002. "Rewriting Ethiopian History." *Annales d'Éthiopie* 18 (18): 37–54.

Debray, Régis. 1991. *Cours de médiologie générale*. Paris: Gallimard.

Dulin, John. 2016. "Intelligible Tolerance, Ambiguous Tensions, Antagonistic Revelations: Patterns of Muslim-Christian Coexistence in Orthodox Christian Majority Ethiopia." PhD diss., University of California, San Diego.

Eickelman, Dale F., and Jon W. Anderson. 2003. *New Media in the Muslim World: The Emerging Public Sphere*. 2nd ed. Bloomington: Indiana University Press.

Eisenlohr, Patrick. 2011. "The Anthropology of Media and the Question of Ethnic and Religious Pluralism." *Social Anthropology* 19 (1): 40–55.

———. 2012. "Media and Religious Diversity." *Annual Review of Anthropology* 41:37–55.

Ephraim Isaac. 1995. "The Significance of Food in Hebraic-African Thought and the Role of Fasting in the Ethiopian Church." In *Asceticism*, edited by Vincent L. Wimbush and Richard Valantasis, 329–42. Oxford: Oxford University Press.

———. 2013. *The Ethiopian Orthodox Täwahïdo Church*. Trenton, NJ: Red Sea Press.

Hannig, Anita. 2013. "The Pure and the Pious: Corporeality, Flow, and Transgression in Ethiopian Orthodox Christianity." *Journal of Religion in Africa* 43 (3): 297–328.

Haustein, Jörg, and Terje Østebø. 2013. "EPRDF's Revolutionary Democracy and Religious Plurality: Islam and Christianity in Post-Derg Ethiopia." In *Reconfiguring*

Ethiopia: The Politics of Authoritarian Reform, edited by Jon Abbink and Tobias Hagmann, 159–76. London: Routledge.

Hermann, Yodit-Judith. Forthcoming. "Sida et religion en Ethiopie: Socio-anthropologie des formes de lutte contre le Sida." PhD diss., University of Aix-Marseille.

Hirschkind, Charles. 2006. *The Ethical Soundscape: Cassette Sermons and Islamic Counterpublics*. New York: Columbia University Press.

Hirschkind, Charles, and Brian Larkin. 2008. "Introduction: Media and the Political Forms of Religion." *Social Text* 26 (3): 1–9.

Keane, Webb. 1997. *Signs of Recognition: Powers and Hazards of Representation in an Indonesian Society*. Berkeley: University of California Press.

———. 2007. *Christian Moderns: Freedom and Fetish in the Mission Encounter*. Berkeley: University of California Press.

Khan, Naveeda. 2011. "The Acoustics of Muslim Striving: Loudspeaker Use in Ritual Practice in Pakistan." *Comparative Studies in Society and History* 53 (3): 571–94.

Larkin, Brian. 2013. "The Politics and Poetics of Infrastructure." *Annual Review of Anthropology* 42:327–43.

Oosterbahn, Martijn. 2008. "Spiritual Attunement: Pentecostal Radio and the Soundscape of a Favela in Rio de Janeiro." *Social Text* 26 (3): 123–45.

Samson Bezabeh. 2015. "Living across Digital Landscapes: Muslims, Orthodox Christians, and an Indian Guru in Ethiopia." In *New Media and Religious Transformations in Africa*, edited by Rosalind I. J. Hackett and Benjamin F. Soares, 266–83. Bloomington: Indiana University Press.

Schulz, Dorothea E. 2008. "Soundscape." In *Key Words in Religion, Media and Culture*, edited by David Morgan, 172–86. New York: Routledge.

Shelemay, Kay Kaufman. 2012. "Rethinking the Urban Community: (Re)mapping Musical Processes and Places." *Urban People* 14 (2): 207–26.

Triulzi, Alessandro. 2002. "Battling with the Past: New Frameworks for Ethiopian Historiography." In *Remapping Ethiopia: Socialism and After*, edited by Wendy James, Donald L. Donham, Eisei Kurimoto, and Alessandro Triulzi, 276–88. Athens: Ohio University Press; Addis Ababa: Addis Ababa University Press,.

Weiner, Isaac. 2013. *Religion Out Loud: Religious Sound, Public Space, and American Pluralism*. New York: NYU Press.

PRAYERS FOR CARS, WEDDINGS, AND WELL-BEING: ORTHODOX PRAYERS EN ROUTE IN SYRIA

ANDREAS BANDAK

Tony talks on his cell phone as I come walking westward on Straight Street in Damascus on a hot August day in 2009.[1] We shake hands while he ends his conversation, which revolves around renting an apartment for a month from late August into September. Tony and his fiancée, Hanan, are getting married later this month and are in the midst of all sorts of preparations. We exchange kisses and Tony says, "There is so much to do here before the wedding. I am so busy!" and goes on to show me his brand-new car: a Subaru Legacy, white and shiny, 2.5 injection, I am told.

He smiles as we get in the car. Tony turns on the AC, and a quite different experience can be enjoyed with the coolness of just twenty-one degrees centigrade, a rather stark contrast to the forty degrees outside. Soon after, we drive through the eastern gate of the old city, Bab Sharqi, and toward the predominantly Christian parts of Damascus, al-Qassaʿ, and al-Qusour to do some errands.

The car interior has several markers of Tony's Christian identity as Greek Orthodox. From the central mirror hangs a large crucifix, a wooden one about ten centimeters tall. On the panel in the front of the car, a prayer card with the Virgin Mary occupies a central location. And a pearl armband adorned with a cross, this one made of metal, is attached to the ignition keys. Around his wrist, Tony has a white woolen thread, a typical Christian marker of either a blessing received or a vow made in the famous monastery of Our Lady in Saydnaya.

"So what do you think of Syria?" he asks as we pass the wall surrounding Bab Touma. I respond that things seem to change, that there are some political openings. "Do you think that? I think the opposite," he continues. "I think things are tighter now. People are more radical. I mean not just here but in the whole of the Middle East," he says while pointing at a veiled person with his hand.

Tony returns again to the topic of the wedding. "There is just so much to take care of! I have been a bit stressed, you know, not relaxed." I ask him about his family, whether they are coming. "They aren't coming. That is what makes me nervous."

He explains some of the details of the strained family relationships, and I ask whether his brother will attend the wedding. "You see, Andreas, he is actually the one who caused all the troubles! He always wants to be the center of attention and to have everybody else hold him in high regard. He wants to control everybody." Tony sighs. "He wants to be the one everybody respects, and when he had a falling out with Hanan, he wanted me to break up with her! You know, he started talking with my parents and with the whole village." He makes small movements with the fingers of his right hand to indicate that such talking goes on unceasingly. "You know how people are in the villages—they are restricted and very stubborn, indeed; Syrians are very stubborn. But what to do?" he says with seeming frustration. "I tried for almost a year to do all kinds of things, but my family does not talk with me."

Eventually Tony takes the car into the old city. The street is packed. "I really don't like to drive here," he says. Tony drives sensibly, but even so his side mirror hits a pedestrian. He hastens to give his apologies, rolling down the window before we turn to the right over the hill named after the famous Saint John of Damascus.

It turns out to be difficult finding a suitable place to park. We drive all the way down to Bab Sharqi before Tony decides to turn left into the narrow streets of the old Christian quarter. "This is the first time I have driven here; hopefully it will work," he says as we continue our slow pace in the extremely narrow street. He decides to park behind two other cars. After two attempts by Tony to maneuver the Subaru into a suitable parking position just next to the wall without scratching it, I get out to direct. We manage but are uncertain if it is enough to let other vehicles pass by without sustaining scratches. Tony eventually opts for driving farther down the alley. He manages to get the car clear, but a loud and horrific sound comes from the right front. The noise of the new car meeting the old wall is not pleasant. I run to the front side, where the paint is scratched off the bumper. Worse, though, a dent was left between the bumper and the chassis. "How bad is it?" Tony asks as he gets the car clear and drives forward.

At first he does not say a word while he looks at his vehicle. "It is the bumper. It will be all right. It is all right," he says, while his fingers examine the plastic front of the headlight, which has a scratch. He then proceeds to the dent left above the bumper. "I think I can fix this," he says, opening the trunk of the car and finding some tools in his kit box. As an engineer he is an expert on these kinds of issues, and he manages to get the dent straightened. The scratches are, however, left as visible markers of his first attempt at driving in Bab Touma.

"Come, let us drive!" Tony says with determination. "I don't want to park here anymore, and I should never have tried!" I apologize for not being attentive enough, even though I felt I did the best I could to direct him. No need for doing so, however. Tony relieves me of any burden of responsibility: "It is not your fault, Andreas. It happened because I didn't pray today! I always pray before I drive, and I didn't do it today. It was a mistake."

Tony then recounts his story. "Andreas, you know how I was really poor when I studied? I had a hard time getting by. Then at one point I was in Deir Mar Musa, and I there surrendered everything to God. I told him that I don't need much, but I needed him. And you know what, the day after a man gave me the possibility of going to Kuwait!" He continues, "God has a plan for everything! You remember the icon I had in my room. I still have it with me in Kuwait." And he concludes, "You see, I need to pray. The incident with the car happened because I didn't pray! God wants to teach you things. He has a purpose for everything."

A couple of days later I receive a call from Tony, who invites me to drive to Deir Mar Musa with him and Hanan as they want to pray for their upcoming wedding and obtain a blessing for their marriage. He says that besides Hanan and himself, her cousin Ilyas will join us on the trip. And so it happens that the following day we meet to drive off to the famous monastery.

As we sit in the car ready to leave, Tony says, "I will just pray before we drive!" This is followed by a long pause where he and Hanan both close their eyes and pray. Ilyas keeps quiet, and I do as well. The prayer takes around a minute, long enough to feel like it is lasting for a while. Ilyas comments, "It was a long prayer. I thought I was going to die with its length!" Everybody laughs.

As we drive, Hanan finds Tony's hand and holds it gently, caressing it. Soon after, Ilyas starts to joke. "Really, I am going to church now for the second day in a row. I can't remember when I did that the last time." Hanan and Tony laugh and are convinced it will do him much good. Ilyas suggests that we listen to some music, and when popular Arabic music streams out of the car's stereo, he immediately shouts "Aiwa!" (yes), taking on a very masculine Arabic posture. "Turn it up." Hanan laughs. Tony turns the music up. "Dom-tik-tikke-dom-dom-tikke-tik." The rhythm goes on and on. Ilyas starts clapping. Hanan starts dancing Arabic-style with her hands. Tony does his best to drive the car and to be part of the dancing. One of the songs is the typical one used for *dabke*, a form of folk dance, which is highly popular in Syria and the Levant more widely. The dance in various local versions is used for festive occasions privately and as part of venerations of popular saints' days or days of the Virgin Mary.

The spirit is elevated in the car as Ilyas starts shouting "Al-'arīs . . . aiwa . . . al-'arīs . . ." (the groom . . . yeah . . . the groom. . .) as one of the songs praises the groom. Tony and Hanan are infected by his words, and Tony starts dancing with the whole upper part of his body. Ilyas makes trills with his tongue. "*Lelelelelelelele*," it goes, while all but Tony are clapping as he still keeps tabs on the steering wheel.

After several songs have been enjoyed by everyone in the car, suddenly Tony says, "I think we should find something different . . . I mean, we are going to pray in the monastery. It is not fitting to come driving like this." He finds a CD with a Christian hymn chanted in a church: "This is a Serbian Orthodox Christian hymn." The devotional music instantly creates a different atmosphere in the car. "I really like this!" Tony comments. "It is so beautiful. I have searched for more like this on the internet. I mean, I would like to understand the words. It is beautiful, isn't it?" Hanan and I both find the music conducive to a more meditative mode. Ilyas, however, is of another opinion. "I don't like it particularly. I prefer what we just listened to." The energetic atmosphere is subdued by the music. Ilyas lets his body fall back in the seat. "Isn't it enough that we are going to the monastery?" he says playfully. Not too long after, the Serbian hymn is finished, and it appears to be the only track of its kind available on this particular CD. Soon we are back to popular music, which again brings Ilyas upright in his seat.

When we arrive at the monastery, we still have a kilometer and a half to walk. Up. This in practice means ascending steep steps made of stone in the middle of the desert. We drink some water, preparing for the walk. Tony takes a Bedouin-style scarf and wraps it around his head to protect it from the sun. Hanan tells Ilyas and me just to start walking up. This naturally leads to Tony and Hanan walking up together as a couple, and when they walk a bit slower than Ilyas and I, the distance between us ends up being rather large.

"I don't really get why people are coming here," Ilyas starts wondering. "I mean, why here in the middle of the desert? What is there to come for?" A little later Ilyas continues, "It is something new with a place like this, where so many different people are coming." Ilyas seems to imply that despite a Syrian legacy of sharing sacred places, a place like this did not exist in the past. He pauses and tries to catch his breath and then adds, "In many respects things remain the same. But this idea of unity they preach here is new." He goes on to explain to me how Christians from various faiths such as Greek Orthodox, Greek Catholics, Maronites, and various other forms of Orthodox and Catholic Christians intermarry today. One boundary persists, however: the boundary between Christians and Muslims. "There is Muslim pressure on Christians today in this country," he says. "We need security—indeed, we need more security, not less!" Ilyas reflects. "See to the neighboring countries. We need security!" as we continue the steep walk, and I can hear Ilyas's exhaustion as he walks and talks at the same time.

When we arrive at the monastery, we are rewarded with a spectacular view. The colors of the landscape and buildings are light yellow and reddish, the sky is dusty, and the sun is shining. Both of us are sweating. Ilyas takes a seat on the low wall besides the monastery and fetches a cigarette from his pocket. I sit next to him. We both enjoy the shade after the massive exposure to the Middle Eastern sun. After a while, Tony and Hanan join us. However, they soon enter the monastery, while Ilyas waits a couple of minutes more to follow suit after finishing off yet another cigarette. Several persons can be seen making their way up the steps to the monastery.

The entrance is a little door carved out of the rock. One can enter only in an awkward position since the first step is level with your knee, or at least some forty centimeters high, and then you have to kneel since the door is no more than one meter and twenty. At the same time, it is not just a doorstep; you have to twist your body in and then turn right to pass through the entrance, the distance being one meter and a half before you can stand up again. Ilyas seems to be puzzled by the construction.

Inside Tony and Hanan have found some plastic chairs in the shade as well as some tea and ripe green grapes.

Tony addresses the purpose of the trip, namely that we are here to pray. Ilyas is hesitant to pray in the church, though. "I was like a devil in the car, I don't know. I made fun of it fifteen times or so. I mean, I don't know if I should do it." Tony and Hanan urge him to pray. Tony gives his explanation of how he started to pray more sincerely. "For me it was difficult in the beginning as well. I didn't mean anything serious when I was here the first time. I just did the sign of the cross but felt it was strange. But while I was here it changed. It started to mean something to me." He continues, "After that I began to come to church more and more, and it has become natural, like a blessing to me." Ilyas is still hesitant. But as we have finished eating, all of us go to the church and pray.

Outside the church a signpost indicates you have to take off your footwear to enter. Several pairs of shoes have already been left there. Each of us leaves his or her shoes and goes into the dimly lit church. The floor is covered with rugs, which adds to the atmosphere of its resemblance to a mosque. The room is decorated with many different icons, ranging from Christ to Saint George over the icon of the Holy Trinity to locally venerated icons of Our Lady of Soufanieh to calligraphies and paintings on the walls. Some of the painted icons on the walls are very old, but their condition could be better. Candles are placed on trays, and alongside one wall Bibles in numerous languages can be found. The altar is somehow half-hidden or secluded behind a wooden fence. And behind the altar is the only window in the church. It is small but lets rays of light enter the room. We all sit in the back of the church. Tony and Hanan start praying, which at times can be heard as whispers escaping their lips.

After half an hour of sitting, Ilyas gets up and walks out of the church. The rest of us continue sitting for a while but then rise up as in unison, me to have a closer look at the icons, Tony and Hanan to kneel in front of the altar and pray together. They both kneel, and whispers can be heard as they have their heads bowed to the ground. A monk explains to four Syrians about Musa al-Habashi, the founder the monastery, of how he left fortunes behind to become a monk.

I meet Ilyas outside. "I fell asleep," he reveals. "I mean, I couldn't concentrate." He continues, "Shame on me! If there is no focus in the prayer, then you should not pray at all." We continue talking. Ilyas gets us some tea and asks me to join him sitting outside the monastery, where he can have a cigarette.

After some time, Tony and Hanan come out to us. They have been praying for at least an hour and a half. Ilyas instantly comments about this. "Did you pray all the time? How is that possible?" Tony explains they have been talking to Abuna Ibrahim as well. Ilyas continues, "Ouiih, still it is a long time. Did you pray for two hours?" Hanan and Tony heartily disagree, saying it was much less.

We drive on, and Tony and Hanan opt for paying the monastery of Our Lady in Saydnaya a visit on the way back to Damascus. Ilyas falls asleep again in the car, which later makes him ask somewhat hopefully if we had already prayed in Saydnaya. Eventually he admits he had never visited Saydnaya before, much to the surprise of Tony and Hanan. Also here, Hanan and Tony take their time praying for their future before the trip back to Damascus.

Back on the road again, Tony decides to stop the car to go to a shop. Ilyas is making jokes about the prosperity of Hanan and her coming husband while Tony buys some soft drinks and snacks. Hanan laughs at these remarks but seems to like to hear words such as "See how smart he is, a big car, work in Kuwait, and so gentle." Ilyas continues, "Let us see whether you will stay with him." Hanan just laughs.

Some years later, Syria looks rather different. On February 10, 2012, Tony writes this:

Dear Andreas,

I hope you are also fine and happy. As for our family, all are OK for now but the situation is becoming bad, day after day, with the Islamist fighters who are brought in from Afghanistan, Iraq, Libya and the Gulf countries. They are targeting the petrol and gas lines, kidnapping people from the minorities, raping women and children and cutting them to pieces, and then they take photos to send to TV stations, claiming the army did it. We are very afraid of the attacks on Christians. These freedom fighters kidnapped a priest and his brother from my village, attacked [the] Saydnaya Monastery with anti-armor rockets. We don't know what will happen, but if they are able to win and bring down the government, I'm sure they will force us out—if they let us live—and will take all our property [...]. Attached you will find pictures of the blast that happened in Aleppo today, Hanan's cousin serves in the army there and he was lucky to be out of the center on a patrol near the borders. Pray for us, we don't want to become refugees and lose our own country. They are forcing us to feel this is a place for Islam only.

Tony's prayers changed over time. His prayers changed as his own life as well as the life of Syria changed. Like all war reports, his words above represent a partial vision, driven by very particular fears, justified in this case by direct experience, media reports, rumors, and pro-regime propaganda. Tony's prayers may therefore not reveal the true nature of things but rather one situated perspective and more clearly his affective dispositions toward his dear ones, the future, and the stakes in life as such. The prayers bespeak how different the preoccupations of Syrian Christians have become in just a few years. For a person like Tony, in contrast to Ilyas, prayer can be seen as a relatively sedimented and continuous practice. But a severe crisis, such as the one we witness unfolding in Syria since the beginning of 2011, may afford new and different ways for all to address what the human condition is and how God, Mary, Jesus, and the saints may possibly intervene.

ANDREAS BANDAK is Assistant Professor in the Department of Cross-Cultural and Regional Studies at the University of Copenhagen. He is co-editor of *Politics of Worship in the Contemporary Middle East* and editor of "The Social Life of Prayers" (special issue of *Religion*).

NOTE

1. Thanks are due to Sonja Luehrmann for the invitation to participate in this fascinating project and for comments on an earlier draft of this text. Likewise, I would like to thank Regnar Albæk Kristensen and colleagues at the Centre for Comparative Culture Studies for comments. All interlocutors have been anonymized.

7 STRUGGLING BODIES AT THE CROSSROADS OF ECONOMY AND TRADITION

The Case of Contemporary Russian Convents

DARIA DUBOVKA

A<small>NYONE WHO HAS EVER LIVED</small> in a contemporary Russian rural monastery would have initially been amazed by the conditions of life in monastic cells. The cause of amazement would not have come from the ascetic interiors; contrary to expectation, there are no empty rooms with thin mats. Instead, the rooms are strewn with old furniture, used clothing, and blankets riddled with holes. The windows are dirty and the cracked ceilings covered with cobwebs. The cheap paper icons stuck to the walls are intended to remind visitors of the spiritual aims of monastic inhabitants, but instead the icons merely add to the unpleasant atmosphere. These cells resemble a warehouse where any and all goods donated to monasteries find their final abode.

The discomfort from these dusty rooms increases when a pilgrim learns that there is no running water in the cloisters. Sometimes in the corridor there is a washbasin, which often ices over in winter. Once a week the permanent inhabitants wash themselves in a bathhouse, but for temporary visitors this does not fully alleviate the problem. Access to hot water only once a week contradicts the habits of both permanent inhabitants and pilgrims: the overwhelming majority of modern inhabitants of Russian rural monasteries were urban dwellers in their past, with an ingrained habit of a daily bath. If a daily bath is a customary practice, why does it cause so many difficulties in a modern monastery? Often the nuns answer that life in a monastery requires asceticism.

In many cultures, austerity is understood as an inevitable property of religious virtuosi (Durkheim [1912] 1995, 313–21). Certainly, practices of asceticism may differ and depend on an image of the natural and desired body in variable historic and cultural contexts. Over the centuries of Orthodox tradition, the understanding of the sinful and the saintly body has changed on numerous occasions.[1] Looking at the canonical examples of saints, one may see an abundance of convenient methods of handling one's own body. Saint warriors, martyrs, passion bearers, holy fools, holy hierarchs, canonized monks (*prepodobnye*)—all these types of sainthood offer different body role models on the way to heaven. What is specific to monastic holiness is a declarative rejection of the body.

According to the mystery of tonsuring, a person who takes monastic vows becomes like a newborn. The new monk's or nun's role models should now be angels, who are fleshless creatures (Lestvitsa 1998). But being corporeal while pretending to be incorporeal is a great tension within the idea of Christian monasticism.[2] Monks and nuns who realized it in practice did it in a different way. I briefly mention only the case of medieval Russian monasticism, because at that time many monasteries were founded in northwest Russia; now they have been renewed, and their new inhabitants especially venerate the founders of their cloisters whose examples they use as a point of orientation for their own piety.[3] Medieval monks, many of whom are now canonized with the title *prepodobnyi* (Old Church Slavonic, literally "most similar"), imitated Christ by bringing direct harm to their bodies. The hagiographies tell about heavy chains worn by saints and amazing feats of fasting performed in the extremely harsh conditions of the Russian north.[4] There are even more eccentric examples of austerity: Nikita the Stylite and Savva Vysherskii are glorified as ascetics who lived for extended periods of time atop pillars (Zhitiia sviatykh [1907] 2005a; [1907] 2005b). The legend about Nikita the Stylite includes a fragment about his early feats: he went to a swampland and allowed his body to be eaten by mosquitoes (Moroz 2009).

This concern with the body and its potential to be transformed into something else can be approached in different ways. Neither fasting nor suppression of the flesh by chains is typical of modern cloisters.[5] Nuns today find the sources of inspiration for changing one's body in patristic literature, which is mainly devoted to the virtue of obedience and the hesychastic tradition. Besides the fact that sources offer quite different conceptions of the body itself and the methods to improve it, today's nuns have a perspective far removed from that of the medieval period, during which these techniques were developed. This chapter focuses on the following questions: to what extent has today's conception of the body changed, and what kind of human body is suitable for a contemporary monastery? I try to untangle the knot composed of hygiene practices and poor living conditions in contemporary convents, as well as the wider economic situation and the current understanding of religious asceticism. This focus on the human body throws light on the problems of the function and understanding of prayer in modern monasteries.

THE ECONOMIC CONDITIONS OF RURAL MONASTIC REVIVAL

At the end of the nineteenth century, Russian convents experienced an unprecedented influx of sisters and pilgrims. This was due to a variety of factors, including the abolition of serfdom and the subsequent opportunity for peasants to leave rural communities and participate in pilgrimages or take monastic vows; the increase of piety among the nobility; and the general process of modernization in the country, such as railroad construction, which facilitated access to distant cloisters (Kenworthy 2010; Robson 2007). Monasteries that had housed about two dozen sisters and been quite poor at the beginning of the nineteenth century increased tenfold, becoming major economic centers by the end of the century. Some of them happened to be well adjusted to the new conditions of advancing capitalism (Wagner 2003). A description of a particular monastery at century's end depicted cloisters with several hundred inhabitants, sizable tracts of arable land, a large garden, a brick factory, and multiple farm buildings.[6]

All this wealth was expropriated by the Soviet authorities in the 1920s and 1930s. During the next seventy years, these monastic buildings would be used as childcare centers, museums, storage areas for collective farms, houses of culture, state archives, and so on (Kelly 2013). Naturally, monastic constructions were rebuilt to the needs of the current owners; churches were deprived of crosses, cupolas, icon screens, and all interior decorations. The same destiny was shared by Orthodox monasteries in other countries that became Socialist after 1917. The regions that were annexed on the eve of World War II (the Baltic countries, West Ukraine, and West Belarus) were able to keep some functioning cloisters.

After the collapse of the Soviet Union, the state began to return former churches and monasteries to the Russian Orthodox Church. But these returned buildings were no longer suitable for either church services or housing nuns. The churches and monastic cells were in need of major repairs, as well as the restoration of interior decorations. All this required a large financial investment. Sometimes the state, appreciating ancient churches as architectural monuments, supported their renewal. At other times the church authorities facilitated the restoration of a monastic complex, but only a few rich eparchies could afford this. Most rural monasteries were restored with the help of a small number of enthusiasts (Tocheva 2011b). In some places, local leaders facilitated the restorations. Elsewhere, urban intellectuals took the lead in restoring rural shrines; these intellectuals had, as far back as the 1960s, considered religious monuments to be embodiments of national ideas (Brudny 1998). This method of restoration via hard manual labor was considered morally blameless, whereas financial sponsorship is often thought of as morally dubious (Köllner 2011). But if the churches, especially those situated in cities, were reconstructed through manual labor, restoring the numerous and remote rural monastic complexes was beyond enthusiasts' power. Volunteers—who as a rule were urban dwellers—restored city churches after work or in their spare time. But the time needed to reach a village made this type of restoration nearly impossible for rural areas.

As a result, a deficit in money and manpower prolonged the time needed to repair monasteries. A small number of nuns (rarely more than ten to twenty) could not maintain housing designed for hundreds. Neither could they cultivate vegetable gardens at pre-revolutionary levels. The cloisters were as a result forced to accept voluntary temporary workers. These workers had unclear status because they were not officially included in the sisterhood, although they were expected to follow a way of life very similar to that of the sisters; in addition, to be a temporary worker was a necessary precursor to becoming a nun. However, since the number of temporary workers was difficult to predict, monasteries had to store more clothing, tools, and food than needed for the sisters alone. These stocks consisted of donations made by local villagers as well as pilgrims.[7]

The economic situation explains the poor condition of the cells, as well as the neglect of hygiene. Indeed, plumbing was not usually installed in pre-revolutionary monasteries. As for contemporary renovations, such redevelopment would be very expensive. Even more prosperous monasteries, which have new hostels for temporary workers and pilgrims, often restrict access to hot water. They may provide good meals, but they still have only a single bathroom with one hot water heater, capable of providing about twenty minutes of warm water for dozens of people. While hot water is certainly an expensive resource and as such is controlled, why are monasteries so very stringent with it in particular? How do monasteries' restrictions on hygiene practice help us understand what kind of body is suitable for a convent?

THE AUTOMATIC BODY

I will begin with a particularly striking case, which resulted in the dissociation of a convent. This was a small convent of twelve inhabitants in the Vologda region. The head of this cloister, Mother Evfaliia, was about sixty years old. She had been a medical assistant in a village until she decided to enter the monastery in her thirties. It was the Soviet period, so active convents were found only in the Ukraine, Belarus, and the Baltic states. Evfaliia came to a Ukrainian convent near the town of Cherkassy, and over the next fifteen years she climbed the hierarchical ladder from novice to monastery administrator (*blagochinnaia*). In those years, the cloister supported itself mainly through farming, and in the 1990s it expanded its farmland and endeavored to have the state return its pre-revolutionary church buildings. In 1995, the bishop of Vologda had Mother Evfaliia return to her native region in order to help restore the Goritskii convent. Many of the Goritskii buildings were either destroyed or abandoned or had been turned into a museum or taken over by local residents.[8] Mother Evfaliia, reproducing Soviet-era patterns of survival, focused the initial restoration efforts on the large farms, which required considerable investment of labor. The nuns and volunteer workers toiled twelve hours a day with no days off. Due to the nuns' exhaustion, church services were held only on Sundays and holy days, and private prayer was not observed. Although the monastery gained a good farm, garden, and cattle yard, this success came at the cost of the dissatisfaction of many sisters. They began to struggle in 2012. I learned about this confrontation by a text message from a novice: "We want a monastic life in the monastery!" What did this mean? They wished to reduce the time of labor obedience (*poslushanie*) and create a special time for prayer.

There are two meanings of the word "obedience." First, obedience is a way of life, in which a nun constantly subordinates her will to the will of another person and through this person to the will of God. Second, obedience is necessary in everyday duties, and in this sense it becomes synonymous with work. The complexity of the analytical category of obedience lies in the fact that it may refer to both the field of theological reflection about inner spiritual work (obedience as a virtue needed for the salvation of the soul) and to the field of economy. In the latter case, obedience is particular to the performance of certain duties. This meaning has been used for a long time within Russian monasteries. A pre-revolutionary list of the Goritskii convent nuns contains information about first names, year of birth, date of admission to the monastery, tonsure date, the estate (*soslovie*) to which each nun belonged, and their obediences, which included seamstress, arch-chanter, and baker (Glyzina 2009).

The work necessary for the restoration of returned buildings was also termed obedience. Apparently, the word "obedience" was chosen in order to stress the continuity of traditional monastic life. However, obedience in the current historic and economic context has a different connotation.

How does obedience work in monasteries today? My informants conceptualize obedience as a spiritual gift from God. But like any reciprocal relationship, this tie implies a degree of mutuality. For establishing this connection, God is not necessarily the original donor. The person can initiate this relationship. But what can a human being present to God? The person's gift as part of this exchange can be his or her voluntarily alienated free will. It requires an extreme self-sacrifice for a person to surrender his or her will to another.

> What does true obedience mean? In fact, that a person "in obedience" relinquishes his will. And why is this most precious to the Lord, when a person relinquishes his will? The thing is that everything comes to us from God, all our virtues are from our God, all from God, that's what the Lord gives us; all talents even, hands, legs, eyes are all from God; the language that we speak, think, everything comes from God. And it is only the will that is just ours. We, humans, are endowed with this free will. We finally give it all to the Lord, sacrifice everything. It's the supreme sacrifice.

According to this excerpt from an interview with a nun who serves as administrator of the Goritskii convent, free will is initially the property of God, who gives it to the person. The believer should in turn return it to the Giver, because one can expect salvation only when living according to God's will. If the will remains a person's property, it will lead to ruin. One cannot be guided by one's own will, because it can be "treacherous": people usually estimate their own deeds in a favorable light. "Everyone is very deceitful and sometimes it seems that the motive of your actions is very noble, but if one looks deeper into oneself, more often the motives come from selfishness," this nun explained.

In spiritual literature by the church fathers, searching is necessary but must be done with caution because "we read the books, but our mind is infected, our mind is sinful; it does not understand anything and cannot see anything." According to this logic, the more that individuals do not own themselves, the more they are owned by God, and thus the more certainly they are saved. By handing over the will through obedience to another, one restores a desired safety and balance.

For monastic work, this means that obedience serves as a moral sanction for daily work. A typical workday in the monastery is twelve hours. The duties for the majority of inhabitants involve cooking, cleaning, simple renovations, working in the vegetable garden, and so on. Such work, while often monotonous, is not considered humiliating because many contemporary monastery inhabitants performed similar work at home or in their summer cottage. At this point the contemporary understanding of obedience begins to depart from the previous interpretation of this virtue as it was described in the older Orthodox texts.

The most famous classical text glorifying the virtue of obedience is *Practical Teaching on the Christian Life* (Dushepoleznye poucheniia) by Abba Dorotheus, an Egyptian hermit from the sixth century. This book begins by telling about a young man of noble birth who demonstrated amazing humility in the monastery, unquestioningly following all instructions and performing any distasteful work (Avva Dorofei 2005). Many similar stories put a nobleman or prince in the center of the plot, likely because, in feudal society, to be subordinated to a lower social position was regarded as a special kind of virtue.[9]

A similar discrepancy concerning the modern understanding of obedience can be observed in the popular histories of the Paterikon, in which a character is given orders to plant cabbage with the roots pointing upward or to water a stick to turn it into a living tree. In these stories, obedience is associated with irrational labor. However, modern monasteries cannot afford the luxury of wasting labor power in this way.

Most probably, the social imagination underlying contemporary ideas of obedience has another origin besides patristic literature. Reading these old legends, contemporary believers understand them through a more familiar cultural grid that includes a knowledge of totalitarian states, with little respect for feudal virtues. The emphasis on the rejection of the person's own will and complete submission to the will of another is more reminiscent of dystopian novels—with strong state power and people like cogs in the system, striving for a brighter future on this earth or in heaven—than of medieval stories about noble humility or irrational labor.

The dystopian storylines elaborate on another popular older idea: belief in the end of days. In the eschatological narratives collected in famous contemporary Orthodox monasteries, one can see a clear parallel to the motives of the well-known dystopian novels of the twentieth century: *We* by Yevgeny Zamyatin, *1984* by George Orwell, and *Brave New World* by Aldous Huxley (Akhmetova 2010, 176–214). However, for those who were training themselves in the virtue of obedience, the old and popular image of the malevolent and omnipotent power, leading to apocalypse or to a depersonalized society, brought up a quite practical question: how to determine the right spiritual leader to receive the gift of their will.[10] Dystopian narratives told stories of people consciously or unconsciously rejecting their own will in favor of the state or an unspecified collective. Strictly speaking, the very difference between utopia and dystopia resides exactly in this point: by whom, and how, these people's wills would be used. For nuns, this choice distinguishes true obedience from false. The task was to find a spiritually gifted leader who could direct his pupils to God. The concern with finding a spiritual leader was not shared by old hermits, who feared false pride as the most dreadful sin. But modern nuns were more afraid of following the wrong leader. The history of the twentieth century, readings of utopian/dystopian movies and books, and contemporary conspirological folklore taught people that their will and consciousness could be subdued. It is a person's own responsibility to choose the right spiritual authority.

By contrast, if individuals give their own will to a saint, they would not need to think about their salvation anymore. Their duty would be only to properly follow the instructions of the saint. For many members of contemporary monastic communities, such dedicated obedience allows one to surrender attachment to ordinary feelings and desires and become instead a completely docile laborer performing rational obligations. As one nun described the ideal obedience, it should be a chain of simple and direct tasks, one following another, so that one need not think at all but only obey instructions. Thus, the contemporary ideal of obedience is of a person who carries out all tasks correctly and without reasoning, much as a robot would. On the one hand, it is clear that such an ideal has recent origins and connects with utopian narratives. On the other, this ideal expresses one of the ancient postulates of monasticism, which is incorporeity. Thus through this mechanistic body, many moods (tiredness, sexual desire, weakness, affliction) can be downplayed or ignored. Whether ancient or recent, robotization helps transform the problematic human body into something more convenient and efficacious, in an economic sense, to monasteries.

Returning to the history of the Goritskii convent's schism, it is clear that in this case prayer existed only as common ritual, that is, as part of the church liturgy. Mother Evfaliia, more managing director than spiritual leader, did not understand the demands to provide time for personal prayer. She regarded any doubt about the wisdom of labor obedience as evidence of laziness. She told me that sisters are allowed to pray as much as they want during their labor obedience, that such was not prohibited. Mother Evfaliia claimed that most labor in the garden, cattle yard, and kitchen required certain skills but that over time these were becoming routinized operations; therefore, during those tasks the sisters' minds remained unoccupied and they were able to pray. In this case, to pray meant to repeat memorized prayers without any additional sensory support, such as kneeling, crossing oneself, or bowing. The priest who acted as confessor to the convent said that sisters are required to perform work but that prayer was a personal matter. If someone painted a fence or cooked a borscht, he said, then the result was obvious, but how to measure prayer? According to the priest, prayer in the monastery was the private affair of each nun.

THE TRANSFORMED BODY

Many sisters, however, did not see prayer as merely an appendix to labor. Some understood prayer as their main transformative practice. They often considered the words of the apostle Paul, "Pray without ceasing" (1 Thess. 5:17, ESV), as the basis of a spiritual life. Their reflection was devoted to analyzing the phrase "without ceasing." How was such possible under the conditions of everyday life? In the imagination of many, monasteries were unique places where people would be free from economic worries so that they could devote themselves to prayer. Often this group of nuns included people with a higher education who had lived in Moscow and Saint Petersburg and begun a religious search in the 1980s and 1990s. Many began their search with Eastern religious traditions and acquired some experience in practicing yoga and meditation.[11] Orthodoxy attracted them with the performance of the Jesus Prayer.

There is a powerful tradition in Orthodoxy called hesychasm. These ideas were developed, between the tenth and fourteenth centuries, by Symeon the New Theologian, Gregory the Sinaite, and Gregory Palamas. According to their doctrine, the godlike state of *theosis* is achievable in this life through contemplation of the divine energies (divine light). For this they offered a special technique to achieve the desired state for the performance of the Jesus Prayer (Pop, this volume). To find the divine light that people had inside, all external sensory impressions had to be limited. A hesychast must sit in a fixed posture, slide the knees to the chest, turn the gaze inward, follow the breath, and silently utter the Jesus Prayer. Exercising the imagination at this time is not recommended. Ideally, such detachment and minimization of external bodily sensations may be found in cave monasteries. However, despite the fact that some monasteries have good conditions for practicing the Jesus Prayer, they are in no hurry to revive this kind of monasticism. In contemporary monastic prayer discourse, a certain hierarchy exists, with liturgical prayer during church services at the very bottom and the Jesus Prayer at the top. The head of the monastery often does not approve of the practice of the Jesus Prayer among monks or nuns, considering the monastic community to be unprepared for the highest spiritual practice.

Thus, the abbot of the Archangel Michael's monastery in the Caucasus does not rush to develop the performance of the Jesus Prayer in such a form, though the monastery's caves were evidently used for that purpose by pre-revolutionary hermits. His doubt is related to the theological distinction between internal and external action (Russian *delanie*), which underpins to a great extent the practice of monastic prayer. External action is considered to be the physical performance of the prayer: kneeling, bowing, reading out loud or in silence. Inner action describes the accompanying emotional mood. If a person undertakes to fulfill the highest virtue but is not ready, then at best he or she will only imitate the external action and at worst will fall into the sin of pride. The abbot spoke about what may happen if he encourages performing the Jesus Prayer: "It is clear how to build up this brand: that I have hermits. The cave, hermits, an Athonite-type monastery, the abbot visiting Mount Athos. These can build up a brand, but we do not want it. We do what we are able to do and what we know right now: we read the morning and evening prayers. Well, now that is the foundation for us."

Some features of the modern understanding of the hesychasts make their teachings particularly attractive to a specific group of monks. This is the doctrine of the light of Mount Tabor. In the hesychasts' teaching, the transfiguration of Christ on Mount Tabor, accompanied by bright light, is used symbolically to demonstrate that invoking the name of Jesus brings internal illumination. In the consciousness of modern monks, this connects with the idea of energies. In the Orthodox tradition, Gregory Palamas developed some ideas about the energies of God (Meyendorff 1974). But contemporary fascination with hesychasm likely has its roots in widespread New Age views in post-Soviet territory rather than in knowledge of the theological debates of the fourteenth century. Energies are a popular quasi-scientific concept, used by some New Age movements. Some of my informants at first told me stories about Indian yogis who did not require the usual sustenance of sleep or food and were able to achieve complete transformation of the body through meditation. Then it turned out that my informants held exactly the same ideas in their understanding of Orthodoxy. For my informants, the Jesus Prayer called the Holy Spirit (that is, the divine energy) to the worshipper, and this energy transfigured humans "cell by cell."

If we look again at the Goritskii convent, the conflict between prayer worshippers and obedience worshippers becomes more obvious. Given the special techniques that are required for the performance of the Jesus Prayer and the physical labor required for sheer survival, it is very difficult for contemporary admirers of hesychasm to integrate this practice into modern institutionalized monasteries. The Jesus Prayer is a very time-consuming practice that not many monasteries can afford.

Novice Maria, who left the Goritskii convent precisely because she was looking for prayer, told the story of her friend, a hieromonk, who practiced the Jesus Prayer. She explained why he considered the current monastic life not conducive to the transfiguration of a person.

> When he came to the monastery, he had already been keeping the Jesus Prayer almost constantly. And he said that everything in the monastery was against the Jesus Prayer. . . . All dwellers labored so much that it was nearly impossible to keep the Jesus Prayer. Now he is released from prayer services and brotherly meals and he prays at night and constructs his day as he wants, except for his obedience, which he bears in the temple. So, when I began to ask him about the little prayer (*molitovke*), he showed me how three fingers add up to pray, so he put them to himself and I put my fingers to myself, and I immediately felt responsive fire at the point of touch. First, I realized where this point is located. Second, because he was standing right by me, with his great energy reserve, the fire was immediately transmitted to me. What I mean is that a person in prayer emanates something like that. Well, but there are now very few such persons.

The idea that the performance of prayer releases a certain energetic force, rebuilding not only the soul but also the body, can be confirmed by the examples of the incorruptible relics and hagiographic histories about the extraordinary light produced by devotees of Christ (Greene 2010). Improvement in this way is accessible to people independent of institutional support. This is what happened in the case of Maria. She returned to her Moscow apartment, where she continued to train in prayer at her own pace. Several other Goritskii nuns and novices preferred to go to another monastery that had many more nuns and a reputation of being more prayerful. Another friend of mine with a biography similar to Maria's also chose the monastic way, but instead of a convent she went to a male monastery. There she carries out the obedience of an accountant, but apart from that her schedule is very different from the rest of the brotherhood, leaving her time for private prayer. Finally, there are those who take on jobs as temporary workers in different monasteries, having come to the conclusion that one can become a monastic in order to avoid thinking about one's economic situation, thus freeing oneself to focus on spiritual affairs and a life of discipline. Yet if a person has no economic problems, modern life in a megalopolis will provide better opportunities for the practice of the Jesus Prayer than will current conditions in monasteries. Indeed, the anonymity and alienation of life in large cities have become proverbial. If, as in Maria's daily routine, a person is retired, owns an apartment, visits the nearest store, and watches an online broadcast of the church liturgy, her conditions would be the envy of any hagiographic hermit, left in the remote Vologda forest of northern Russia or in the Syrian desert for the practice of prayers.

The notion of a monastery as a place of individual prayer is rarely recognized in contemporary Russian convents. The Goritskii priest disagreed with Maria's opinion, because Maria's way of transforming herself implied personal autonomy and attention to her own internal states. The priest did not consider contemplation of one's inner state to be spiritual work; rather, as seen in his comment, he thought it a sentimental and romantic impulse without support by everyday actions: "The Goritskii convent could well become a kind of elite monastery for ladies disappointed in life. And I think it would meet demand, in the sense that there would be a lot of nuns fluttering around as butterflies, not sowing, not reaping, but recollecting themselves in solitary prayer and dreams of Heavenly Jerusalem. Mother Evfaliia provided an earthly monastery, from the plow, a kind of agricultural work team [*artel'*]; thus labor combines with prayer and this shapes the form of a monastic life." Different sensory regimes accord with different meanings of prayer. The performance of the Jesus Prayer implies very strong ties between prayer and the body of the worshipper and at the same time requires isolation from other people, while for Mother Evfaliia, prayer is simply a pronunciation, out loud or silently, of memorized texts. Contrary to the robotization of the human body in contemporary monastic labor, people do not easily imagine themselves as docile mechanisms. This framework contradicts the diverse personal and bodily experience of everyday life.

Another framework seems to be more sustained. The work on the body ("cell by cell") is intended to transform the human person and bring it closer to the divine. This process of transformation is understood in quasi-scientific terminology as "sensitivity to invisible energies." Given their attention to the body, the group of inhabitants who wanted more prayer could not leave without reflecting on the hygiene situation in monasteries. Unexpectedly, they accepted the idea that little access to bathing would lead to self-renewal and self-purification of the body. Moreover, they viewed water as a substance with a memory that can transmit negative information to a bather.[12] The novice Maria, for example, believed that if for two months a person did not wash his or her hair, it would arrive at a natural balance. Her beliefs incorporated both the idea of a golden age before modernization and civilization, when humanity was in a natural state, and the concept of self-transformation through the Jesus Prayer.

UNCLEANED BODIES AND MODERNIZATION

The theme of modernization is a very important one for monasteries. Since the world, according to biblical eschatology, never changes for the better, cloisters should be rooted in tradition, meaning a habitual way of life as well as imitations of exemplars from patristic literature. In a world where technological innovations are happening at a rapid pace, however, the traditional lifestyle is called into question. Even such monasteries as those on Mount Athos, with a thousand years of uninterrupted history, are forced to argue about acceptable and unacceptable inventions (Fajfer 2012). Such things as electricity, roads, and mobile phones have become the subject of serious debates. Even if these things were not the cause of disagreements, they become a means of pointing out one's opponent's lack of spirituality, as happened in two monasteries of Athos: Vatopedi and Esfigmenou (Paganopoulos, n.d.).

Russian Orthodox monasteries have had a seventy-year break in their history, during which there have been significant changes in the infrastructure and technology of the state. The tradition of monastic life, on which the current dwellers rely, stopped at the technological and social level of early twentieth-century society, and patristic literature does not offer any advice about using modern devices. In conditions when it is impossible to rely on tradition, monastery inhabitants are trying to decide on their own the degree of modernization within their cloister. This gives rise to inconsistent-combinations: in one case, laptops are prohibited but mobile phones permitted; in another case, central electricity is intentionally not installed, but dwellers have laptops, which are powered by the generator; in a third convent, laptops, mobile phones, and TV are forbidden, but the convent has its own tractors, harvesting machines, and cars. However, in this kaleidoscope it is possible to trace an economic logic of what is permitted and what is prohibited. Monasteries usually tolerate those innovations that help them to survive. Loopholes for innovations are possible even if a monastery is firmly convinced of the inadmissibility of certain items in its territory. For example, many monasteries prohibit the use and even the presence of a computer, but some work that requires a computer is performed by members of the laity, who are often voluntary helpers at the monastery.

The issue of modernization seems to be most apparent via the example of the use of electronic devices. Nevertheless, this topic refers to wider questions, including the restoration of monastic buildings and the interior decoration of a cell. These questions are not left unconsidered by the nuns. I had a conversation with a cantor of the Goritskii convent who was still practicing obedience at the time but would a couple of years later leave for another monastery in search of prayer. She told me that the large, rebuilt, pompous monasteries did not attract her; she preferred the cloisters with cracks in the walls. I asked, "These cloisters are more correct, aren't they?" The cantor answered, "They are traditional." She went on to say that when Trinity-Sergius Lavra near Moscow was being renovated, the leadership decided to do European-style remodeling. A number of inhabitants did not agree with this type of restoration. They called the renovated monastery Euro-Lavra.[13] In spite of this renovation, however, the life of the monks has not changed much: windows of ascetic schemamonks still look out over the dustbins.

The cantor, who graduated from a Moscow university with a specialty in sound production, belonged to the metropolitan intelligentsia, just like the novice Maria. This group is most appreciative of the aesthetics of ancient Russia: the icons of Andrei Rublev, the *znamenny* chant, the medieval architecture of northern churches, all of which create an image of the solitary monastery, alien to economic and other worldly troubles.[14] The aesthetics of imaginary ancient Russia resonates more with picturesque ruins than with rich monasteries serving as production centers. According to this cultural code, the dilapidation of monastic buildings is regarded as proof of their authenticity. Thus, some degree of damage to objects or buildings is not considered negative but on the contrary serves to demonstrate their merits. At the same time, this group may exhibit even more aversion to ordinary rubbish than is usual in Russian society. So, for the cantor, the unpleasant view from the schemamonk's windows serves as a sign of irrational modernization, where what should be left alone gets repaired and what needs to be cleaned up gets ignored.

The heads of the monasteries usually hold different beliefs. For them a tidy facade is more important than the preservation of antiquities, because a renovated facade gives the authorities the most obvious proof of success. Therefore churches are the main structures repaired, since they are the primary buildings observed by diocesan authorities, pilgrims, and tourists. The interior and the internal infrastructure of these buildings are renovated last of all. The question remains, however: if economic constraints are at the heart of monastery hygiene practices, why does this kind of relation to the body meet with support from the rest of the monastery inhabitants?

People with different aesthetic views and understandings of the practice of salvation may in fact have a similar relation to the body if they agree with one idea: the cloister should be inhabited by monastics seeking to establish a connection with God, not with other people. Lives of northern Russian monastic saints are full of stories about how the future saints left their communities and settled in the dense forests in order to devote their whole life to God. The image of a similarly solitary monastery is ideal for almost all the nuns. This ideal was demonstrated in an interview with the Goritskii administrator who supported the practice of obedience in everyday life:

> I imagine Saint Zosima Verkhovskii, who lived in the wilderness in Siberia, where the frost is deeper; he lived in an earth house with no wood. Do you know how they prepared their food?[15] During a week in the fall, they baked bread consisting of half flour, half grass, and then they froze it and froze vegetables and cooked some soup and froze it too so that they didn't need to cook in winter. Every winter they lived in their cells; I don't know how warm they were, but they prayed. Since they didn't want to spend time on cooking, they cut off a piece of the frozen bread and soup and continued their prayer.

It is noteworthy that her image of the ideal monastery does not mention obedience. In fact, this image emphasizes the relationship of a person with God as it is expressed by prayer. The denial of relationships with laypeople, as is required of Orthodox nuns, leads to the rejection of public life and public presentation of the self. Before the monastery inhabitants arrived, they were familiar with a very modern form of public life, closely related to the development of a new cultural body, which became less tolerant of a variety of smells and more demanding in terms of hygiene (Elias [1939] 2000; Foucault 1973; about the Russian situation, see Pirogovskaya 2014). Smells, or rather their absence, serve as a marker of both the level of culture and the safety of the environment; hence deodorants and various means of hiding the body's natural smells are very popular in contemporary society.

Despite the monastic idea of transforming the human body into something incorporeal, it is in the monasteries that the sweaty, dirty human body receives the right to exist.[16] This kind of austerity, in which hygiene practices are severely curtailed, contrasts with the increased desire to clean that is the contemporary norm. At the same time, monastery inhabitants' neglect of cleanliness calls for neglect of the usual standards of public behavior. The desire to create a nonsocial society, where every nun would, in the first place, take care of her relationship with God rather than her relationship with other people, correlates well with the reverse concern for one's body, where an unclean and unkempt body is more highly valued.

CONCLUSION

Contemporary Russian monasteries are very young, in contrast to the centuries-old monastic communities of Mount Athos and other parts of the Orthodox world. Most contemporary monasteries were under restoration during the 1990s. Today it is rare for a monastic community to be older than twenty years. The people who came to monasteries in those early years were faced with a situation in which nobody knew exactly what to do. The principal aim of those who went to the cloisters was the salvation of their souls, but the Orthodox textual tradition, as well as the millennial history of Russian monasteries, offers very different strategies for reaching heaven or building a proper monastery. So during this period, the chief questions were these: which practices lead a person to God, and which practices are most preferable for a spiritual community such as a monastery?

Asceticism is implied as an essential practice for such religious communities, limiting as it does the practitioner's ties with the mundane world (Moore 1987). But in the Orthodox interpretation, this should not be a spontaneous austerity that doesn't follow a traditional model. For Orthodox monasteries, it is important to seek acknowledgment in patristic literature of the activity of their inhabitants. Today's nuns represent themselves as possibly weaker in feats than the ancient saints but as their heirs in terms of grace. Thus both the adherents of obedience and the practitioners of the Jesus Prayer derive their authority from the patristic tradition. However, the traditions they choose, and the interpretation of those traditions, depend on the modern conditions of a revival of monastic life.

I used the example of the relationship to the body to describe the contemporary application of the patristic tradition. Modern nuns and novices are faced with the ancient monastic challenge of the minimization or transformation of the body into something fleshless. The contemporary solution for how to handle one's body in a monastery lies in the appeal to very modern conceptualizations of the body, power, and free will. One path follows plots of utopian/dystopian narratives; another borrows models of individual and self-transformation, ideas that are most popular in New Age groups. Prayer occupies a central place in these debates. It is alternately considered a mental activity, transformative practice, or collective ritual. Consequently, the body may not be given any attention at all (at least on a discursive level), or it may be considered both instrument and indicator of deification.

Actually, economic problems determine many ascetic activities in modern monasteries. These problems of the cloisters can be viewed within the broader context of small, closed, agricultural religious communities under threat within a capitalist economy and secular state. Monastic life in contemporary cloisters is very diverse, as it depends on the availability of buildings in need of restoration, sponsorship aid, the position of local authorities, the number of voluntary temporary workers, and what image of the monastery the abbot, bishop, and inhabitants wish to achieve.

However, even among such diverse monasteries, there is a need to deal with common key issues: they must become part of the modern world while at the same time emphasizing their difference from it. The latter is in part accomplished via austerity in hygiene practices. Hygienic practices are so deeply ingrained in modern society that they are hardly noticed. The impossibility for contemporary monasteries to live up to citizens' hygienic standards leads to new ascetic potentialities.

DARIA DUBOVKA is a postgraduate student at Peter the Great Museum of Anthropology and Ethnography, Russian Academy of Sciences, Saint Petersburg.

NOTES

1. For Catholic tradition, see, for example, a brilliant description of attitudes regarding crippled bodies (Orsi 2006, 19–47) or about female physicality in Roman theological works (Bynum 2007).

2. Nowadays there is a movement in the Catholic tradition, called new monastic communities, that rejects this angelic image as theological doctrine. This movement considers the human body bestowed by God as something that makes humans sacred (Palmisano 2015).

3. Materials for this article came from my fieldwork in some convents in this region. This region is associated by many believers with Holy Russia: a mythical golden age of prosperity, Orthodoxy, and morality.

4. Clearly these hagiographical narratives have complicated links with reality, but for the aims of this article it's enough to point out that the medieval body demanded the apparent presence of God or demons or the king's power (Foucault 1975).

5. Of course, meats and some other products are prohibited, and all fast days are kept, but cooks always aspire to provide variety and abundance for the permanent dwellers. The idea of the value of fasting is quite common, but it isn't realized in practice. This fact is especially interesting because many monasteries experience a shortage of funds. In that case, cooks sacrifice the quality but not the quantity of food.

6. Such descriptions may be found in monasterial booklets that were published in the late nineteenth century and recently reprinted. See, for example *Mikhailo-Afonskaia Zakubanskaia pustyn'* ([1897] 1999).

7. On the popular image of Orthodox churches as centers for redistributing objects, see Detelina Tocheva (2011a).

8. Before the revolution, this convent was inhabited by seven hundred sisters.

9. In the Cistercian Order, physical labor was considered an exercise for achieving humility. Such work was assessed as undignified for members of the upper class from which the order drew most of its membership (Asad 1993, 147–53).

10. Many booklets circulating in Orthodox monasteries and churches are also devoted to this question.

11. Apparently, such people can be found across post-Soviet spaces (Naumescu 2012).

12. Some of these ideas may have been acquired through television. In 2006, the "Russia" TV channel showed a quasi-scientific film, *Water*, in which viewers were told that water has the ability to perceive and transmit information, thoughts, and emotions. See http://russia.tv/brand/show/brand_id/10258.

13. Trinity-Sergius Lavra is one of the most important and famous Russian Orthodox monasteries. In the *lavra* are an ecclesiastical seminary and a cantor's school, where my interlocutor studied before taking her monastic vows. In the post-Soviet era, the *lavra*, like many monasteries, was being repaired. The *lavra* was restored using the most prestigious repair method, known as "Eurorepair" (Evroremont), which means the repair has been done according to European standards. This type of repair is also used in homes and offices. In most contexts, this renovation serves as a sign of the owner's status. Quality was attributed to the high cost of the repair as well as to the prestige of the European materials. In the Orthodox world, however, the nickname "Euro-Lavra" has distinct negative connotations, for Europe is generally considered to be a violation of conservative Orthodox traditional values.

14. The *znamenny* chant is the main type of liturgical singing in ancient Russia. It disappeared from churches in the nineteenth century. At the end of the twentieth century, the *znamenny* chant began to be revived.

15. She generalizes the way of life of ascetics in Siberia.

16. A description of littered cells and an unpleasant smell coming from the saint is characteristic of a new type of modern hagiography: life stories of female elders (Kormina and Shtyrkov 2014).

REFERENCES

Akhmetova, Mariia. 2010. *Konets sveta v odnoi otdel'no vziatoi strane: Religioznye soobshchestva postsovetskoi Rossii i ikh eskhatologicheskii mif.* Moscow: OGI.

Asad, Talal. 1993. *Genealogies of Religion: Discipline and Reasons of Power in Christianity and Islam.* Baltimore: Johns Hopkins University Press.

Avva Dorofei. 2005. *Dushepoleznye poucheniia*. Sergiev Posad: Lod'ia.
Brudny, Yitzhak M. 1998. *Reinventing Russia: Russian Nationalism and the Soviet State, 1953–1991*. Cambridge, MA: Harvard University Press.
Bynum, Caroline Walker. 2007. "Women Mystics and Eucharistic Devotion in the Thirteenth Century." In *Beyond the Body Proper: Reading the Anthropology of Material Life (Body, Commodity, Text)*, edited by Margaret Lock and Judith Farquhar, 202–12. Durham: Duke University Press.
Durkheim, Emile. (1912) 1995. *The Elementary Forms of Religious Life*. New York: Free Press.
Elias, Norbert. (1939) 2000. *The Civilizing Process*. Oxford: Blackwell.
Fajfer, Lukasz. 2012. "The 'Garden of the Virgin Mary' Meets the Twenty-First Century: The Challenge of Technology on Mount Athos." *Religion, State and Society* 40 (3–4): 349–62.
Foucault, Michel. 1973. *The Birth of the Clinic: An Archaeology of Medical Perception*. London: Routledge
———. 1975. *Discipline and Punish: The Birth of the Prison*. New York: Random House.
Glyzina, L. I. 2009. "Poslushaniia nasel'nits Goritskogo monastyria v nachale XX-go veka." *Kirillov: Kraevedcheskii al'manakh* 7:104–19.
Greene, Robert N. 2010. *Bodies Like Bright Stars: Saints and Relics in Orthodox Russia*. DeKalb: Northern Illinois University Press.
Kelly, Catriona. 2013. "From 'Counter-revolutionary Monuments' to 'National Heritage': The Preservation of Leningrad Churches, 1964–1982." *Cahiers du monde russe* 54:1–34.
Kenworthy, Scott. 2010. *The Heart of Russia: Trinity-Sergius, Monasticism, and Society after 1825*. New York: Oxford University Press.
Köllner, Thobias. 2011. "Built with Gold or Tears? Moral Discourses on Church Construction and the Role of Entrepreneurial Donations." In *Multiple Moralities and Religions in Post-Soviet Russia*, edited by Jarrett Zigon, 191–213. New York: Berghahn Books.
Kormina, Jeanne, and Sergey Shtyrkov. 2014. "Staritsa i smert': Zametki na poliakh sovremennykh zhitii." *Gosudarstvo, religiia, tserkov' v Rossii i zarubezhom* 1 (32): 107–30.
Lestvitsa. 1998. *Prepodobnogo ottsa nashego Ioanna igumena gory Sinaiskoi lestvitsa*. Kyiv: Kievo-Pechers'ka Uspens'ka Lavra.
Meyendorff, John. 1974. *St. Gregory Palamas and Orthodox Spirituality*. Crestwood, NY: St. Vladimir's Seminary Press.
Mikhailo-Afonskaia Zakubanskaia pustyn'. (1897) 1999. Krasnodar: Krasnodarskie Izvestiia.
Moore, Barrington, Jr. 1987. "Austerity and Unintended Riches." *Comparative Studies in Society and History* 29 (4): 787–810.
Moroz, Andrei Borisovich. 2009. *Sviatye Russkogo Severa: Narodnaia agiografiia*. Moscow: OGI.
Naumescu, Vlad. 2012. "Learning the 'Science of Feelings': Religious Training in Eastern Christian Monasticism." *Ethnos* 77 (2): 227–51.
Orsi, Robert. 2006. *Between Heaven and Earth: The Religious Worlds People Make and the Scholars Who Study Them*. Princeton: Princeton University Press.
Paganopoulos, Michelangelo. n.d. "The Concept of 'Economy' in Two Monasteries of Mount Athos." Paper presented at the Third Panhellenic Conference, Volos, Greece,

2012. Last accessed April 10, 2017. Retrieved from https://www.academia.edu/2349875/_The_Concept_of_Economy_in_Two_Monasteries_of_Mount_Athos.

Palmisano, Stefania. 2015. *Exploring New Monastic Communities: The (Re)invention of Tradition*. Farnham, UK: Ashgate.

Pirogovskaya, Maria. 2014. "The Plague at Vetlyanka, 1878–1879: The Discourses and Practices of Hygiene and the History of Emotions." *Forum for Anthropology and Culture* 10:133–64.

Robson, Roy R. 2007. "Transforming Solovki: Pilgrim Narratives, Modernization, and Late Imperial Monastic Life." In *Sacred Stories: Religion and Spirituality in Modern Russia*, edited by Mark Steinberg and Heather Coleman, 44–60. Bloomington: Indiana University Press.

Tocheva, Detelina. 2011a. "An Ethos of Relatedness: Foreign Aid and Grassroots Charities in Two Orthodox Parishes in North-Western Russia." In *Multiple Moralities and Religions in Post-Soviet Russia*, edited by Jarrett Zigon, 67–91. New York: Berghahn Books.

———. 2011b. "Ot vosstanovleniia khrama k sozdaniiu obshchiny: Samoogranichenie i material'nye trudnosti kak istochniki prikhodskoi identichnosti." In *Prikhod i obshchina v sovremennom pravoslavii: Kornevaia sistema rossiiskoi religioznosti*, edited by Alexander Agadjanian and Kathy Rousellet, 277–97. Moscow: Ves' Mir.

Wagner, William. 2003. "Paradoxes of Piety: The Nizhegorod Convent of the Exaltation of the Cross, 1807–1935." In *Orthodox Russia: Belief and Practice under the Tsars*, edited by Valerie A. Kivelson and Robert H. Greene, 211–38. University Park: Penn State University Press.

Zhitiia sviatykh sviatitelia Dimitriia Rostovskogo. (May 1907) 2005a. *Pamiat' prepodobnogo ottsa nashego Nikity Stolpnika, Pereiaslavskogo chudotvortsa*. Moscow: Lestvitsa.

———. (October 1907) 2005b. *Zhitie prepodobnogo Savvy Vysherskogo*. Moscow: Lestvitsa.

COMPETING PRAYERS FOR UKRAINE

SONJA LUEHRMANN

In november 2013, citizens of Kyiv and other Ukrainian cities took to the streets in protest against the government of President Viktor Yanukovych and in support of policies that would bring the country in closer alliance with the European Union. The movement, which quickly became known as Euromaidan (after the principal place of demonstrations in Kyiv, Independence Square or Maidan Nezalezhnosti), successfully toppled the government. However, the conflict escalated as neighboring Russia annexed the Crimean Peninsula and pro-Russian and pro-Kyiv militias started fighting in Eastern Ukraine. The conflict has complex religious dimensions (Wanner 2014), as Ukraine is home to a large number of Russian Orthodox congregations that belong to the Moscow Patriarchate but also boasts its own Kievan Patriarchate, a Ukrainian Orthodox Autocephalous Church (neither of them recognized by most other Orthodox churches), and a large Greek Catholic Church that observes Eastern liturgical rites but recognizes the supreme authority of the pope in Rome. Evangelical Protestants are also highly represented in Ukraine's public life and took an active part in the protests. Since 2014, both the Russian Orthodox Church of the Moscow Patriarchate and the Ukrainian Orthodox Church of the Kievan Patriarchate include prayers for peace in Ukraine in the Divine Liturgy, drawing on shared biblical formulas but with subtle differences in content and language.

The "Prayer for Peace in Ukraine" is recited in Ukrainian during the so-called fervent litany in Kyiv's Transfiguration Cathedral, a newly constructed church belonging to the Kievan Patriarchate. Drawing on the language of the Psalms, it includes images of military strength as well as images of peace, framing those who pray as under attack from outside enemies:

> Lord Our God, strong and steadfast in battle, we, though undeserving, call for Your help and pray: stretch out Your hands in mercy and save our country from war, bloodshed, and suffering. We do not place our trust in our own bow, and our own weapons will not protect us, but we hope for Your almighty help: keep our Fatherland in peace, soften by Your mercy the hardened hearts of enemies, avert their evil intentions, we pray to You, Almighty King, hear us and have mercy upon us.
>
> Look down from heaven, Lord, and do not let our enemies lift their swords and string their bows to subdue us, Your undeserving servants, who praise You faithfully. Make haste to change our sorrows into joy, and calamity into stable peace. Do not allow the suffering of mothers and tears of children, but accept their prayers for us sinners and useless ones as incense before Your Great Throne, giving our Ukraine peace and quiet; we pray to You from our hearts, Merciful Benefactor, hear us and have mercy upon us.[1]

The Church Slavonic "Prayer for the end of internecine strife, to be read during liturgy in the fervent litany," was issued by Patriarch Kirill of Moscow in June 2014, to be recited in all churches of the Moscow Patriarchate, in Russia as well as in Ukraine. Significantly, it was first introduced on June 22, 2014, the Sunday that marked the seventy-third anniversary of Hitler's attack on the Soviet Union. The date simultaneously served to remind Orthodox faithful of a powerful pull to unity with other post-Soviet countries and reinforced attempts in the Russian media to portray the new Ukrainian government and its supporters as "Fascists." At the same time, the text of the prayer avoids overtly taking sides, asking instead for an end to "internecine strife." This reflects both the conciliar tone of Orthodox liturgy and an awareness that the clergy and faithful of Moscow Patriarchate congregations within Ukraine could be placed in a vulnerable position by openly pro-Kremlin positions emanating from their hierarchy. As has often happened in the history of Orthodox churches, a language that is open to multiple interpretations serves to bridge internal differences and project a unified, if underdetermined, vision of the church's political persona.

Lord Jesus Christ our God, look with Your merciful eyes upon the sorrow and painful cries of Your children in the Ukrainian land.

Deliver Your people from internecine strife, quench the spilling of blood, avert imminent disasters. Bring those deprived of shelter into houses, feed the hungry, comfort those who mourn, and reunite those who were separated.

Do not let Your flock decline, who were put into misery by their kin, but in Your generosity bring reconciliation soon. Soften hardened hearts and turn them to knowledge of You. Give peace to Your Church and her faithful children, so that in unity of hearts and unity of mouths we may praise You, our Lord and Savior, forever and ever.[2]

These contemporary prayers show a difficult dance between visions of territorial jurisdiction, awareness of conflicting political commitments within the church, and claims to maintaining a transnational vision of Orthodox Christendom at times of war.

NOTES

1. See http://www.preobraz.kiev.ua/prayers/peace_in_ukraine/, posted April 2015, last accessed November 21, 2016.

2. See http://www.patriarchia.ru/db/text/3675026.html, posted June 17, 2014, last accessed November 21, 2016.

REFERENCE

Wanner, Catherine. 2014. "'Fraternal' Nations and Challenges to Sovereignty in Ukraine: The Politics of Linguistic and Religious Ties." *American Ethnologist* 41 (3): 427–39.

8 ORTHODOX REVIVALS

Prayer, Charisma, and Liturgical Religion

SIMION POP

CONCERNED ORTHODOX

I met Elena, an Orthodox woman in her sixties, in 2010 in the Romanian city of Cluj, in Transylvania, while I had been doing ethnographic research on post-Socialist Orthodox revival activities and movements in urban settings. A retired worker, Elena was dedicated to deepening her personal life of prayer and becoming closer to God by attempting to practice the virtues that the Orthodox Church was preaching. Several years ago, she had decided to leave her district parish, where she previously attended weekly services, and join a community gathered around a small wooden church located on a university campus and led by a young Orthodox priest, Father Mihail, having the mission to provide pastoral care for the Orthodox student population in the city. Over time this community had become frequented not only by students but also by Orthodox believers of all ages and from all walks of life who were mainly attracted by the young priest's pastoral vision and style of worship. Father Mihail's approach to pastoral care emphasized the necessity of a conscientious cultivation of the Christian virtues through sustained spiritual guidance and catechization and through active and frequent participation in the sacraments (*taine* in Romanian, translated as "mysteries").

More than anything, Father Mihail insisted on the necessity of "a personal encounter and a sincere relationship with God, with Christ and his saints." Only the unabating practices of virtue, prayer, fasting, and purification through confession and receiving communion make believers capable of that. For the young priest this entailed, first and foremost, the restoring of an authentic Orthodox tradition and the rejection of the presumably invented traditions ("new traditions," as he called them) that have accumulated in the church's life in the last few centuries and have driven away believers from continual participation in the sacraments. His call for restoring the "true tradition" seemed to resonate with the deep concerns of many lay Orthodox, among them Elena, who aspire to have a genuine *viață duhovnicească* ("spiritual life" in English, *pneumatikos bios* in the language of the Greek church fathers). Their main concern was that today, especially after several decades of communism—a political regime hostile to religion—the authentic Orthodox tradition was in need of being rediscovered in the Romanian lands and to a greater extent in Transylvania, which historically was also exposed to long-lasting Catholic and Protestant influences.

I recall the exasperated exclamation of one of my Transylvanian Orthodox interlocutors: "It seems we lost the authentic tradition. We need teachers [of faith] to guide us!" This sense of loss present among these lay Orthodox was heightened by the fact that often, they believed, the ordinary parish life, the immediate environment of their religious lives, seemed to show the unfortunate adaptation of the church to "the ways of the world" rather than make manifest "the ways of God." And the ways of the world were acutely and upsettingly discernible, by the concerned Orthodox I encountered, not simply as putative moral failings and lack of spiritual purpose (of clergy and parishioners alike) but in their experience pertaining to the everyday in an ordinary parish.

Social interactions between clergy and parishioners, among parishioners themselves, both men and women, and between clergy and civil authorities and politicians; styles of chanting and iconography; architecture; organization of the liturgical space and the church's surroundings; the quality of preaching and styles of worship; priests' and parishioners' casual conduct and their way of speaking and dressing—all of these often evinced a *lumesc* (mundane) ethos that the concerned Orthodox had meticulously learned to sense and discern in the minutiae of their everyday life and of their liturgical practice as potentially estranged from the *duh Orthodox* (the Orthodox spirit). Often, the adjective *duhovnicesc* ("spiritual" or "Spirit-filled") was used to describe the presence of the right "spirit." *Duhovnicesc* can be applied to the qualified performance of an Orthodox ritual, to the priest's conduct, and more generally to the quality of one's religious life but also to persons, events, social relationships, conversations, theological exegeses, or states of mind—ultimately to everything that seems to make manifest the ways of God and the presence of the Holy Spirit.

The concerns were manifold. For instance, for the concerned Orthodox, the widespread (if seemingly insignificant) custom of hanging a clock on the wall, especially in rural churches, for presumably practical reasons, close to the sanctuary so that the entire congregation could see it, showed a lack of understanding of the special quality of time and space promoted in the Orthodox liturgy. A liturgical space that was exposed to too much light (especially to electric light) was also seen as not very conducive for spiritual states. A certain kind of liturgical chanting with folkloric influences, widespread in Transylvania, stirred discordant emotions and thereby inhibited concentration and the prayerful detachment from mundane concerns. The charity work and donations that were transformed in mere social occasions for displaying social status were considered as lacking spiritual content and as a lost opportunity for practicing the virtues of humility and hospitality. Addressing the priest in everyday interactions with the formula "Father, Sir" (*domnule părinte* in Romanian), especially in Transylvania, betrayed a misperception of true spiritual (*duhovnicească*) authority. The additional "Sir," indicating a mundane status, was judged as incompatible with an Orthodox notion of "spiritual fatherhood." A priest who did not wear his cassock in daily interactions outside church also showed a worldly attitude. Often, politicians and representative of civil authorities visited parish churches. In fact, civil authorities and secular rulers were habitually commemorated during the Eucharistic liturgy. The political mobilization involving the parish priests as a way of reaching out to the ordinary citizens always triggered questions among the concerned Orthodox about the proper relationship of religion to politics.

There were also more elusive concerns. An Orthodox believer, a young engineer, told me that he decided to leave his district parish, as did Elena, because over time he felt estranged from his fellow congregants, especially during services. He came to believe that this was the result of the infrequent confession practiced in that parish. He then started attending the services at the student wooden church. Here, besides frequent confession that, in his opinion, nurtured a true fellowship and a sense of purified relationships, the young engineer participated in the Eucharistic liturgy where the ancient "kiss of peace" was shared not only among concelebrating clergy, which was the widespread liturgical protocol, but also among the lay congregants. The ancient liturgical gesture was stylized in the form of three rounds of embracing concelebrating fellows standing nearby (sources indicate that early Christians kissed each other on the lips), accompanied by the words "Christ is in our midst—he is and shall be." This engendered, for my interlocutor, the sense of an active participation in the mysterious creation of the living body of Christ, that is, the Eucharistic community as the ultimate Christian fellowship. Reviving the "kiss of peace" in a form that involves the entire congregation, Father Mihail claimed to restore a pristine Orthodox practice belonging to the authentic tradition, facilitating an enhanced personal and active participation in the sacramental mystery.

I have suggested that for the concerned Orthodox I met, such as Elena, the young engineer, and Father Mihail, discerning "the ways of God" from "the ways of the world," the "true tradition" from accumulated, invented traditions, is mostly an ongoing praxis, a way of sensing and making sense, predicated on discursive and embodied Orthodox traditions (Asad 2015; see Luehrmann's introduction in this volume). Such discernment is fostered in what I call a "revival milieu," a network of persons, social relationships, and communities committed to restoring what they consider to be authentic and timeless Orthodoxy. This praxis, as a way of doing and experimenting, involving discipline and inspiration, is nonetheless embedded in social-historical, institutional, and material relationships and is fraught with contradictions, unintended consequences, and potential failure and misrecognitions.

REVIVAL MILIEUS

In this chapter, the inclusive notion of revival milieu is meant to foreground activities and communities driven by a perceived sense of discontentment with the extant state of affairs, in church and in society at large, and purposefully oriented toward precipitating social and personal transformation in accordance to renewed religious aspirations and expectations. In the case of Christianity, and other religious traditions, a fluid vocabulary of overlapping terms is used, both by the observer and observed, to describe and interpret aspects and manifestations in history of these revival activities and communities: revival, renewal, revitalization, restoration, reform, pious, devotional, utopian, enthusiastic, nativistic, charismatic, millenarian. The difference in using one term or another, or a cluster of terms, comes from the predilection for particular analytical frameworks as well as from the diversity of the actual claims of those involved in such revivalistic activities (Burridge 1987). In the case of Eastern Orthodox Christianity, foundational reference to the "holy tradition"—to the sacraments and liturgical practices (Bandak and Boylston 2014; Naumescu 2013; Pelikan 1998; T. Ware 1993)—gives the notion of revival a certain specificity in comparison with other religious traditions.

The revival milieu in contemporary Romania, with its own social and political ramifications, represents the socioreligious (material and symbolic) space wherein the religious and ethical aspirations of the concerned Orthodox are claimed, embodied, and practiced. This milieu links everyday lives and institutional settings, personal commitments and liturgical engagements, self-formation and social outreach. It accommodates the social reality of variable levels of religious commitment among the Orthodox faithful and the encounter between lay and clerical initiatives. Orthodox revival is simultaneously a popular, bottom-up movement and a top-down institutional process, and sometimes clerical attempts claimed as forms of restoring tradition go against lay revivalist expectations. Revivalist initiatives often strive to emancipate themselves from power structures apparently dominated by clericalism in hope of legitimizing alternatives to existing authority. However, the activities and discourses within the revival milieu cut across institutional markers and social boundaries, aggregating members of the clerical hierarchy, parish priests, monks, nuns, and laypeople in competing communities and national and transnational networks facilitated by social mobility and media technologies.

For instance, it is rather common to meet believers belonging to the Romanian revival milieu referring to practices and exemplary persons from monasteries in Mount Athos or from some monastery or parish in Greece or the United Kingdom. Some of them have even visited those places. One can contend that the religious aspirations and practices within the revival milieu have thrived in post-Socialism, amid the typical parochial Orthodox life, precisely because of these translocal connections that could be developed once Romanian society became reconnected to the global circulation of ideas, things, and persons. For instance, for a parish priest belonging to the revival milieu to propose more frequent confession and communion or an all-night prayer vigil in his parish, he has to rely on authoritative traditional arguments and practices that are almost nonexistent in the immediate religious environment of his parishioners but might be reinforced by examples from abroad.

Overall, revival activities point to a dissatisfaction among some Orthodox believers with the current configurations of their tradition that seem to be, on the one hand, incapable of nurturing the personal commitment and interiorization of faith and, on the other, ineffectual in dealing with the challenges of contemporary secular lifestyles (for example, the case of family, parenting, and gender relationships). This motivates attempts to retrieve traditional Orthodox discourses and practices that were presumably nurtured by a genuine Orthodox spirit and effective in making manifest "the ways of God." Thus, the past becomes a confrontational terrain where competing claims and practical resources were deployed in various projects of reviving personal lives and communities. Which historical practices and discourses embodied the "true tradition"? Should one privilege a particular epoch? What are the criteria for restoring one practice or another as belonging to the authentic tradition?

For instance, authoritarian imperial legacies (Byzantine or Tsarist Russian) and the supposedly more democratic early Christian communal aspirations, with their eschatological undertones, are concomitantly revisited to support new Orthodox communal experiments with forms of leadership and styles of worship and to elucidate the relations between the church and the nation-state that are adequate to the social transformations of the present time. Monastic ways of living and worshipping are reconsidered to provide strategies of ethical self-formation and corporate worship. The religious activities within the revival milieu turn to the Orthodox discursive tradition as a space of argumentation and reasoning about the function, scope, and apt performance of certain traditional practices but adapt it by reference to the present and the future.

During my ethnographic fieldwork in Romania, I analyzed multiple ways in which religious practices within the revival milieu oriented toward creating and sustaining appropriate environments for worship and social action. Attempts at reforming and reviving parish life and at creating alternative communities of practice have been also identified in many other parts of the Eastern Christian world (Agadjanian 2013; Halemba 2015; Hann and Goltz 2010; Naumescu 2007; Steinberg and Wanner 2008). The revival impetus seems to be a modality of tradition, the built-in way in which the Orthodox tradition maintains its revelatory capacities for the present time and future expectations.

In this chapter I explore activities within the revival milieu to point out their specificity in a comparative perspective. More specifically, I consider the role of prayer practices within the revival milieu and their capacity for connecting the everyday and ritual performance and for creating a communal arena for self-formation through enhancement of interiorization and personal commitment.

ECONOMIES OF PRAYER

In one of our conversations that took place in 2013, I asked Elena to share more about her daily routine of prayer. She promptly responded that her actual prayer life was far from what she wanted because, even though retired, she was busy taking care of her grandchildren and as a result was left with too little time to dedicate to prayer. Nevertheless, she insisted that she could not imagine her life without prayer and church attendance. Although she would be always eager to help her family, she seemed convinced that ultimately only a prayerful life would make anyone capable of navigating the hardships of life without losing sight of God and his saints' mercy and intervention. As a result of my insistence that learning about her day-to-day practice was important to my research and that I would not regard her words as showing unjustified pride, Elena meticulously started to describe what she had done when one of her sons, working abroad, had gone through some difficult times several weeks prior to our conversation.

I sum up Elena's rich account by pointing up the diversity of prayer practices she engaged in. As soon as she learned about her son's difficulties, she began praying intensely to one of her favorite contemporary saints, Father Arsenie, to intercede for her son.[1] She would use one of the methods of prayer that the saint himself recommended to those who needed his intercession especially in difficult times. The petition should be preceded by the recitation of the Lord's Prayer nine times, presumably for reminding the petitioner that the saint is only the favorable intercessor who supports one's prayer in front of God. Elena added her own contribution: while she prayed to the saint, she would keep several pebbles in her hand that she had taken from the saint's grave, which had been a pilgrimage site for some time. She explained to me that she asked for her invisible companion's protective presence every day, but there were certain times when a more sustained prayer was needed (Pop 2017).

At the same time, she asked her priest-confessor and spiritual father, Father Mihail, to begin commemorating her son's name in the Divine Liturgy for forty days in a row. Elena pointed out to me that the commemoration of someone's name in the Eucharistic liturgy was "very powerful" because the liturgical prayers were more powerful than any personal prayer. The entire community prays together with the celebrating priest. These commemorations were done during the Prothesis or Proskomedia (the preparation of the Eucharistic gifts). This ritual sequence represents the introductory part of the Eucharistic liturgy, which takes place in the sanctuary as the priest prepares the Eucharistic offerings. At that moment, the priest removes small particles, each of them representing the commemorated living and dead, from the loaf of leavened bread (prosphora), carefully prepared as a Eucharistic gift. Those particles representing the commemorated persons would be carefully placed by the end of the liturgy, after the communion rite, in the Eucharistic chalice containing the leftover consecrated wine and bread so that the commemorative particles would eventually be in contact with Christ's body and blood. The priest would then say the following prayer: "Wash away, O Lord, the sins of all those here commemorated, by thy precious blood, through the prayers of thy saints."

Although Elena participated regularly in the Divine Liturgy, receiving communion fairly frequently, during those difficult times she would confess and receive communion even more often. During her confessions, she would pray together with her spiritual father that God's will be done in her son's case, and she would ask for a word of advice that would help her and her son make sense of the entire situation. Elena maintained throughout our conversation that only God knows what is best for everyone and one should accept his will manifested into the trials of life. Almost every time she mentioned "God's will" or "God's mercy," she made the sign of the cross on herself. She also told me that she encouraged her son to pray as much as he could, although she was aware that his considerable workload and daily stress were not much conducive to praying.

Elena considered that intense participation in the sacramental life of the church together with regular periods of fasting would purify her life and strengthen her own capacity to pray and ask for intercession. She emphasized that nobody can learn to pray at home lying in bed. Prayer is much more powerful and effective in the church's sacred space. However, at home she tried keeping to her daily rule of prayer as her spiritual father urged her to do, especially mornings and evenings, when she would use her prayer book. Also, preparation for communion entailed reading a certain order of prayers. At his suggestion, she had also started several years ago to practice the Jesus Prayer (also called "Prayer of the Heart"), consisting in the mental repetition of the formula "Lord Jesus Christ, Son of God, have mercy on me, a sinner." She would do that amid her daily duties or even while walking on the street. This mental prayer helped her do away with the evil thoughts that would get in her mind during the day— for instance, when in a state of despondency concerning the situation of her son. She discreetly hinted at the fact that over time she had some intense experiences (the virtuosi of this special prayer, spiritually improved monks known as hesychasts, mentioned in their accounts the rare mystical moments when they "descend with the mind into the heart," leading them "from earth to heaven") while repeating the Jesus Prayer, but she refrained from any further comment. For her, commenting on that would be a sign of pride and self-complacency that would drive her away from experiencing the work of prayer. She insisted that true prayer was a state of grace that would break into our lives for short moments of time. Most of the time, she thought, we were incapable of focusing on God's presence. However, she would always add, "God's mercy is great, and I try as much as I can to keep remembering him all day."

Orthodox tradition is saturated with prayer practices, individual as well as collective. Elena was not my only Orthodox interlocutor referring to a simultaneous involvement in such diverse practices. Moreover, I noticed that the constant pondering, tacit or stated, of such an involvement was a steady and widespread preoccupation of my interlocutors and not necessarily of those professing a more methodical prayer life. I encountered such questions as these: Why should I pray in church as much as possible considering that I already pray at home? Why is liturgical prayer more powerful? How should I pray during the Divine Liturgy? Is sincerity the only condition for an effective prayer? How can repentance and purification strengthen my prayer? What does it mean to pray unceasingly? Is this possible for a layperson? Is the Jesus Prayer reserved to monastic life? Outside church, should I pray with my own words, or should I use a prayer book? When is the proper moment for praying during a day? Should I use in my personal prayer those Psalms that contain curses? What does it entail to pray for somebody dear, and what is the meaning of liturgical commemoration? What is the point of paying a prayer service to be done by a priest? Why do I need to pray to the saints? How do they intercede for me? Do we have to use the hymn dedicated to the saint? Is my personal prayer not worthy? Why do we need icons to pray? Can I pray in a Catholic or Protestant church? Why is the spontaneous and exalted prayer of Pentecostals, for instance, considered inappropriate and even devilish?

One can identify within Orthodox tradition numerous attempts (Krueger 2014; Taft 1986) of the ecclesiastical authorities to organize the life of prayer (both in monastic and parochial settings) by integrating the individual and liturgical prayer in coherent disciplinary programs articulated through sound pedagogical and theological arguments and suited for daily use and specific periods of the liturgical year (for example, Lent). Attending to the specificity of each of these disciplinary programs throughout history can offer us important insights not only into the formation of Orthodox subjects (Krueger 2014) but also into the ways in which ecclesiastical authorities envisaged the insertion and orientation of the Orthodox communities within society at large (see, for example, Kenworthy 2008). However, leaving aside the complicated (and often conflictual—see, for instance, the idiorhythmic versus cenobitic debate within the context of monasticism) history of the constitution and codification in liturgical and prayer books of these ideal programs of prayer, one can assert that, within the Orthodox tradition, the monastic models had become dominant, especially after the Byzantine iconoclasm. Since then the organization of the liturgical life of parishes has been and still is an abbreviation of and adaptation to parochial conditions of the monastic programs (scripted in the Typikon, for example).

Father Mihail was aware of the contradictions that came with the fact that any attempt at intensification of prayer life in his community inevitably resorted to monastic ways of organizing individual and liturgical prayer in the context of a lay community consisting of persons who had not taken monastic vows but instead had families and jobs. Revival communities, such as that of Father Mihail, are thus confronted with the difficult and unexpected task of creating their own way nonetheless, predicated on Orthodox discursive and embodied traditions. As I already mentioned, Elena was consciously dedicated to her own ethical cultivation and spiritual improvement. To achieve that, she had decided to join Father Mihail's community, where she found a religious environment sustaining her efforts. This decision had placed her within a specific field of prayer practices demanding disciplinary efforts and participatory resources and generating, at the same time, an arena for self-formation and ethical responsiveness. Although I noticed Elena's fascination with the great charismatic monks of tradition, the heroes of "unceasing prayer," her choice to talk about a certain period of intensification of prayer triggered by her son's difficult times, instead of presenting her aspirations to an ideal program of prayer, conveyed the notion that her prayer life was necessarily intertwined with the daily domestic responsibilities. There would be no ideal conditions of withdrawal from the flow of everyday life in order to cultivate improbable monastic disciplines and virtuosities. She insisted explicitly, "We [laypeople] cannot pray as monks do!"

To understand the complex predicament of self-formation and prayer within the revival milieu and to capture the transformative dynamics within these communities and their insertion and orientation within the larger religious field, I propose the analytical notion of "economy of prayer."[2] This notion represents a distinct approach to studying Orthodox prayer. Elena's account suggests that prayer life can be regarded as a participatory field of practice. Instead of presupposing clear-cut taxonomies that isolate specific prayer practices in categories such as individual and collective, spontaneous and formulaic, mental and bodily, personal and vicarious, situational and ritualized, this approach sees Orthodox prayer life as a capacity of acting and participating within economies of prayer shaped by the Orthodox discursive and embodied traditions. Economies of prayer are predicated on matrices of power relations and authorizing processes (Asad 1993)[3] and on specific conceptions of self-formation and agency, human and nonhuman (Keane 2007). They involve ritual performances, exemplary persons, and constitutive social relationships and include persuasive and disciplinary practices, bodily and sensory engagements, material and textual resources. The plural "economies of prayer" indicates the historical generation and local embeddedness of various participatory fields of practice within the Orthodox tradition, each of them entailing specific ways of integrating individual and liturgical lives of prayer, connecting the everyday and ritual events and producing a complex, non-individualized prayerful agency. Indicating open-ended and contingent ways of organizing prayer life and depending on the ongoing praxis of actors involved (clergy and laypeople alike), they reflect more than mere exemplification of ideal disciplinary programs of prayer under specific historical and social conditions. In this sense, the constitution of revivalist economies of prayer enhances participatory capabilities and personal commitment and creates new forms of belonging, with far-reaching and unintended consequences for the orientation and insertion of the Orthodox communities within the church and society at large.

ORTHODOX REVIVALS, MYSTERIES, AND CHARISMA

One fundamental question that has become apparent in the case of Orthodox revivals concerns the ways in which a hierarchical, liturgical religion such as Eastern Orthodox Christianity is able to permeate believers' everyday lives and foster interiorization of faith and personal commitment. This question opens up broader problematics concerning the modernity of this branch of Christianity. The notions of interiorization and personal reform are not necessarily products of modernity but rather belong to the historical core of apostolic Christianity (Ladner 2004; Krueger 2014; Stroumsa 2009; Taft 1986). However, the historical and institutional configurations of these processes changed dramatically over centuries. It is well known that Eastern Orthodox Christianity did not undergo something similar to or as radical as the Protestant Reformation, although historians have identified, especially in the domain of liturgical life, recurrent attempts at reform and revival (Denysenko 2015; Pott 2010; Meyendorff 2014; Zhuk 2004; Wybrew 2013). Scholars such as Charles Taylor (2007), Webb Keane (2007), and Talal Asad (1993), following Max Weber's early exploration (1985), have produced accounts of convergence between complex historical processes of reform and revival within Western Christianity and "moral narratives of modernity" (Keane 2007). They tell the story of the attempts to displace liturgical, outward, sacramental religion in favor of a more personal, sincere, inward commitment. Consequently, sacred times, spaces, and vocations lost importance in comparison with the affirmation of ordinary life as the locus of religious accomplishment. This story of displacement reveals complex processes of dematerialization and deritualization, mainly based on semiotic ideologies (Keane 2007) and authorizing processes (Asad 1993) embedded in languages and practices of purification and interior belief, that is, on forms of disengagement of the self from materiality of religion. Nonetheless, these accounts point out that there are necessary limits to processes of purification and interiorization: semiotic forms and materialities of a religion, however transcendental and interiorized, are integral to its constitution. Beyond the historical trajectory of Western Christianity, to become moral imperative and practicable possibility in everyday life, reforms and revivals attempting to create a certain religious self and community still have to be predicated on material practices and pragmatic conceptions capable of connecting bodies, words, and things, human and nonhuman agents, and communal events and social relationships.

In the case of Orthodox revival that I discuss below, interiorization and personal commitment seem to be intensified, as in Elena's case, by the enhanced believer's capacity to act and participate in the material and social practices made possible by sacramental rituals that are the liturgical and institutional core of the Orthodox tradition and not necessarily by creating alternative forms of ritualization outside of them (see, for example, the case of Catholic charismatic revivals, Csordas 1997). How can holy mysteries and the accompanying economies of prayer become the locus of revival transformations? To approach this question, I propose a framework based on understanding the relations between charisma, ritual, and self-formation.

Anthropologists of religion working all over the globe have recurrently revisited Weber's (1978) notion of charisma (Csordas 1997; Feuchtwang 2010; Feuchtwang and Mingming 2001; Kirsch 2008; Reinhardt 2014; Tambiah 1984). These contributions have reasserted the analytical value of charisma as referring to the source, locus, and object of certain transformative potentialities and creative interventions recognizable within religious traditions. They also have attempted to overcome the temptation (reinforced partially by the theological origins of the notion, Riesebrodt 1999) to reify charisma in persons, objects, or events and proposed instead to see it as potentiality, process, and activity. Moreover, where Weber focuses on exceptional personalities and the necessary historical and organizational transformation of charisma from original and unstable to conventional and institutional, these scholars open the way for a more sustained investigation of how charisma is produced and transmitted through daily disciplines and ritual practices connected to processes of self-formation.

A revised notion of charisma can help us identify, conceptually and empirically, situations, conditions, and means within a religious tradition by which it resourcefully and recurrently generates its own transformative expectations (Feuchtwang and Mingming 2001, 19). "Charisma is the name for the innovative and restorative potential of tradition," remark Stephan Feuchtwang and Wang Mingming (2001, 19). In this sense, Eastern Orthodox Christianity, and more specifically the contemporary revival milieu, can be treated as a "tradition of charisma" that is not routinized charisma, as in a classical Weberian perspective, but rather "a tradition of break with routine" that "contains a strand of hope for transformation, which legitimizes an alternative to existing authority, or for innovation even though it presents itself as restoration" (19). In some cases this "hope for transformation" (for example, the unrestrained work of the Holy Spirit—in terms of tradition) can annihilate the very conditions of its emergence, as in the case of the Protestant Reformation and the myriad of revival movements it spawned. In Eastern Orthodox Christianity, charisma can be approached as an authorizing and persuasive process (Asad 1993; Csordas 1997) defining tradition in its generic potentiality, maintaining revelatory and transformative capacities for each historical generation and creating responsive subjects.

In the remainder of the chapter, I examine how holy mysteries and accompanying economies of prayer can become charismatic authorizing processes in revivalist personal and collective transformations. In the case of Father Mihail and Elena's community, the frequent and active participation in sacraments, especially in confession and Holy Communion, was the main source and locus of an Orthodox self-formation sustaining *viața duhovnicească*. Confession and communion, conventionally among the seven most important sacraments instituted by the church as privileged channels of grace and of the effective presence of the triune God, are the two mysteries that can be administrated frequently and integrated into a quotidian program of spiritual improvement. The frequency and modality of their administration (Kizenko 2012; Meyendorff 2014) has been an issue of ongoing debate in the Orthodox world. Such debates are connected to the ways the ecclesiastical authorities have framed religious self-formation (in monastic and parochial settings alike) but also have far-reaching social and political ramifications for the insertion of Orthodox communities within wider society. In post-Byzantine Orthodoxy, especially, the ritual connection between confession and communion has become a contentious issue because of two significant historical processes. On the one hand, since the Middle Ages, private, auricular confession, based on an ancient model of a personal conversation between monastic novices and their spiritual fathers but adapted to priestly, sacramental authority, gradually replaced the public penitential system of the early church oriented toward the reintegration of those who had lapsed in the Eucharistic community (Demacopoulos 2007; Meyendorff 2014). On the other, following certain liturgical and ecclesiastical transformations (for example, the recognition of Christianity as a public religion in Constantine's time), the practice of lay communion became infrequent from the fourth century onward (Taft 1992, 2007; Wybrew 2013), meaning that the faithful started to participate in the Eucharistic liturgy without receiving communion.

Today, the widespread situation in the Orthodox world is that the frequency of sacramental participation, in confession and communion, among many of the Orthodox faithful in ordinary parishes is rather low. Typically, the Orthodox faithful are advised to confess and partake of communion at the same time during the main four fasting periods of the liturgical year. There are variations in practice in different Orthodox countries: in Russia and Romania, the tie between confession and communion is usually strictly observed, although on rare occasions priests will allow people to take communion without having confessed that day or the evening before. Easter week, for example, can be such a more "generous" time. In Greece, by contrast, there is a practice closer to that of many Catholic churches, where people confess once a month or more rarely and can then take communion as often as they wish until the next confession. Not all priests in Greece are entitled to hear confession and to function as spiritual fathers. In Russia and Romania, though, the entitlement to hear confession almost automatically comes with ordination. Practically, Lent is the privileged time for confession and communion for those Orthodox believers who try to regularly participate in the Sunday liturgy. When some life crises occur, they tend to confess and communicate more often. In many parts of the Orthodox world, most of the faithful confess and communicate only a few times during their entire life.

In the Romanian revival community that I present here, the intensification of sacramental life through frequent and active participation generates an economy of prayer that incorporates more and more of believers' daily life and demands interiorization and personal commitment. These ritual transformations are connected to processes of charismatization of the sacramental tradition.

In the Orthodox tradition, all sacraments are accomplished through prayer (Meyendorff 1979). The ritual of confession thus contains specific prayers and liturgical gestures. The penitent confesses his or her sins privately to a priest (sins often read from a confessional manual by the priest himself) in a private place near the sanctuary and usually in front of an icon of Christ and then receives a formal absolution from the priest through a priestly prayer. The ritual involves specific bodily gestures on the part of the priest and penitent: the penitent kneels, and the priest places the stole on the penitent's head. At the moment of absolution, the priest puts his hand on the stole, making the sign of the cross on the penitent's head and reciting the prayer of remission. The ritual is framed to indicate that God's forgiveness is a response to the priestly prayer made in the name of the penitent. The ritual of confession sometimes contains a short conversation where the penitent is advised how to avoid the confessed sins and requires the penitent to perform an *epitimia* (a formal penance) consisting of prayers, prostrations, readings, or fasting.

In the revival community, without downplaying the importance of sacramental absolution, Father Mihail significantly accentuated the spiritual guidance aspect of the ritual, entailing the inauguration of a specific relationship between the penitent and his or her priest-confessor: discipleship. The practice of confession is now determined by the need, on the part of the disciple, for an increased spiritual intimacy and constant supervision from the spiritual father and not necessarily by formal requirements of confessing sins several times in a year. The ritual is thus particularly infused with practices of spiritual fatherhood (eldership) that originally developed in monastic milieus (Demacopoulos 2007; Paert 2010, 2014; K. Ware 1974). Practices such as "the disclosure of thoughts," the "unquestioning obedience" (or "cutting off the will") on the part of the disciple (see Dubovka, this volume), and "discernment of spirits" and "the utterance of prophetic word" on the part of the spiritual father establish an intense interpersonal relationship that is missing altogether from the brief and formalistic ritual of confession in an ordinary parish.

The Orthodox notion of spiritual guidance implies that discovering and following God's will is the main way of overcoming one's sinful nature and of achieving gradually the communion with God, deification (*theosis*; see Naumescu, this volume). God's will is not simply a rule to adhere to, presented in scripture or tradition, but more of a personal relationship, a form of communion, to uniquely embody in one's life, with consequences for ethical conduct. The confession and absolution of sins should not be considered ends in themselves but rather the necessary means in the constant struggle for personally discerning God's will and for becoming responsive to it. The ethical self-formation and spiritual improvement involve not only the retrospective confession of sins but also the prospective disclosure of intimate thoughts and passions that potentially hide temptations from the evil spirits and disrupt the self in his or her aspiration for communion with God. The constant self-examination and search for God's will should occur in each situation of one's life (domestic, professional, or strictly religious) because each of them has the potential to bring one closer to or alienate one from God. Within the Orthodox revival milieu, the ritual of confession and spiritual fatherhood have become the privileged means to search for God's will, often more important than one's conscience and close reading of scripture. I often heard in the revival milieu that "there is no true Orthodox without a spiritual father."

There is a widespread expectance within the revival milieu that under certain conditions, one's spiritual father can be charismatically endowed by God to become a prophet for his disciple.[4] He is able to utter "God's word," "the prophetic word" that is not the fruit of his human wisdom or conventional teaching and addresses, by disclosing God's will, the current spiritual situation of the disciple. The mysterious personal relationship inaugurated between the disciple and his or her spiritual father is essentially a prayerful relationship. Disciples have the confidence that their spiritual father prays for them constantly, and the spiritual father expects sustained and committed prayer from his disciples. Only prayer can open the spiritual father's heart for it to be inhabited by "the prophetic word." As I was told by many of my interlocutors, prayer could acquire sometimes unscripted, emotional forms during the ritual of confession when the penitent and the spiritual father start praying together in a common attempt to discover God's will for a specific situation (without, nonetheless, expecting a response on the spot). Moreover, many believers told me that they mentally pray (usually they say the Jesus Prayer) during confession in waiting for "God's word." Confession, seen as a privileged locus for discovering God's will and not only for speaking out one's sins, involves also an intense program of prayerful preparation outside the frame of the ritual performance. The ethical disposition to receive and submit to the spiritual father's "prophetic word" and to act accordingly within the world is nurtured by prayer.

Not every confession and spiritual advice calls for "the prophetic word." Nor does every life situation. Usually God's will can be discerned through the meaningful conversation with the spiritual father taking place within the ritual frame of the sacrament, "where the devil can't enter," as I was often told. However, there are moments in life when the transformative power of "the prophetic word" is expressly needed. The capacity of the disciple to discern (and then to obey) in the spiritual father's words the providential word from God, disclosing God's will at the right moment, is enhanced by intense personal prayer on the part of the disciple as well as of the spiritual father. There is always the possibility that the spiritual father's message represents only his human wisdom and experience. The priest as a sinner himself is prone to fail in delivering the divine word and imposing his human will onto the disciples. In the Orthodox tradition (Paert 2010), the prophetic guidance has been usually performed by stellar charismatic elders possessing thaumaturgical powers and exerting their prophetic gift in a sovereign way even for sporadic visitors who were not necessarily their disciples.

Today, frequent visits to charismatic elders found in monasteries are made almost impossible by the lifestyle of an urban member of the revival milieu. Believers search for solutions at hand, that is, for urban priests, such as Father Mihail, willing to responsibly engage in spiritual fatherhood. Those priests are recognized as having an exemplary life dedicated to the church and certain spiritual qualities that make them apt for the task. For example, Father Mihail was regarded as a "man of prayer" with a special gift for guiding young people. However, these qualities are decisively amplified by the power of the mystery of confession. In monastic tradition, the spiritual father did not have to exert his guidance in the context of sacramental confession; his own charismatic endowment was enough for establishing a relationship of spiritual guidance. In the case I present, one witnesses an interesting reconfiguration of the Orthodox tradition of charisma, where the dynamic spiritual guidance of monastic type is combined with the institutionalized authorizing process actualized in the priestly performance of the mystery. The efficacy of the sacrament of confession is extended from the priestly prayer of absolution to include the unpredictable fruits of discipleship.

Ethical practices of self-examination, obedience, and discernment accompanying the revivalist ritual of confession are thus intertwined with the abilities to pray and identify the works of prayer in the mysterious quality of discipleship. The incentives and effects of personal prayer are inscribed into an ethical relationship that should be nurtured and cultivated: God chooses to utter "prophetic words," personally addressed, through the mouth of another person (in this case, one's spiritual father), and this is ultimately a humbling experience. Trust, intimacy, responsibility, and loyalty are all intertwined with one's attempt to pray well and discover God's will at the right moment (*kairos*). In the revival milieu, spiritual fatherhood is a privileged way, instituted by the church through the ritual of confession, to develop personal prayer as an ethical way of encountering and accepting the other and, ultimately, God. As with any other relationship, the relationship with the spiritual father can be superficial, treacherous, and insincere. It could fail because of both parties involved.

However, in this case, the failure to engage in sustained personal relationships represents also a failure of prayer as ethical practice.

In addition to frequent confession and spiritual guidance, another unusual feature of revivalist congregations such as that led by Father Mihail is that participating in the Divine Liturgy without receiving communion is regarded as a failure to complete the ritual.[5] In this case, the sacramental change of the offerings effected by priestly prayers and then clergy communion do not represent the completion of the ritual. Only the transformation of the entire congregation and individual Christians through the ingestion of the Eucharistic Christ accomplishes the mystery. The steady decrease in the frequency of lay communion started in the fourth century, and the current shape of the Divine Liturgy ritually downplays the significance of receiving communion (Taft 1992, 2007; Wybrew 2013). Lay faithful spend much of the ritual praying in front of icons and looking at the icon-screen (iconostasis), which blocks the sight of the sanctuary where the Eucharistic action takes place. The importance of prayerful commemorations during the liturgy and the distribution of the antidoron (pieces of blessed but not consecrated prosphora received by believers at the end of the liturgy) indicate the necessity of substitutes for the Eucharistic communion. Ecclesiastic authorities also legitimized various forms of "spiritual communion" and "mystical contemplation" during the Divine Liturgy to replace physical ingestion and developed ascetic models of preparation for communion that emphasized more and more the "unworthiness" of the ordinary believer for a frequent communion and the Eucharist as a dreadful mystery especially dangerous for those "unclean" (Taft 2007).

In revivalist congregations, there are several ritual modifications that I discuss here meant to accommodate and enhance the practice of frequent communion: the audible recitation of the Eucharistic prayer, open sanctuary, and modified practices of preparation for communion. They show and produce the intensification of interiorization and personal commitment while drawing people into enhanced participation in a traditional ritual, thus indicating a charismatization of the Eucharistic mystery.

One of the salient features of the Orthodox liturgical space is the presence of the iconostasis that separates the nave of the church from the sanctuary (Taft 2007; Wybrew 2013). The iconostasis consists of several rows of icons arranged in a precise way and two lateral and one central door (with curtains) covering the entrances to the sanctuary and the sight of the altar. In the standard liturgy of Byzantine rite, the main acts of the Eucharistic ritual enacting the Lord's Supper take place in the sanctuary behind the iconostasis with doors closed at crucial times. The fundamental prayer of the Divine Liturgy, the Eucharistic prayer (*anaphora*, offering), is read silently by the celebrant priests in the sanctuary in front of the altar (Krueger 2014; Woolfenden 2007). In this prayer, the celebrant narrates the biblical story of redemption, utters the "words of institution" (*anamnesis*), and invokes the Holy Spirit (*epiclesis*) to change the Eucharistic gifts and to sanctify the participant community to properly receive the body and the blood of Christ. The Byzantine text of the Eucharistic prayer still in use today recounts what Jesus did at the Last Supper when he instituted the Eucharist and the entire salvation history actualized by Christ's Incarnation and Resurrection but also mentions explicitly the "fruits of communion" with the Eucharistic Christ, communion that refers to the whole participant community, clergy and laypeople alike. Behind the iconostasis, the celebrating priest necessarily receives communion at every liturgy he performs, and then he emerges in front of the iconostasis to show the consecrated gifts, Christ's body and blood, to the congregants and to offer communion to those who come forward. As already mentioned, very few adult believers communicate in a regular Sunday liturgy.

Father Mihail, in his community, started to read aloud the Eucharistic prayer and to keep open the doors and curtains that obstruct the sight of the altar, especially during the recitation of the Eucharistic prayer. By doing so, he claimed to retrieve early Christian practices. His explicit intention was to enhance the experience of communion that should be considered the climax of the liturgical participation. The recitation of the Eucharistic prayer was made audible for the entire congregation (technology is also part of this: an audio-system discreetly enhances the voice in the sanctuary).[6] The prayer is also punctuated at certain moments by a loud "Amen" uttered by the entire congregation. This way of reciting the Eucharistic prayer signals that the priest prays together with the congregation instead of merely representing it silently before God. As a matter of fact, the text of the prayer suggests that the "we" of the congregation led by the priest is the originating and performing subject. The shift toward an audible Eucharistic prayer and the open sanctuary emphasizes the necessary unity between the liturgical text and the ritual action and the fact that the Eucharistic ritual is completed by believers' desire and need for communion. In this sense, the authority of Eucharistic prayer does not lie in its internal semantic structure as sacramental formula but in its specific ritual enactment by the entire community led by the priest. The open sanctuary allows congregants to see the priestly gestures of preparation of the sacred food and intensifies the sense of participation in a sacred meal. The Eucharist thus can be perceived as the mystery of the actual "food" and "drink" for those in need, for the entire congregation, and not only of word and priestly recitation of a sacramental formula effecting the mysterious change of the offerings to be seen from a distance. Congregants are actively engaged in the Eucharistic action and do not only passively contemplate the sacred objects in a play of veiling and unveiling. Note here the departure from notions of purification through entextualization that are associated with religious revivals in the Protestant and Muslim worlds (Keane 2007, 2015). In Orthodox revivals, words and their embeddedness within ritual actions do become more important, in this case through loud recitation of the Eucharistic prayer and through ingestion of the Eucharist. Through communion the drama of redemption enacted on the altar, for seeing and hearing, is eventually transferred from the altar into the faithful bodies (see Flood 2014 for the power of ingestion of the sacred in Christianity and Islam). The material referent of the words, the Eucharistic Christ, embodied in the sacred food, becomes endowed with more intrinsic power to transform persons and communities, rather than remaining the iconic Christ contemplated by the faithful in scriptural texts and holy icons.[7]

The act of frequent communion (for example, every Sunday) can easily become routine, and that is a major concern for believers in the revival community. I was often told that nothing can show the danger of routine better than priests' continuous communion, which for many has become a mere ritual act to be accomplished. The preparation for communion and the act itself should break with routine. Because of infrequent communion, the standard preparation involves a set of ritual purity requirements that are expected to make the "unworthy" believers worthy of receiving the terrifying sacrament: confession of sins (mortal sins, such as murder, adultery, and apostasy, but also fornication, despondency, pride, envy, and anger would prohibit someone from communion), several days of fasting and sexual abstinence, and private recitation of an order of prayers for preparation. In the case of frequent communion, the believers do not discard the ritual preparation but apply it in a different way. They fast especially on the day of communion, and that often includes sexual abstinence (with the condition that they observe the usual Orthodox days of fasting on Wednesdays and Fridays). They also try to read, in the days before, the specific order of prayers, even though they communicate weekly.

Nevertheless, the daily preparation of a sincere and pure conscience appropriate for receiving the sacraments becomes the main focus in the revival community. Again, confession is not only a ritual requirement but also the place where the sincere conscience is forged through spiritual guidance and purification from evil thoughts and passions. "Nobody would ever be worthy of communion, so it is important to have a prepared conscience and a true desire to encounter the living Christ," I was told. "The Divine Liturgy itself is the best preparation for communion, but you have to maintain your spiritual watchfulness and prayerful attention." Ultimately, the spiritual father decides if one is aptly prepared for frequent communion. He gives his blessing, in each case, after familiarization with the spiritual state of his disciple and not based on applying strict rules, emphasizing again the preparation of a sincere conscience. Receiving the Eucharist is a tremendous personal and transformative encounter with Christ that should be intensely expected at every Divine Liturgy one participates in and that reverberates in the everyday life through the power of believers' ritualized, eucharized bodies. These fragments from standard prayers used in preparation for communion evoke this well: "I tremble, taking fire, lest I should burn as wax and hay. O dread Mystery! O Divine Compassion! How can I who am clay partake of the divine Body and Blood and become incorruptible!" Or "The Lord is good. O taste and see! For of old He became like us for us, and once offered Himself as a sacrifice to His Father and is perpetually slain, sanctifying communicants." Or "Let these Holy Things be for my healing and purification and enlightenment and protection and salvation and sanctification of body and soul, for the turning away of every phantasy and all evil practice and diabolical activity working subconsciously in my members, for confidence and love towards Thee, for reformation of life and security, for an increase of virtue and perfection, for fulfillment of the commandments, for communion with the Holy Spirit, as a provision for eternal life, and as an acceptable defense at Thy dread Tribunal, not for judgment or for condemnation." These are authoritative prayers ascribed to great church fathers, and through their frequent recitation with heightened attention, revivalist believers strive to bring the sense of mystery and self-interrogation before God into their everyday lives and to enhance their prayerful attendance of the ritual.

CONCLUDING REMARKS

In this chapter I have mapped out the social and ritual space of the Orthodox revival milieu as I encountered it in my fieldwork in Romania. Drawing on that, I have proposed a comparative framework for approaching revival activities in other cases belonging to the Orthodox tradition. Charismatization of tradition, as intensified engagement with the authoritative relationships and materialities of ritual, enhances believers' capacity to act and participate in their social and religious world and sustains interiorization of faith and personal commitment.

In conclusion, I tentatively address the political and social consequences of the emergence of revival milieus within the Orthodox tradition. One can identify two apparently contradictory impetuses triggered by revival activities. On the one hand, as in the case of other revival movements belonging to different religious traditions, the Orthodox revivals tend, in their own ways, toward a totalizing vision of religious life that attempts to bring together separate social domains (religion, education, law, politics, aesthetics) under an all-encompassing religious ethics. Charismatization of tradition articulating this totalizing vision of "ethics as piety" (Keane 2015) connects self-formation and collective transformative expectations. The social and political actions of individuals and communities within the revival milieu are thus prone to be oriented toward creating and sustaining social (at local and national level) environments in which this totalizing impulse can be enacted. For instance, promotion of pro-life legislation, Christian family values, and religious education in public schools can politically mobilize the revival milieus. On the other hand, revival milieus have a pluralizing effect. They are capable of subverting steady polarizations that divided the social embodiment of the Orthodox tradition between virtuoso and demotic religiosities, between clerical and lay reformers, between inner-worldly and other-worldly orientations, and between the temptations to save the world or renounce it (Kenworthy 2008).

Historically, the monastic milieu with its internal variations has been the benchmark social project where the totalizing impulse within the Orthodox tradition was enacted in elaborated disciplinary programs. The contemporary revival milieus have become a space for experimenting with the various resources of the Orthodox tradition in the secular world, bridging creatively active social engagement and a preoccupation with spiritual improvement. All the revival communities I studied in Romania, without exception, were engaged in some sort of social outreach and networks beyond strictly religious observance because they put lay vocations and the ordinary life at the center of their formative efforts. Some of the revival communities are more spiritually oriented; others are much more politically driven (for example, by promoting politicians with a conservative agenda). Others engage in various social projects (charity, education, counseling, social care, various NGO activities). In one way or another, all are preoccupied with religiously shaping lay lives without removing them from "the world" but through active constitution of religious environments to accommodate their religious aspirations. In this way, the charismatization of tradition creates a dynamic link between sacramental participation and everyday life, fueling new disciplines and new politics.

SIMION POP is a PhD candidate in the Department of Sociology and Social Anthropology at Central European University, Budapest.

NOTES

1. I discuss in detail Elena's prayerful engagement with Arsenie Boca, a contemporary saint not yet canonized, elsewhere (Pop 2017). Besides the ritual changes that I approach in this chapter, the ethical orientation toward "contemporary saints" is another significant feature of the Romanian revival milieu and part of what I call bellow "the charismatization of tradition."

2. Saba Mahmood (2001) introduced the notion of "economy of prayer" to analyze the ritual prayer (*salat*) in the case of Islamic revival and to make sense of different configurations of the self, body, discipline, and authority enabling the practice of prayer within the same cultural milieu (contemporary Egypt). I expand this notion to include various concomitant practices of prayer and go beyond a certain individualization of *salat* in Mahmood's case while maintaining her preoccupation with self-formation, discipline, and embodiment.

3. The authorizing processes actualize matrices of power relations and give meaning and embody concrete events (utterances, practices, and dispositions) in disciplinary programs and institutions belonging to a tradition (Asad 1993)

4. In *The Sayings of the Desert Fathers,* the famous monastic compilation, the visitor or the disciple says to the elder, "Speak a word to me, how I may be saved!"

5. While the practice of spiritual fatherhood is widespread within the Romanian revival milieu, the practice of frequent communion remains controversial. Besides examples from tradition and a few authoritative voices within the Romanian Orthodox Church, Father Mihail has been influenced in promoting this practice by examples of Orthodox communities (monasteries and parishes) belonging to the Western Orthodox diaspora and by the revival of this practice in several monasteries of Mount Athos.

6. In Romania, the liturgical language is the vernacular language so that the text of prayer is understood by all.

7. It is worth noting here that the practice of frequent communion and the accompanying renewed Eucharistic piety—without displacing the role of the iconic piety that has dominated the Orthodox tradition, especially after the Byzantine iconoclasm—is able to produce a reconfiguration of the Orthodox modalities of embodiment and engagement with materiality.

REFERENCES:

Agadjanian, Alexander. 2013. "Reform and Revival in Moscow Orthodox Communities." *Archives de sciences sociales des religions* 2:75–94.

Asad, Talal. 1993. *Genealogies of Religion: Discipline and Reasons of Power in Christianity and Islam*. 2nd ed. Baltimore: Johns Hopkins University Press.

———. 2015. "Thinking about Tradition, Religion, and Politics in Egypt Today." *Critical Inquiry* 42 (1): 166–214.
Bandak, Andreas, and Tom Boylston. 2014. "The 'Orthodoxy' of Orthodoxy: On Moral Imperfection, Correctness, and Deferral in Religious Worlds." *Religion and Society* 5 (1): 25–46.
Burridge, Kenelm. 1987. "Revival and Renewal." In *The Encyclopedia of Religion*, edited by Mircea Eliade, 12:368–74. New York: Macmillan.
Csordas, Thomas J. 1997. *Language, Charisma, and Creativity: The Ritual Life of a Religious Movement*. Berkeley: University of California Press.
Demacopoulos, George E. 2007. *Five Models of Spiritual Direction in the Early Church*. Notre Dame: University of Notre Dame Press.
Denysenko, Nicholas E. 2015. *Liturgical Reform after Vatican II: The Impact on Eastern Orthodoxy*. Minneapolis: Fortress Press.
Feuchtwang, Stephan. 2010. *The Anthropology of Religion, Charisma, and Ghosts: Chinese Lessons for Adequate Theory*. New York: Walter de Gruyter.
Feuchtwang, Stephan, and Wang Mingming. 2001. *Grassroots Charisma: Four Local Leaders in China*. London: Routledge.
Flood, Barry Finbarr. 2014. "Bodies and Becoming: Mimesis, Mediation and the Ingestion of the Sacred in Christianity and Islam." In *Sensational Religion: Sensory Cultures in Material Practice*, edited by Sally M. Promey, 459–93. New Haven: Yale University Press.
Halemba, Agnieszka. 2015. *Negotiating Marian Apparitions: The Politics of Religion in Transcarpathian Ukraine*. Budapest: Central European University Press.
Hann, Chris, and Hermann Goltz, eds. 2010. *Eastern Christians in Anthropological Perspective*. Berkeley: University of California Press.
Keane, Webb. 2007. *Christian Moderns: Freedom and Fetish in the Mission Encounter*. Berkeley: University of California Press.
———. 2015. *Ethical Life: Its Natural and Social Histories*. Princeton: Princeton University Press.
Kenworthy, Scott M. 2008. "To Save the World or to Renounce It: Modes of Moral Action in Russian Orthodoxy." In *Religion, Morality, and Community in Post-Soviet Societies*, edited by Mark Steinberg and Catherine Wanner, 21–55. Washington, DC: Woodrow Wilson Center Press; Bloomington: Indiana University Press.
Kirsch, Thomas G. 2008. *Spirits and Letters: Reading, Writing and Charisma in African Christianity*. New York: Berghahn.
Kizenko, Nadieszda. 2012. "Sacramental Confession in Modern Russia and Ukraine." In *State Secularism and Lived Religion in Soviet Russia and Ukraine*, edited by Catherine Wanner, 190–217. Washington, DC: Woodrow Wilson Center Press; New York: Oxford University Press.
Krueger, Derek. 2014. *Liturgical Subjects: Christian Ritual, Biblical Narrative, and the Formation of the Self in Byzantium*. Philadelphia: University of Pennsylvania Press.
Ladner, Gerhart B. 2004. *The Idea of Reform: Its Impact on Christian Thought and Action in the Age of the Fathers*. Eugene, OR: WIPF and Stock Publishers.
Mahmood, Saba. 2001. "Rehearsed Spontaneity and the Conventionality of Ritual: Disciplines of Ṣalāt." *American Ethnologist* 28 (4): 827–53.
Meyendorff, John. 1979. *Byzantine Theology: Historical Trends and Doctrinal Themes*. 2nd ed. New York: Fordham University Press.

Meyendorff, Paul. 2014. "Confession and Communion in the Orthodox Church: A Modern Dilemma." *St. Vladimir's Theological Quarterly* 58 (3): 253–79.
Naumescu, Vlad. 2007. *Modes of Religiosity in Eastern Christianity: Religious Processes and Social Change in Ukraine*. Berlin: Lit.
———. 2013. "Old Believer's Passion Play: The Meaning of Doubt in an Orthodox Ritualist Movement." In *Ethnographies of Doubt: Faith and Uncertainty in Contemporary Societies*, edited by Mathijs Pelkmans, 85–119. London: IB Tauris.
Paert, Irina. 2010. *Spiritual Elders: Charisma and Tradition in Russian Orthodoxy*. DeKalb: Northern Illinois University Press.
———. 2014. "Mediators between Heaven and Earth: The Forms of Spiritual Guidance and Debates on Spiritual Elders in Present-Day Russia." In *Orthodox Paradoxes: Heterogeneities and Complexities in Contemporary Russian Orthodoxy*, edited by Katya Tolstaya, 134–54. Leiden: Brill.
Pelikan, Jaroslav. 1998. "The Eastern Orthodox Quest for Confessional Identity: Where Does Orthodoxy Confess What It Believes and Teaches?" *Modern Greek Studies Yearbook* 14/15:21–37.
Pop, Simion. 2017. "'I've tempted the saint with my prayer!' Prayer, Charisma and Ethics in Romanian Eastern Orthodox Christianity." *Religion* 47 (1): 73–91. doi:10.1080/0048721x.2016.1225908.
Pott, Thomas. 2010. *Byzantine Liturgical Reform: A Study of Liturgical Change in the Byzantine Tradition*. Crestwood, NY: St. Vladimir's Seminary Press.
Reinhardt, Bruno. 2014. "Soaking in Tapes: The Haptic Voice of Global Pentecostal Pedagogy in Ghana." *Journal of the Royal Anthropological Institute* 20 (2): 315–36.
Riesebrodt, Martin. 1999. "Charisma in Max Weber's Sociology of Religion." *Religion* 29 (1): 1–14.
Steinberg, Mark D., and Catherine Wanner, eds. 2008. *Religion, Morality, and Community in Post-Soviet Societies*. Washington, DC: Woodrow Wilson Center Press; Bloomington: Indiana University Press.
Stroumsa, Guy G. 2009. *The End of Sacrifice: Religious Transformations in Late Antiquity*. Chicago: University of Chicago Press.
Taft, Robert. 1986. *The Liturgy of the Hours in East and West: The Origins of the Divine Office and Its Meaning for Today*. 2nd ed. New York: Liturgical Press.
———. 1992. *The Byzantine Rite: A Short History*. New York: Liturgical Press.
———. 2007. "The Decline of Communion in Byzantium and the Distancing of the Congregation from the Liturgical Action: Cause, Effect, or Neither?" In *Thresholds of the Sacred: Architectural, Art Historical, Liturgical, and Theological Perspectives on Religious Screens, East and West*, edited by Sharon E. J. Gerstel et al., 27–49. Washington, DC: Dumbarton Oaks Research Library and Collection.
Tambiah, Stanley J. 1984. *The Buddhist Saints of the Forest and the Cult of Amulets: A Study in Charisma, Hagiography, Sectarianism, and Millennial Buddhism*. Cambridge: Cambridge University Press.
Taylor, Charles. 2007. *A Secular Age*. Cambridge, MA: Belknap Press.
Ware, Kallistos. 1974. "The Spiritual Father in Orthodox Christianity." *CrossCurrents* 24 (2/3)296–313.
Ware, Timothy. 1993. *The Orthodox Church*. London: Penguin.
Weber, Max. 1978. *Economy and Society: An Outline of Interpretive Sociology*. Berkeley: University of California Press.

———. 1985. *The Protestant Ethic and the Spirit of Capitalism*. 20th ed. Translated by Talcott Parsons and with an introduction by Anthony Giddens. London: HarperCollins.

Woolfenden, Gregory. 2007. "Praying the Anaphora: Aloud or in Silence." *St. Vladimir's Theological Quarterly* 51 (2–3): 179–202.

Wybrew, Hugh. 2013. *The Orthodox Liturgy: The Development of the Eucharistic Liturgy in the Byzantine Rite*. London: SPCK Publishing.

Zhuk, Sergei. 2004. *Russia's Lost Reformation: Peasants, Millennialism, and Radical Sects in Southern Russia and Ukraine, 1830–1917*. Baltimore: Johns Hopkins University Press.

EPILOGUE

Not-Orthodoxy/Orthodoxy's Others

WILLIAM A. CHRISTIAN JR.

THE ESSAYS IN THIS VOLUME address the nature of prayer in Orthodoxy. Almost all, directly or in passing, allude to the religions and ideologies that share the human environment with the Orthodox and affect their faith and their prayers. In these essays, Muslims in Ethiopia, Egypt, the Balkans, and Cyprus; Protestants in Egypt, India, and Eastern Europe; Roman and Greek Catholics in Romania and the Ukraine; Paganism in central Russia; and New Age practices everywhere constitute adjacent alternatives that impinge on Orthodoxy, bleed into it, galvanize it, undermine it, reconfirm it.

One way, then, to parse the differences in prayer among the different Orthodox communities is to look at the different religious and political fields in which they are inserted. There is considerable variation in the fields on a nation-to-nation level, ranging from historical near-monopolies in the case of quasi-state churches (Belorussia, Serbia, Greece); dominance in a plural field (Russia, Ethiopia, Romania, Cyprus); close competition (Ukraine); substantial minority (Egypt); and a small minority (India, Western Europe, the Americas). Furthermore, these fields are dynamic, shifting in part on the religious policies of the dominant political power.

A rich ethnographic sense of the range of person and group interrelations in a single community can be found in David Frick's meticulous account *Kith, Kin, and Neighbors: Communities and Confessions in Seventeenth-Century Wilno* (2013). It is an exceptional example of a number of studies of interconfessionalism in early modern Europe—in this case, in Wilno, currently more often known as Vilnius, now in Lithuania, a city that had a significant population of Orthodox inhabitants.

Frick shows that the people of Wilno were involved in a series of nested oppositions/confrontations/mirrors/engagements, so that they came to know themselves as followers of a religion as they were interacting with those of other religions. Perhaps the most intimate of these engagements was an inter-Ruthenian one between the Orthodox and the Uniates (after the recent separation in 1596), in which essentially the same ethnic group engaged, intermarried, served as godparents, and surrounded each other's deathbeds, despite constant bickering and competition at the level of clergy. The next oppositional sphere was that between Greek Orthodox and Roman Catholics, an institutionalized one for which parity was maintained in certain city offices by law (as in some German and French cities for Catholics and Protestants). For the Orthodox of Wilno, as for the rest of its confessions, the Roman Catholics were the official reference group, the one that set the calendar, to whose saints' altars guild dues had to be paid, and the religion set officially by the Polish monarchy that set the rules of engagement.

In these two mutually reinforcing oppositions, between the Orthodox and the Uniates, on the one hand, and between the Orthodox and the Roman Catholics, on the other, the religion of the other was well known: the old calendar versus the new; Cyrillic versus Latin script; Eastern versus Western. In both these engagements there seems to have been a certain amount of fuzzy edges and crossing of boundaries (as for similar reasons there was between Lutherans and Calvinists and between Roman Catholics and Uniates).

A third, yet wider, sphere for the Orthodox included all of Wilno's Christian confessions, Lutherans and Calvinists along with Catholics and Uniates, which engaged with, constrained, and periodically harassed the non-Christians: the Jews and Tatar Muslims. Here the edges were harder, and the ritualized confrontations kept them hard. But many Jews and Christians nevertheless lived in the same houses, and a few belonged to the same guilds, while in other cases Jewish and Christian guilds were in competition, legally recognized by the courts.

Continuous contact with the wider world, including the experiences of the traveling students of the merchant class in foreign institutions, and of course in the presence of teachers and professionals from the rest of Europe, east as well as west, helped to identify what Wilno could be, was, and was not. People were aware of a European spectrum of interconfessional relations running between extreme intolerance, persecution, or exclusion in Spain, personified in Wilno by the more obdurate Spanish Jesuit teachers (Frick 2013, 148, 160), to relative religious freedom in the Netherlands and the New World, exemplified by the

Lutheran physician trained in the Jesuit Academy of Wilno and then in Basel, Paris, and Catholic Louvain and Padua and who married a Calvinist. Orthodox sons sent to study in Western Europe similarly studied in Catholic or Protestant universities, or both (168).

The world beyond Wilno was perhaps just as formative to citizens' identity as their ethnicity or religion. The local Ruthenians might sometimes be referred to as *ruskis*, but when the Tsarist army occupied Wilno from 1655 to 1661, Muscovites became the *ruskis* and were considered quite different from the local Orthodox. As with the Orthodox and Uniates, people from other groups were not considered first and foremost representatives of external powers or faiths but rather citizens of Wilno. As in Wilno, in the other towns of Eastern Europe people had powerful, idiosyncratic identities, the result of centuries of political, social, and religious sedimentation and adjustment.

The essays in this volume point to a similar deep historical sedimentation for interconfessional relations. And on a material level, buildings, boundaries, family names, cemeteries, monuments, and heirlooms bear witness to the past and keep it in the foreground of the present. Perhaps only in a new land with few of these material reminders could a truly new start take place.

And historical geopolitical changes that shifted the relations of power among the confessions still deeply affect the Orthodox and their prayers: whether the Uniate separation of 1592 (Mahieu and Naumescu 2008); the removal of imperial protection for pluralism of the Ottomans in the Balkans (Hayden 2002); the end of Habsburg rule in Transcarpathia, Galicia, Romania, and the former Yugoslavia; the disestablishment of national Orthodox regimes in the Soviet Union and Ethiopia; the Jewish Holocaust of the 1940s; and in many places the establishment of religious freedom in the late twentieth century.

Now widespread migration and the omnipresence of the world beyond through the internet have undermined the particularities of local communities. In this volume, we see the impingement of web-based interconfessional conflict in Afaf and the effect there of stories posted by migrants in Saudi Arabia or brought back by returnees (Boylston, this volume).

In 2006 I accompanied students from Pécs in Hungary to the village of Seuca/Szőkefalva, then a site of religious visions. We found that Seuca's typically Transylvanian mosaic of religions had a host of international ramifications. The Hungarian-speaking Calvinists, a substantial majority in the village, received shipments of secondhand clothes from Calvinists in the Netherlands, which they in turn distributed to the other churches; the Hungarian-speaking

Unitarians had a sister church in Albany, New York, with a system of mutual transatlantic visits; and about half of the town's Roma, many of whom periodically worked in Hungary, had set up a Pentecostal church with the help of a missionary from Norway. The Romanian-speaking Orthodox (in a church that was formerly Greek Catholic) had the institutional support of the Romanian government, but I could not help feeling that its lack of prestigious Western ties left it at a certain disadvantage. In the 1980s a Unitarian minister had brokered a truce among the confessions by which the pastors agreed to attend each other's festivities and not to criticize each other in their sermons.

Since 1995, the visions of Mary by a Roma, Rózsika Marián, had been attracting to Seuca additional international contacts. Rózsika, at first backed by Greek Catholic priests from the adjacent city of Târnaveni/ Dicsőszentmárton, received messages in Romanian, and then, when she became allied with the pastor of the Hungarian-speaking Roman Catholic Church, her messages came in Romanian and Hungarian. The Roman Catholic parish received pilgrims from Catholics in Switzerland, Hungary, Germany, and Poland (Peti 2009; Pócs 2010; Győrfy 2009).

Down the road was a Saxon village where the last remaining German speakers were periodically serviced by Lutheran ministers. In Seuca we met people who spoke English, Spanish, German, and Italian, in addition to Hungarian and Romanian, many as a result of stays as workers in Western Europe, and among some of them an additional religious stance was religious disaffection and indifference. Seuca's international ties had deep roots; villagers of all faiths had migrated to Ohio a century before.

In nearby Târnaveni the synagogue, converted into a social club, and the overgrown Jewish cemetery bore witness to yet other neighbors within living memory. The longtime Jewish "other," now missing, must still somehow be present. And another conspicuous absence in the day-to-day discourse is active, state-sponsored rationalism or atheism. Communism is so utterly eclipsed and discredited in the former Socialist states of Eastern Europe that disbelief has become uncomfortable to voice and atheists maintain a low profile. Yet well within living memory, an entire political system holding that religion was superstition was operated by local people, a good number of whom are still alive (Valtchinova 2002; Luehrmann 2011; Wanner 2012; Naumescu 2016). Furthermore, there has been a deep penetration in Seuca, as throughout the Orthodox world, of more personalized spiritual alternatives or accessories, with pantheistic notions of returning spirits, energies, past lives, and associations with nature.

I did not ask how all these local alternatives have affected the Orthodox of Seuca and their prayers on my short visit, but affect them they surely did. As in seventeenth-century Wilno, there were mixed marriages, neighbors of different confessions who attended each other's rites of passage, and people of different religions who worked together and were aware of differences in beliefs and liturgy. One can imagine interactions ranging from synergy to syncretism to imitation, emulation, conflict, and rigidification in an unstable field vulnerable to agitation and manipulation. In Transylvania, Romanian Orthodox monks are consulted by Hungarian-speaking Calvinists and Unitarians (Komáromi 2010); Latin and Greek Catholics "observed each other's holidays, and popular practices (such as carol singing) could even merge at the local level" (Hann 2008, x); and in the Greek archipelago, Orthodox and Catholics have worked out ways to share shrines (Seraïdari 2010, 2013).

Orthodoxy, like Catholicism and Judaism, is a legacy religion, to which in its home territories people rarely convert unless through marriage, and for whom what little proselytizing there is tends to be directed at reclaiming its own lapsed or indifferent clients. In the legacy mindset, Orthodoxy is the one true religion, at least for its particular place or people, and other religions are the result of schisms, errors, or aberrations or are simply alien. Conversion does become an issue when the Orthodox are the targets of proselytizing, which directly threatens families and parishes. In the twentieth century this threat, aside from the reemergence of Greek Catholicism, has largely come from Protestant missionaries, especially Baptist and Pentecostal, who are seen to present the kind of stark alternatives for the Orthodox that Greek and Roman Catholics do not truly represent.

Catherine Wanner points to the great contrast between the more static, place-based mindset of the Orthodox, for whom "Orthodox identity is geographically defined and automatically inherited," and the more mobile mindset of the Baptists and the Pentecostals: "These are not only 'religions made to travel.' They are religions that make people travel too. The doctrinal belief that 'every believer is a missionary' plants migratory potential in every evangelical" (2007, 136, 12).

For the Orthodox the impingement of these alternatives can provide a way to observe and know oneself. One of Simion Pop's interlocutors in this volume asks, "Why does the spontaneous and exalted prayer of the Pentecostals seem devilish?" A Jacobite woman tells Vlad Naumescu in his chapter that she feels "uncomfortable throughout the liturgical service" when visiting another Syrian church of Protestant influence. A young man who left a Neo-Pentecostal church founded by American missionaries tells Sonja Luehrmann (this volume) he felt that Orthodox prayer, while more repetitive, "took him deeper" over time. In the 1960s the rural people in northern Spain had a set phrase when approached by Jehovah's Witnesses or Mormons: "If I don't even believe in the Apostolic Roman Catholic religion, which is the only true one, how can I believe in yours?"

Indeed, the transformative effect of Protestantism in its many forms on legacy religions is a theme common to almost all the essays in this volume (see also Heo 2013; Luehrmann 2010). It resonates with what we know of Western Europe, where Roman Catholicism in countries with substantial or influential Protestant populations (Ireland [and thence the United States], the UK, France, Netherlands, Germany, Switzerland) tends to have harder edges and is more militant, polemical, and rigorist than that of countries like Spain or Italy where Roman Catholicism has traditionally predominated. It would seem that the active presence of Protestants has set in motion within Catholicism internal mechanisms of vigilance and correction.

Tom Boylston (this volume) uses "galvanization" to describe the arousal of the Orthodox of Afaf in reaction to the new mosque and loudspeakers of Muslims. The word derives from the Bologna physiologist Luigi Galvani, who in the late eighteenth century demonstrated that electricity could provoke a reaction in the nerves of dead animals. The "shaping up" seems to work in two ways: on a theological and practice level, as a kind of purification, and as a stimulus, shocking everyday routine into new activity.

For Roman Catholicism there have been many such moments: the Counter-Reformation, leading to a clergy and believers who were more self-aware, with greater militancy, greater internal cohesion, more international presence, and a strong proselytizing impulse outside of Europe; the rise of atheistic communism in the Soviet Union and imposed on Eastern Europe, leading to a wave of religious visions, starting in Portugal and culminating in a series on both sides of the Iron Curtain in the 1940s and 1950s; and more recently, worldwide competition from Protestant Pentecostals leading to the spread of charismatic, Pentecostal Catholicism.

The repercussions on prayer of these galvanizations have varied. In the case of the Counter-Reformation, the strengthening of systems of internal control led to a suppression of more spontaneous public visions and free-form inspirational prayer. The reaction to communism was spurred by a wave of seers who delivered messages from the divine that instructed the use of penance and the repetitive prayer of the Rosary (Kselman 1982; Christian 1984; Halemba 2015; Shaw 2003; Ventresca 2003; Scheer 2006, 2009; de la Cruz 2015).

The charismatic movement has broken out from Tridentine devotions but with a strong emphasis on parish and clergy-centered groups.

The historical process most at work in Eastern Europe is the breakup of state socialism and the freeing up of religious competition of all kinds. One reaction within Orthodoxy is a back-to-the-Byzantine movement, evident from these essays on Russia, Romania, and Greece, and not dissimilar to a revival among lapsed Jews in Hungary or the reenergizing of Orthodox in rural Ethiopia.

One is tempted to refer to confessional "significant others." This notion, which originated in psychology referring to persons who serve as examples, is useful for thinking about religious groups in plural configurations. More and more the world is made up of this looking-over-the-shoulder environment, where everyone is aware of a complex force field. Even in local mono-religious contexts, the religious "others" are present through the news, the internet, correspondence, and migrants. The notion of others is especially germane to the subject of prayer, for prayer involves contact with divine, nonhuman others. The participants in these complex force fields are aware not only of the others who are humans but also of these other humans' nonhuman others. The participants are all, all the time, forming and understanding themselves through interaction (Mead 1934).

The essays in this volume in fact raise questions for any religion, not just Orthodoxy:

1. What are the immediate and relevant cohabiting faiths and practices, and what is the particular configuration? The essays in the present volume show they range from more homogeneous to dominant to more dual to more plural and to small minority.

2. How is this set of groups nourished and informed by international networks? Much of the world is saturated by missionaries of one kind or another. American Presbyterians under British protection who founded the Coptic Evangelical Church in Egypt provoked an expansion of Orthodox education programs as a defensive measure (Heo 2013). Ukraine has a long tradition of charismatic and evangelical Protestantism, nurtured by missionaries and financial support from the diaspora, and Ukrainian Protestants in turn send missionaries into Russia and Central Asia (Wanner 2007, 146; Naumescu 2007, 65). Luehrmann (2011) describes a Pentecostal group in her largely Orthodox/Pagan Mari locality established by a missionary from Beaumont, Texas, who, when he moved on, was replaced by a Russian from Moscow, who in turn adapted sermons downloaded from the internet by a charismatic preacher from

Nigeria. The Syrian Malankara church in South India had to defend its heritage against Anglican missionaries (Naumescu, this volume). Increasingly, not just clergy but individual migrants themselves, in person and by means of social media, are linking local believers to international networks and conflicts and communicating their interconfessional experiences to their home communities (Boylston, this volume). Hann (2008, x) found that some of his Eastern European Greek Catholic informants had formed their notions of "a pristine version of Byzantine Christianity" during extended stays in the United States and Canada.

3. What are the less organized trends and techniques of spirituality and self-formation, which may enhance or compete with traditional prayer? Daria Dubovka describes, for instance, how in Russia, New Age energy theories and yogis who do without food or sleep serve to validate methods of Orthodox prayer.

4. What are institutionalized challenges to faith in general, through atheism and rationalism? Tom Boylston mentions the disestablishment of the Orthodox Church in Ethiopia under the Socialist Derg regime, and Jeanne Kormina discusses the gradual reidentification of secularized Russians (see also Luehrmann 2010).

5. And what are the challenges of a more diffuse drift toward secularism? Jeffers Engelhardt alludes to the competition represented by Facebook, the morning news on the car radio, and "the unbeneficial noise of urban life." And Simion Pop mentions an antimodernist element of the Orthodox revival.

6. How do all these impinge on practices of prayer? As we have seen, people who experience prayer in different religious liturgies find by comparison which kind feels more right, comfortable, or profound. In Ethiopia the amplification of Muslim and Orthodox prayer in the public sphere has "significant effects on how people experience their religious allegiances, connections, and claims to shared space" (Boylston, this volume). Liturgies increasingly emphasize vigilance about remaining in the true faith (Luehrmann, this volume). Perhaps the intensification of ascetic and prayer practices in the Orthodox revival milieu may be related to the un-Orthodox world around it, with, as Luehrmann (personal communication) suggests, "modernity conceptualized as distraction, standing in opposition to the mood of concentration that prayer is supposed to entail."

It is clear from the essays here and the literature they cite that the various significant others in the religious field stimulate, affect, condition, and place limits upon the practices of Orthodoxy. Icons are also not-statues, spoken or chanted prayers are also not-silent-meditations, and not-short, repetitive, formulaic prayer is also not-spontaneous-glossolalia, silent meditation, or imaginative identification. Orthodoxy itself, after all, like other great traditions, arose defining itself against what it was not.

WILLIAM A. CHRISTIAN JR. teaches anthropology at the Universitat Autònoma de Barcelona. He is author of *Visionaries: The Spanish Republic and the Reign of Christ*.

REFERENCES

Christian, William A., Jr. 1984. "Religious Apparitions and the Cold War in Southern Europe." In *Religion, Power and Protest in Local Communities: The Northern Shore of the Mediterranean*, edited by Eric R. Wolf, 239–66. Berlin: Mouton.
de la Cruz, Deirdre. 2015. *Mother Figured: Marian Apparitions and the Making of a Filipino Universal*. Chicago: University of Chicago Press.
Frick, David. 2013. *Kith, Kin, and Neighbors: Communities and Confessions in Seventeenth-Century Wilno*. Ithaca: Cornell University Press.
Győrfy, Eszter. 2009. "'That Is Why Miracles Happen Here': The Role of Miracle Narratives in the Legitimation Process of a New Shrine." In *Passageways: From Hungarian Ethnography to European Ethnology and Sociocultural Anthropology*, edited by Gábor Vargyas, 339–58. Pécs and Budapest: l'Harmattan.
Halemba, Agnieszka. 2015. *Negotiating Marian Apparitions: The Politics of Religion in Transcarpathian Ukraine*. Budapest: Central European University Press.
Hann, Chris. 2008. Preface to *Churches In-between: Greek Catholic Churches in Postsocialist Europe*, edited by Stephanie Mahieu and Vlad Naumescu, x. Berlin: Lit.
Hayden, Robert M. 2002. "Antagonistic Tolerance: Competitive Sharing of Religious Sites in South Asia and the Balkans." *Current Anthropology* 43 (2): 205–31.
Heo, Angie. 2013. "The Virgin between Christianity and Islam: Sainthood, Media, and Modernity in Egypt." *Journal of the American Academy of Religion* 81 (4): 1117–38.
Komáromi, Tünde. 2010. "Crossing Boundaries in Times of Personal Crisis: Seeking Help from Orthodox Clergy in Transylvania." In *Religion and Boundaries: Studies from the Balkans, Eastern Europe and Turkey*, edited by Galia Valtchinova, 155–66. Istanbul: Isis Press.
Kselman, Thomas A. 1982. "Our Lady of Necedah: Marian Piety and the Cold War." Working Paper 34, Cushwa Seminar on American Religious History, Notre Dame.
Luehrmann, Sonja. 2010. "A Dual Quarrel of Images on the Middle Volga: Icon Veneration in the Face of Protestant and Pagan Critique." In *Eastern Christians in Anthropological Perspective*, edited by Chris Hann and Hermann Goltz, 56–78. Berkeley: University of California Press.
———. 2011. *Secularism Soviet Style: Teaching Atheism and Religion in a Volga Republic*. Bloomington: Indiana University Press.
Mahieu, Stephanie, and Vlad Naumescu, eds. 2008. *Churches In-between: Greek Catholic Churches in Postsocialist Europe*. Berlin: Lit.

Mead, G. H. 1934. *Mind, Self, and Society*. Edited by Charles W. Norris. Chicago: University of Chicago Press.

Naumescu, Vlad. 2007. *Modes of Religiosity in Eastern Christianity: Religious Processes and Social Change in Ukraine*. Münster: Lit.

———. 2016. "The End Times and the Near Future: The Ethical Engagements of Russian Old Believers in Romania." *Journal of the Royal Anthropological Institute* 22 (2): 314–31.

Peti, Lehel. 2009. "The Marian Apparition from Seuca/Szőkefalva in the Context of Religious and Ethnical Interferences." Working Papers in Romanian Minority Studies 24. Institutul pentru Studierea Problemelor Minorităților Naționale, Cluj. / "Apariția Fecioarei Maria de la Seuca, în contextul interferențelor religioase și etnice." Studii de atelier. Cercetarea minorităților naționale din România 24. Institutul pentru Studierea Problemelor Minorităților Naționale, Cluj.

Pócs, Éva. 2010. "Seers, Visions and Shrines: Divine Interventions in Crises of Private and Public Affairs." In *Religion and Boundaries: Studies from the Balkans, Eastern Europe and Turkey*, edited by Galia Valtchinova, 196–225. Istanbul: Isis Press.

Scheer, Monique. 2006. *Rosenkranz und Kriegsvisionen: Marienscheinungskulte im 20. Jahrhundert*. Tübingen: TVV.

———. 2009. "Taking Shelter under Mary's Mantle: Marian Apparitions in the Early Cold War Years, 1947–1953." In *The "Vision Thing": Studying Divine Intervention*, edited by William A. Christian Jr. and Gábor Klaniczay, 195–218. Workshop Series No. 18. Budapest: Collegium Budapest Institute for Advanced Study.

Seraïdari, Katerina. 2010. "The Virgin between Orthodox and Catholics: Religious Mediations on Tinos." In *Religion and Boundaries: Studies from the Balkans, Eastern Europe and Turkey*, edited by Galia Valtchinova, 97–117. Istanbul: Isis Press.

———. 2013. "Negotiating Religious Differences in the Cyclades: Discourses of Inclusion and Exclusion." In *Sites and Politics of Religious Diversity in Southern Europe: The Best of All Gods*, edited by R. L. B. José Mapril, 309–30. Leiden: Brill.

Shaw, Tony. 2003. "Martyrs, Miracles and Martians: Religion and Cold War Cinematic Propaganda in the 1950s." In *Religion and the Cold War*, edited by Dianne Kirby, 211–31. Basingstoke, UK: Palgrave Macmillan.

Valtchinova, Galia. 2002. "Orthodoxie et communisme dans les Balkans: Réflexions sur le cas bulgare." *Archives de sciences sociales des religions* 119:79–97.

Ventresca, Robert. 2003. "The Virgin and the Bear: Religion, Society and the Cold War in Italy." *Journal of Social History* 37 (2): 439–56.

Wanner, Catherine. 2007. *Communities of the Converted: Ukrainians and Global Evangelism*. Ithaca: Cornell University Press.

———, ed. 2012. *State Secularism and Lived Religion in Soviet Russia and Ukraine*. Washington, DC: Woodrow Wilson Center Press with Oxford University Press.

GLOSSARY

acrostic (Greek). Poetic device where each line of a poem starts with a consecutive letter of the alphabet. Used in a number of Byzantine and Byzantine-inspired prayer texts.

akathistos (Greek; Old Church Slavonic *akafist*). Literally, "without sitting down." A hymn of twelve parts glorifying the Virgin Mary, Jesus, or a saint, performed either as part of a liturgical service or in private lay prayer. The original akathistos was a hymn to the Virgin Mary composed in the seventh century, in praise of her aid in fending off a Persian attack on Byzantium.

analogion (Greek; Old Church Slavonic *analoi*). Slanted stand on which icons or the Gospel are placed for veneration in church.

anaphora (Greek). Literally, "carrying up, offering." The prayer of consecration over the bread and wine performed by the presiding priest during the Orthodox Divine Liturgy to transform these elements into the sacramental body and blood of Jesus Christ.

antidoron (Greek). Literally, "instead of gifts." Prosphora (loaves of bread) that are consecrated in the sanctuary during Divine Liturgy but not consecrated to become the Eucharistic body of Christ. Antidoron is distributed to the faithful at the end of the liturgy and can also be sent home to sick or housebound congregants.

apechema (Greek). In Byzantine chant, an introductory musical phrase that is chanted by the cantor to establish the mode and pitch for the choir.

avtobusniki (Russian). Literally, "bus people." A colloquial term for pilgrims who travel by chartered bus.

"*Axion Estin*" (Greek; Old Church Slavonic "*Dostoino est*'"). Literally, "It is truly meet," a short prayer-hymn in praise of the Virgin Mary, performed as part of liturgical services and as a closing prayer at many Orthodox gatherings.

Axumite Empire. Kingdom in the area of today's northern Eritrea and Ethiopia that existed from about 100 to 940 AD. The empire became Christian in the fourth century.

baraka (Arabic). A term used by Arabic-speaking Muslims and Christians to denote blessing, holiness, or a power inherent in sacred places and objects.

blagochinnyi, blagochinnaia (Russian). In a church organization, a dean overseeing a number of parishes. In a monastery, a monk or nun whose duty is to manage the economic life of a monastic community.

blagodat' (Russian). Grace; a quality of a sacred place or object comparable to the Arabic baraka.

blagoslovenie (Russian). Blessing, understood both as approval, commission, and permission to do something. The corresponding verb is *blagoslovit'* (to bless).

catharsis (Greek). Purification.

cenobitic. A monastic community centered on communal life and following a common rule (as opposed to an eremitic community, where hermits live in isolated cells or caves and devote themselves to more individualized prayer lives).

Chalcedonian churches. The churches that accept the dogma of the dual nature of Christ (divine and human) as adopted at the Council of Chalcedon in 451 AD. These include the Orthodox churches of Byzantine derivation as well as the Roman Catholic Church and its Protestant offshoots.

chrism. Holy oil, used for anointing during services, after baptism, and for the sick.

Divine Liturgy. The Orthodox Eucharistic Mass.

duhovnicesc (Romanian; Greek *pneumatikos*; Russian *dukhovno*). Spiritual, Spirit-filled, spiritual realm. A term used in phrases such as "spiritual life," "spiritual person," "spiritual father," and "spiritual guidance," denoting that in Eastern Orthodoxy a reality is qualified as "spiritual" through the perceived presence of the Holy Spirit.

eparchy. From Greek *eparchia* (rule, jurisdiction). An Orthodox diocese, ruled by a bishop or archbishop.

epitimia (Greek). Penance imposed after confession.

fervent litany, litany of fervent supplication (Greek *ektenés ikesía*; Old Church Slavonic *sugubaia ekteniia*). Prayer litany marked by a special supplicatory tone, underlined by the choir responding "Lord have mercy" three times after each petition. In the Divine Liturgy, it occurs after the Gospel reading, not long before the beginning of the Eucharistic canon. It may be augmented by special prayers reflecting the need of the congregation or the local or national community.

filioque (Latin). "And from the son": a phrase inserted in the Nicene Creed by Western churches from the ninth century onward to assert that the Holy Spirit proceeds not only from God the Father but also from the Son, Jesus Christ. To this day, this phrase marks a difference in the recitations of the creed between Eastern Orthodox and their Catholic and Protestant counterparts.

Ge'ez. The classical language of Ethiopia, now mainly used as a liturgical language and studied by religious specialists.

guru (Sanskrit). Teacher; term used for a spiritual guide by Hindus as well as by Christians in India.

hesychasm. From Greek *hesychia* (stillness, silence). A mystical tradition of meditative prayer perfected in thirteenth-century Byzantium. Following the rhythm of their breath, hesychasts strive to constantly recite the Jesus Prayer and focus their attention on their navel or stomach.

hieromonk. A tonsured monk who is also an ordained priest, able to serve the Divine Liturgy, take confession, and administer other sacraments.

hypostasis (Greek). Enduring entity, fundamental reality. In Christian theology, each of the three persons of the Trinity (Father, Son, and Holy Spirit) is one hypostasis.

iconoclasm. A movement, receiving support from the Byzantine emperors in the seventh and eighth centuries, against the veneration of icons. It found its ending in the second Council of Nicaea (787 AD), where veneration, but not worship, of icons was affirmed.

iconostasis. A screen with several rows of icons, separating the sanctuary from the nave in post-Byzantine Orthodox churches.

Irmologion (Greek). A liturgical book containing *irmoi*, that is, melodic models for chanting odes during matins.

íson (Greek). The low drone that accompanies Byzantine chant.

Jesus Prayer. A short prayer invoking the name of Jesus, repeated in the rhythm of the breath, most commonly "Lord Jesus Christ, son of God, have mercy on me, a sinner."

koinonia (Greek). Community.

kontakion (Greek). First part of each stanza of an akathistos, containing a narrative account of the saint's life or other event that is glorified in the hymn.

lavra (Greek/Old Church Slavonic). A particularly renowned and respected monastery.

matins (Anglicized Latin). Morning service. In many parish churches in Slavic Orthodox countries, matins are served in the evening immediately following vespers, following the Jewish custom of beginning a new liturgical day at sunset.

metropolitan. The church hierarch who presides over a cluster of dioceses.

Miaphysite. Also referred to as Monophysite, both derived from Greek terms for "one nature." Churches that do not accept the dogma on the dual nature of Christ established by the Council of Chalcedon and instead insist on the indivisible mixing of humanity and divinity in Jesus Christ. These include the Syriac Orthodox, Coptic Orthodox, Ethiopian Tewahedo, and Armenian Apostolic churches.

mode. Also referred to as "tone." In Byzantine liturgical chant, a system of eight core melodies used in divine services, each of which in turn dominates one week of the church calendar. The eight-mode system is known as *oktoechos* in Greek and *osmoglasie* in Old Church Slavonic.

moleben (Russian). A short prayer service for a particular need, such as curing a disease or bringing good crops, or for giving thanks. It may be addressed to a saint or to an icon of the Virgin Mary and served inside or outside of church.

molitvennik (Russian). Literally, "one who prays." A person particularly skilled in prayer, able to intercede effectively for others.

Monophysite. See Miaphysite.

Mount Athos. Also known as "Holy Mountain." Peninsula in Greece that has been home to monasteries since at least 800 AD. Currently there are twenty monasteries that form an autonomous monks' republic within Greece; they can be visited only by male pilgrims. In many parts of the Orthodox world, the monasticism of Mount Athos is considered to be a standard to follow.

muqaddas, muqadassa (Arabic). Title for a Christian who has made pilgrimage to Jerusalem.

mysterion (Greek; Old Church Slavonic *tainstvo*; Romanian *taină*). Literally, "mystery." Orthodox term for the sacraments, generally counted as seven: baptism, chrismation (anointing with oil after baptism), Eucharist, confession, marriage, ordination, and holy unction of the sick or dying.

neumes (Greek). Literally, "sign, gesture." Byzantine system of musical notation.

oikos (Greek; Old Church Slavonic *ikos*). The second part of each stanza of an akathistos hymn, consisting of several lines that usually start with "Rejoice" or, more rarely, with "Have mercy on me."

parádosis (Greek). Literally, "handing over." Tradition, seen as the source of legitimacy and ongoing revelation within the Orthodox Church.

paraklesis (Greek). Service of supplication for the needs of the living, addressed to the Virgin Mary or a saint, analogous to the *moleben* of Slavic practice. In many Greek churches, the *paraklesis* to the Virgin Mary is served in conjunction with vespers; those addressed to various saints may be served as stand-alone services according to need.

Paterikon (from Greek *pater*, father). Collection of saints' lives.

Philokalia (Greek). Literally, "love of goodness" or "love of beauty." A collection of spiritual writings by Christian church fathers from the fourth to the fourteenth century. It was compiled on Mount Athos in the eighteenth century.

phýsis (Greek). Nature. In Christian theology, this refers to the divine and human natures united in the person of Christ.

pomiannik (Russian, plural *pomianniki*). "Book of commemoration," record of names of living and deceased people to be commemorated in private or communal prayer.

poslushanie (Russian). Literally, "obedience." In monasteries, both the virtue of obedience and the tasks assigned to each monastic, novice, or volunteer.

prepodobnyi (Old Church Slavonic, plural *prepodobnye*). Literally, "most similar." Title of a saint who was a monk or nun in life.

Prester John. In western European medieval legend, a priest-king said to rule over an isolated land of Christians in the Orient. Chroniclers and explorers have variously situated it in India, Central Asia, or Ethiopia.

Proskomedia (Greek). Preparation of the gifts to be used for communion at the beginning of the Divine Liturgy. Prayers for the sick and for the dead that are said in the sanctuary at this time are considered to be particularly powerful by many Orthodox Christians and often serve as a substitute for actually taking communion.

prosphora (Greek). Small loaves of leavened bread used for communion.

Qurbana (Malayalam; Syriac "Qurbono qadisho"). Divine Liturgy.

schemamonk/schemanun. An advanced monastic rank where a monk or nun takes on a new name and begins a life exclusively devoted to prayer and asceticism instead of to a mix of prayer and labor. Schemamonks and schemanuns wear robes that are reminiscent of those in which corpses are dressed at funerals.

s'elot (Amharic). Prayer.

shahid, shahida (Arabic). Martyr.

shirk (Arabic). Idolatry or polytheism, worship of anything other than God.

sigdet (Amharic). Worship, surrender, obeisance; also the full-body kneeling bow that expresses these attitudes.

silet (Amharic). Vow.

soslovie (Russian). Feudal rank. In imperial Russia, clergy and monastics represented their own *soslovie*.

starets (Russian, plural *startsy*). Literally, "elder." A monk or priest who is considered to have special spiritual gifts, such as the ability to foresee the future or to know the personal concerns of his followers. The abstract noun *starchestvo* (elderhood) refers both to the qualities of these spiritual elders and to the phenomenon of laypeople turning to them for spiritual guidance.

Starovery (Russian). Russian Old Believers, a group that separated from the Russian Orthodox Church after the seventeenth century schism; also known as Old Ritualists (Russian *staroobriatsy*).

Synaxarium. Book with the lives of saints, organized according to their commemoration in the church calendar.

tabot (Ge'ez). Replica of the tablets of law or the Ark of the Covenant. One resides in the sanctum of every Ethiopian Orthodox Church and is the focus of consecration.

tamgid (Arabic). Coptic hymn glorifying a saint, comparable to the Greek and Old Church Slavonic akathistos.

theosis (Greek). Deification; the restoration of the image of God in oneself that is the ultimate goal of Orthodox spirituality.

Theotokos (Greek; Old Church Slavonic "Bogoroditsa"). God-bearer. Title of the Virgin Mary since the Council of Ephesus (431 AD).

trebnik (Russian). "Book of needs"; book of occasional services used by clergy when conducting baptisms, marriages, blessings, or prayer services.

Typikon (Greek). Liturgical book containing the order and variable parts of the Divine Liturgy and other services.

viață duhovnicească (Romanian; Greek *pneumatikos bios*). "Spiritual life"; the ensemble of prayer, participation in liturgy and sacraments, and consultation with spiritual authorities that advance an Orthodox Christian on a trajectory of personal spiritual growth.

votserkovlenie (Russian). "Enchurching," the process of becoming a practicing Orthodox Christian and learning to participate in Orthodox rites and liturgies.

yenefs abbat (Amharic). Literally "soul father," the priest assigned as spiritual adviser to each individual Ethiopian Christian.

yphos (Greek). In Byzantine chant, the style of interpreting Byzantine musical notation (neumes).

zapiska (Russian). Literally, "note." Sheet of paper on which names of living or deceased people can be written down for commemoration in prayer. Fees collected for accepting these prayer notes are a significant part of the income of many Russian churches.

zikkir (Amharic). Feast in honor of a saint, held on the saint's memorial day in the Ethiopian Orthodox calendar.

INDEX

Page numbers in *italics* refer to photographs

Abanub, Saint, 84, 92
acrostic, 132
akathistos, *115*, 129, 132–35, 136, 159
Aleksii of Moscow, Saint, 157
analogion, 68
Anderson, Jon, 177
Anglican Church Mission Society, 50n7
antidoron, 233
Antuni, Yustus al-, 93, 94, *111*
apechema, 69, 70
Aristotle University of Thessaloniki, 74
Armenian Apostolic Church, 6
Asad, Talal, 15, 226
asceticism, 19, 194, 207
Athanasius of Cyprus, Metropolitan, 70
atheism, 245, 247, 249
Axion Estin, 5, 68
Axumite Empire, 165

baptismal names, 129–31
baraka, 89, 163–64
Basil the Great, Saint, 123
Bawit monastery, Asyut, Egypt, 84
Bishoi, Saint, 96
blagochinnaia, 196
blessing, 11, 148, 160n3, 188; of a pilgrimage, 146–47, 150–51
Bloch, Maurice, 122
Boca, Father Arsenie, 222, 238
Brown, Peter, 93–94, 99n9
Brubaker, Leslie, 87
Byzantium, 17

canonization. *See* Coptic Orthodox Church; saints

catharsis, 59, 60
cenobitic monasteries, 97, 224
Chalcedonian Eastern Orthodox churches, 5, 89, 166
chant, 11, 17, 65, 217, 218; training in, 68, 71; *znamenny*, 18, 205, 209n14
Chapel of Saint Xenia, Saint Petersburg, Russia, *114*
Cherubic Hymn, 36
chrismation, 31
Christ, dual human-divine nature of, 4, 6, 165
Christian-Muslim relations, 163–64, 167–74, 187
Christotokos, 5
Chrysostom, Saint John, 62, 66
church fathers (Orthodox), 13, 18, 59
Church of Greece, 73
Church of Pireaus FM station, 64
Church of the Virgin, Zaytun, Egypt, *110*
Church on the Blood, Ekaterinburg, Russia, 145
Church Slavonic. *See* liturgical languages; Old Believers
Cistercian Order, 209n9
Clement of Alexandria, Saint, 88
Coleman, Simon, 19
communion, 31, 42, 148, 151, 156, 216; confession, 133, 149; church revival and frequency of, 125, 216, 218, 220, 223, 228–33, 235–36; frequency of, *119*, 125, 143, 220, 223, 228, 229, 233, 238n5, 238n7; with other believers, 45, 155; preparation for, 133, 235–36
Constantinople, Ecumenical Patriarchate of, 17
Convent of St. Mercurius, Cairo, Egypt, 93

259

Convent of the Holy Trinity, Sarov, Russia, 153–54
conversion, 246
Coptic Catholics, 98n2, 99n3
Coptic Evangelical Church, 86–87, 89, 99n3, 248
Coptic Orthodox Church, 6, 84, 89, 90, 93, 97
Council of Chalcedon, 6
Council of Ephesus, 5
Council of Nicaea, 6, 22n1
Cyril of Alexandria, 6
Cyril IV, Pope, 89
Cyril VI, Pope, 93, 95, 97

Davie, Grace, 144
deification. See *theosis*
Denisov, Leonid Ivanovich, 133
diakonia, 75
Dimyana the Martyr, Saint, 83–84, 85, 98n1, 109
Diocletian, Emperor, 84
Diveevo, 161n9. *See also* Convent of the Holy Trinity, Sarov, Russia
Divine Liturgy, 36, 42, 104, 133, 149; and communion, 223, 233–36; and prayer, 38, 213, 222, 224
Dorotheus, Abba, 198
Dubovka, Daria, 11

Eickelman, Dale, 177
Eisenlohr, Patrick, 179
elders, 19–20, 31
enchurching, 29–30, 154–59
Epiphany Cathedral, Elokhovo, Moscow, 157
epitimia, 230
eschatology, 198–99, 208
Estonian Orthodox Church, 17
Ethiopian Orthodox Christianity, 6–7, 165–80
Ethiopian Orthodox Tewahedo Church, 165, 166
ethnography, sensory, 10
Evangelical Christians, 42, 43, 50n9, 122–23, 213, 246–48. *See also* Coptic Evangelical Church
exorcism, 43, 44, 92, 163

Ezana, King, 165

Facebook, 171–74, 177, 178, 249
fairs, 113, 129, 144, 146, 159n1
Faith, Hope and Charity, Saints, 133
fasting, 209n5, 216, 223, 229; in Ethiopian Orthodox practice, 167, 175, 176
fervent liturgy, 213, 214
Feuchtwang, Stephan, 228
Fikos, 66
filioque, 7, 22n1
Finnish Orthodox Church, 8
Florovsky, Georges, 15
4E TV, 73, 74
Frick, David, 125, 242–44

Ge'ez. *See* liturgical languages
Gendy, Atef, 86
George, Father K. M., 30, 44, 48, 49n2
George the Martyr, Saint, 92, 96, 163
glossolalia, 121, 122, 128, 136, 250
Gobran, Mama Maggie, 92
Goritskii convent, 118, 205, 206; restoration of, 196–97; schism in, 199–200, 202–4
Gospel of St. John, 42
grace, 88, 153, 155, 207, 228
Great Compline, 70, 74, 75, 76
Great Schism, 7
Greek Catholic churches, 7, 213, 243–44, 246
Greek Orthodox Christianity, 58–81, 183–90
Gregorios, Paulos Mar, 34–35, 39, 41, 47, 49n2
Gregory of Nyssa, Saint, 30
Gregory Palamas, 200, 201
Gregory the Sinaite, 200
Gurianov, Father Nikolai, 115

Hagia Sophia, Istanbul, 17
Hail Mary, 50n7, 153
Haldon, John, 87
Hellenic Broadcasting Corporation, 70
Herzfeld, Michael, 96
hesychasm, 39, 46, 193, 200, 202
hesychast fathers, 48, 200–201

hesychast prayer, 31, 44, 65, 223
Higher Institute of Coptic Studies, 89
Hoffman, Valerie, 92
holy foolery, 48, 96, 97
holy objects, veneration of, 155
Huxley, Aldous, 198
hymns, Amharic, 175–76, 178

iconoclasm, 33, 86–90, 99, 224, 238
iconography, 81–82, 86–87, 90, 99n5, 205, 217
iconostasis, 2, 6, 37, 119, 233–34
icons, 18, 173, 250; as art, 86–87, 89; in Ethiopian Orthodoxy, 176; explanation of, 47, 84, 86, 93, 94; images on, 3, 11, 81–84, 95–96, 123; in Indian Orthodoxy, 38; and liturgy, 230, 233; locations of, 2, 71, 84, 113, 185, 188, 192; Marian, 92, 95, 96, 98n2; and miracles, 92, 148, 151, 152–3; and pilgrimages, 151, 153, 154; veneration with, 6, 37, 85, 88, 90–91, 151–52, 155, 158
Ignatius Brianchanninov, Bishop, 124
Indian Orthodox Church, 6, 34–36, 38, 42, 249
Innocent, Saint. *See* Veniaminov, Ioann
Irenaeus of Lyon, Saint, 30
Irini, Tamav, 93
Irmologion, 59
ison, 58, 69, 71
"It Is Truly Meet." *See* Axion Estin
Ivan the Terrible, Tsar, 134
Iveria, 160n9

Jacobite Syrian Orthodox Church, 34, 37, 50n7
Jehovah's Witnesses, 247
Jesus Prayer, 8, 9, 58; in daily life, 69, 73, 203; as meditative prayer, 18, 74, 200, 223; in monasteries, 201, 202, 207; for spiritual growth, 43, 46, 158, 231
John Chrysostom, Saint, 50n5, 62, 66
John of Damascus, Saint, 6, 87, 99n4, 184
John of Kronstadt, Saint, 9, 125
John the Baptist, Saint, 97

Kamil of Alexandria, Abuna Bishoi, 93, 98
Kazan Cathedral, Saint Petersburg, 160n2

Kazan Theological Academy, 133
Keane, Webb, 180, 226
Kievan Patriarchate, 213
Kirill (Gundiaev), Patriarch, 214
"kiss of peace," 218–19
Konanos, Father Andreas, 73
Konevetz Monastery, 145
Kuraev, Andrei, 161n10
Kyievo-Pechers'k Lavra, Kyiv, 161n9

Leo III, Emperor, 87
Levada Center, 143
liturgical languages: Church Slavonic, 38–39, 120, 126, 134, 135, 214; Ge'ez, 166, 175; Syriac, 38, 103–4; the vernacular as, 103–4, 238n6
liturgy, 174, 177, 203, 224. *See also* Divine Liturgy
Liudogovskii, Feodor, 133, 134
Ljubojevic, Divna, 7
Lord's Prayer, 123, 157, 222
Lossky, Vladimir, 84
Luhrmann, Tanya, 19, 122–23
Lydia FM, 73, 74

Macarius III, 2
MacIntyre, Alasdair, 15
Mahmood, Saba, 238
Makarius, Saint, 123
Malankara Syrian Orthodox Church. *See* Indian Orthodox Church
Manahri, Abuna Abdel-Masih al-, 93, 97, 98
Mari (ethnic group), 126–27
Marina, Saint, 94
Mark, Saint, 96
Maslova, Natalia, 82
mastery, 30–31, 41, 48
Matrona of Moscow, Saint, 148–49
Matthew the Poor, 85
Mauss, Marcel, 9, 35, 36, 45
media, marked, 60–62, 65, 67
media, unmarked, 60–62, 67
media technologies, 58–77, 167, 171, 174–80, 186–87. *See also* Facebook; MP3 files; YouTube
Menas the Wonderworker, Saint, 84, 95

Mercurius, Saint, 84
metanias, 3
Meyer, Birgit, 16–17
Miaphysites, 4, 5, 89, 165–66
moleben, 8, 126, 128–29
Monastery of St. Anthony the Hermit on the Red Sea, 93, 94, *111*
Monastery of St. John the Theologian, Souroti, Thessaloniki, 94, *112*
Mondzain, Marie-Jose, 88
Monophysites. *See* Miasphysites
Mormons, 247
Moscow Patriarchate, 14, 133, 213–14
Moscow University, 133
Mount Athos, 5, 67, 68, 77, 94, 161n9; monasteries of, Esfigmenou, 204; monasteries of, Simonpetra, 69, 73; monasteries of, Vatopedi, 71, 160n2, 204; as an Orthodox model, 3, 65, 201, 204, 220, 238n6
Mount Tabor, 201
MP3 files, 65, 68, 69, 74, 77
music, instrumental, 61
mysteries (Orthodox sacraments), 31, 62, 216, 219, 228, 232
mystery, 30–31, 48, 62, 193

Nestorians, 5
Nestorius of Constantinople, Patriarch, 5
New Age, 201, 208, 242, 249
Nicene Creed, 7, 123
Nicholas the Wonderworker, Saint, 65, 131, 136
Nicholas II, Emperor, 145, 160n7
Nicodemus, 42, 47
Nikephoros of Constantinople, Patriarch, 87, 99n4
Nikita the Stylite, Saint, 193
Nikon, Patriarch, 3
Nikonites, 4
nomads, religious, 144, 154, 158
non-Chalcedonian churches. *See* Oriental Orthodox churches

obedience, 193, 230; as work, 196–200, 202, 205, 206, 207
Old Belief, 32, 33, 39

Old Believers, 4, 48; and liturgy, 32, 38, 39, 125; in Romania, 43, 45, 49n3
Oosterbahn, Martijn, 177
Optina Pustyn' Monastery, Kozelsk, Russia, 132
Optinskii, Lev, 132
Oriental Orthodox churches, 5, 7, 165–66
Ormylia monastery, Greece, 69
Orthodox Christianity, 4–5, 12–19; conversion in; culture of, 4, 12, 13, 44, 58; in Ethiopia, 165, 168; organization of, 4–5, 13–14, 144; post-Socialist revival of, 42, 43, 63, 216–21, 226–28, 249; in Romania, 40, 216–21, 235–37, 238n1, 238nn5–7, 242–44; in South Alaska, 55; worship practices in, 20, 43, 47, 59, 61, 154, 238n7. *See also* enchurching
Orthodox Church of America, 14
Orthodox Syrian Sunday School Association of the East, 35
orthodoxy, 4–5, 34
orthopraxy, 5, 32, 37
Orwell, George, 198
Our Lady of Saydnaya Monastery, Saydnaya, Syria, *117*, 184, 189, 190
Our Lady of Soufanieh, 188
Ouspensky, Leonid, 87, 90

Paisios, Elder, 72, 94, *112*
Pankhurst, Jerry, 23n2
paradosis. *See* tradition
paraklesis, 69, 70, 73, 74
Paraskevi the Bulgarian, Saint, 2
paschal troparion, 31
Paterikon, 198
Paul of Aleppo, Archdeacon, 2
Paul the Apostle, Saint, 70, 131, 200
Peirce, Charles, 85–86
Pentecostals, 128
Philokalia, 46–47, 48
pictures, religious, 176
pilgrimage, 144, 153, 154, 159, 160n4, 194; organized, 146–47, 149, 150; and prayer, 135–36, 155
Pliakin, Maksim, 134
Pokrovskii Monastery, Moscow, 148
pomianniki, 125, 126

praxis, 39
prayer: and baptismal names, 129–31; canonical, 5, 38, 120–21, 123, 127, 203, 235–36, 250; and confession, 229–31; in daily life, 12, 35, 38, 124–25, 127, 185, 221–25, 229; in Ethiopian Orthodoxy, 176–77, 180n1; evangelical, 121, 122–23; and glossolalia, 136; and icons, 81–82, 131, 154, 176; in Islam, 122, 249; in liturgy, 5, 8, 38, 199, 220, 222, 224, 233–36; and media, 128, 168, 171–74, 180, 249; monastic, 194, 196, 201–3, 206–7, 224, 225; in Orthodox Christianity, 20, 41, 46, 121, 123, 135–36, 242, 248; for personal transformation, 200, 202, 208, 216, 233, 248; prayer books, 8, 120–22, 123, 131–32, 135; private, 3, 8, 131, 185–86, 188–91, 232; public, 3, 8, 128–30, 167–68, 177–80, 208; as skill, 12, 19–21, 35, 39, 123, 157; by specialists, 129, 166; topical, 173, 213–15
Presbyterians, 89
Prester John, 168
Pseudo-Dionysios Aeropagitos, 14

Romania. *See* Orthodox Christianity; Old Believers
Rublev, Andrei, 205
Rus, 33
Russian Orthodox Church, 143, 146, 149, 160n7, 194, 213. *See also* enchurching
Russian Orthodox monasteries, 192–95, 198–99, 200, 201, 209n13. *See also* Goritskii convent; obedience

sacraments. *See* mysteries (Orthodox sacraments)
saints, 40, 91, 95, 163; baptismal names and, 130–31; canonization of, 93, 94, 148; Coptic, 97–98; icons and, 84, 86, 91–92, 94; intercession by, 98, 131, 167, 222; relics of, 2, 83
Saint Thomas Christians, 103–4
Sayings of the Desert Fathers, The, 238n4
Seraphim of Sarov, Saint, 44, 48, *105*, 153–54, 160n7
Sergiev, Ioann. *See* John of Kronstadt, Saint

Seventh-day Adventists, 50n9
Shenouda III, Pope, 93
shirk, 91
spiritual fathers, 40, 46, 48, 218; and confession, 228, 229, 230, 231; and pastoral guidance, 74, 76, 232, 233, 236, 238n5
startsy. *See* elders
Steniaev, Oleg, 81, 131
St. George Orthodox Church, Puthuppally, India, 107
St. George's Church, Bahir Dar, Ethiopia, 170
St. Mark's Coptic Orthodox Cathedral, Azbakiya, Cairo, 89
St. Mary and St. Antonious Coptic Orthodox Church, Milwaukee, U.S.A., 99n6
St. Thomas Jacobite Church, Keezhillam, India, 106
St. Trinity-Sergius Lavra, Sergiyev Posad, Russia, 125, 205, 209n13
Sunday of Orthodoxy, 6
Symeon the New Theologian, Saint, 200
Synaxariun, 85, 93
Synod, 133, 134
Syria, 183–91
Syriac Christianity, 7, 33, 34, 49n3, 103–4
Syriac Orthodox Church, Antioch, 34
Syrian Orthodox Patriarchate, 34

tabots, 166
Taylor, Charles, 226
Tawfik, Magued, 94, 95
Theophilus, Emperor, 87
theoria, 39
theosis, 30, 39, 55–57, 59, 60; how to reach, 68, 200, 230
Theotokos, 5, 68, 69, 70, 133; appanages of, 154, 160n9; Holy Belt of, 144, 160. *See also* Hail Mary; Tikhvin icon; Virgin Mary
Thomas the Apostle, Saint, 7, 33, 34, 103
Tikhvin icon, 151–53, 160n6
Tocheva, Detelina, 209n7
tradition, 32, 59
Transfiguration Cathedral, Kyiv, 213
trebnik, 129, 131

Tsiamoulis, Christos, 73
Typikon, 71, 133, 224

Ukraine, 213–15, 248
Ukrainian Orthodox Autocephalous Church, 213
Uniates. *See* Greek Catholic churches
Utkina, Elena, 82

Varus, Saint, 131
Veniamin (Milov), Bishop, 125
Veniaminov, Ioann, 55–57
Verkhovskii, Zosima, Saint, 206
Virgin Mary, 5, 99n2, 163, 172; and akathistoi, 132, 133, 134; appearances of, 83, 245; images of, 6, 96, 173, 183; veneration of, 92, 95, *117*, 186. *See also* Theotokos
Vysherskii, Savva, Saint, 193

Wang Mingming, 228
Ware, Kallistos, Bishop, 30
Weber, Max, 226–28

Youssef, Isaac Fanous, 90
YouTube, 59, 62, 65, 68, 73, 74

Zamyatin, Yevgeny, 198
Zigon, Jarrett, 43
zikkir, 167

www.ingramcontent.com/pod-product-compliance
Lightning Source LLC
Chambersburg PA
CBHW060946230426
43665CB00015B/2081